Promoting Successful Transition to Adulthood
to Adulthood
for Students with Disabilities

WHAT WORKS FOR SPECIAL-NEEDS LEARNERS

Karen R. Harris and Steve Graham, *Series Editors*

www.guilford.com/WWFSNL

This series addresses a significant need in the education of students who are at risk, those with disabilities, and all children and adolescents who struggle with learning or behavior. While researchers in special education, educational psychology, curriculum and instruction, and other fields have made great progress in understanding what works for struggling learners, the practical application of this research base remains quite limited. Books in the series present assessment, instructional, and classroom management methods that have strong empirical evidence. Written in a user-friendly format, each volume provides specific how-to instructions and examples of the use of proven procedures in schools. Coverage is sufficiently thorough and detailed to enable practitioners to implement the practices described; many titles include reproducible practical tools. Recent titles have Web pages where purchasers can download and print the reproducible materials.

Promoting Successful Transition to Adulthood for Students with Disabilities

Robert L. Morgan
Tim Riesen

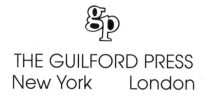

THE GUILFORD PRESS
New York   London

Copyright © 2016 The Guilford Press
A Division of Guilford Publications, Inc.
370 Seventh Avenue, Suite 1200, New York, NY 10001
www.guilford.com

Printed in the United States of America

This book is printed on acid-free paper.

Last digit is print number: 9   8   7   6   5   4   3   2   1

Library of Congress Cataloging-in-Publication Data

Names: Morgan, Robert L. | Riesen, Timothy J.
Title: Promoting successful transition to adulthood for students with
  disabilities / Robert L. Morgan, Tim Riesen.
Description: New York : The Guilford Press, 2016. | Series: What works for
  special-needs learners | Includes bibliographical references and index.
Identifiers: LCCN 2015023335| ISBN 9781462523993 (paperback) |
  ISBN 9781462524136 (hardcover)
Subjects: LCSH: Students with disabilities—Services for—United States. |
  Students with disabilities—Counseling of—United States. | Students with
  disabilities—Vocational guidance—United States. | School-to-work
  transition—United States. | BISAC: EDUCATION / Special Education /
  Learning Disabilities. | MEDICAL / Psychiatry / Child & Adolescent. |
  PSYCHOLOGY / Psychopathology / Autism Spectrum Disorders. |
  SOCIAL SCIENCE / Social Work.
Classification: LCC LC4031 .M648 2016 | DDC 371.9—dc23
LC record available at *http://lccn.loc.gov/2015023335*

About the Authors

Robert L. Morgan, PhD, is Professor in the Department of Special Education and Rehabilitation at Utah State University, where he is also Director of the Severe Disabilities Program, Director of the Transition Specialist Master's Program, and Co-Director of the Institute for Interdisciplinary Transition Services. He has worked in classrooms as a behavior specialist and transition specialist and has consulted to schools and transition programs throughout the United States. Dr. Morgan has published nearly 100 journal articles and book chapters as well as three books, and has assisted in the development of nationally disseminated educational products for students, teachers, and transition specialists.

Tim Riesen, PhD, is Research Assistant Professor in the Department of Special Education and Rehabilitation and a Faculty Fellow at the Center for Persons with Disabilities at Utah State University. He specializes in employment for people with significant disabilities, transition, and adult services. Dr. Riesen has developed and conducted trainings for over 2,000 professionals and parents across the United States, on topics including supported employment, customized employment, work incentives, systematic instruction, transition to employment, and behavior supports in the workplace. His published research has focused on response prompting, school-to-work barriers, and embedded instruction.

Preface

From our experience in schools, we find transition from school to adulthood for youth with disabilities to be one of the most complex of all educational endeavors. And yet, when it works, the rewards far exceed the toil and turmoil. For youth with disabilities and their families, the challenge of moving from school-based special education services to adulthood is immense. However, even in the face of formidable odds, the field of transition is making progress on several fronts. First, we are excited about recent legislative and advocacy efforts that reinforce the importance of integrated employment for all students. Second, we are pleased to see students with disabilities being supported in postsecondary education with greater frequency. Third, we are delighted to see youth with disabilities engaging in integrated community activities. The success of postschool outcomes depends on interrelated factors, including student motivation, the involvement of parents and families, the presence of trained teacher and transition team members (we use the terms *transition educator* and *transition professional*), the use of research-based practices, the willingness of educators to work together (we refer to *transition teams*), and a collaboration of professionals across disciplines in the best interests of the youth. Transition research has established ways to increase successful postschool outcomes. In fact, the resurgence of transition research in recent years, along with the call for *college and career readiness* for youth with disabilities, gives us optimism that we may see significant improvements in the future.

But we remain humble as to the multifarious nature of the transition process. Supporting a youth with disabilities from school to a self-determined career path, a plan for postsecondary education, and a highly valued independent life rich with social and recreational activities is a formidable and painstaking process. When it works, success is celebrated by all stakeholders. In practice, the small successes along the pathway deserve celebration because transition is ultimately a journey, not an outcome.

PURPOSE AND OVERVIEW

The purpose of this book is to describe issues, processes, and outcomes involved in the transition from special education to adulthood for youth with disabilities, with particular attention to:

- Evidence-based, research-based, and promising practices in transition approaches.
- Practices that can be implemented in schools and communities to improve post-school outcomes.
- Methods for involving youth and their families as driving forces in the process of transition.

POINTS OF EMPHASIS

In this book, we address youth who have various disabilities, focusing mainly on low-incidence developmental disabilities (e.g., mild, moderate, and profound intellectual disability; autism spectrum disorder) and high-incidence disabilities (e.g., specific learning disabilities, emotional disturbance). With respect to services for students with profound and multiple disabilities, we recognize the need for specialized transition services and support systems. However, we only touch on transition services for students with profound and multiple disabilities because we do not find a research base sufficient to guide practice. We take the position that a person with a disability is best understood by analyzing his or her unique, individual characteristics and the environments within which he or she operates. The "deficit model" used in some human and medical service approaches is inconsistent with our experience as we work with youth on a daily basis and learn to recognize their strengths, aspirations, and dreams. We use the term *disability* only because it is conventional in the current lexicon.

We use the terms *transition educator* and *transition professional* to refer to specialists who provide transition services. In practice, teachers, secondary service coordinators, career technical educators, vocational rehabilitation counselors, social workers, para-professionals, and others can provide transition services. We use these more general terms as all-encompassing ones. Finally, we use the term *stakeholder* to refer to transition team members (e.g., family members, employers, friends) who advocate for youth with disabilities.

In each chapter, we describe vignettes involving youth in transition and their families. Most of these are distillations of our own experiences over the years. Consistent with those experiences, the vignettes—if one follows the youth from chapter to chapter—represent points along a journey from special education to adulthood. We describe the challenges, barriers, and opportunities experienced by these hypothetical youth and families and hope they might resonate with readers.

Importantly, we have developed deep respect for families and are humbled by the challenges they face when their youth make the transition from school to adulthood. We understand how families face day-to-day struggles of putting food on the table, clothes on kids, and gasoline in the tank. Our vignettes are meant to reflect the challenges that youth and families face in transition. As such, we have tried to be realistic and not "sugarcoat" the process. Throughout the book, we speak to the importance of understanding and respecting family priorities while being stubbornly assertive about planning a youth's transition starting at an early age. A family's day-to-day struggles may obscure the importance of early transition planning. When immediate needs take precedence, it is hard to recognize a future event as critical. But families need frequent reminders of the value of early transition planning. So do educators. Only when a team of committed educators, family members, and the youth dedicate themselves to the career and lifelong learning of the individual involved will transition be successful.

SOME THOUGHTS ON EDUCATION AND CHANGE

Our perceptions of what constitutes progress over time in education depend on our perspectives. We may look at changes in the field of education over a 50-year period and conclude, "Yes, things have changed," but also "No, it is not nearly enough." For example, 50 years ago, special education was in its infancy. Special educators who provided services were just beginning to serve children with disabilities in the least restrictive environment. A free, appropriate public education was an ideal held by special educators and parents. The Education for All Handicapped Act (originally called Public Law 94-142), which provided entitlements for children with disabilities in public schools, was becoming a reality. Yet, most students receiving special education services were housed in a self-contained school or a self-contained classroom. Deinstitutionalization was just beginning as a social movement. State institutions for individuals with disabilities were unlocking the exit doors. Community-based service programs were in their infancy. Many children requiring significant supports were moving from state institutions to community-based intermediate care facilities. Schools that accepted children with disabilities housed them in classrooms away from the mainstream.

Yes, things have changed. But today, self-contained classrooms remain in many schools. In some cases, special education remains a place, not a service. General educators, in some instances, do not participate in teaching students with special needs because they have not been adequately taught how to do so. Inclusion may amount to a student with disabilities sitting idle in the corner of a general education classroom. Many students with disabilities are still far behind their peers in academic knowledge and skills, and the distance widens as they enter secondary schools. No, it is not nearly enough.

More specifically, consider transition from school to adulthood. Fifty years ago, transition was not a part of educational language. The prospect of a young adult with disabilities being selected for employment or enrolling in a course at a postsecondary institution of higher education was unlikely. Adults exiting state institutions for individuals with disabilities were, for the most part, finding their way to sheltered workshops. Those programs consisted largely of vocational, social, and recreational activities. The reasoning was that, once learned, these skills would lead to community integration and employment. Yet, after the program, skilled individuals often stayed put. Segregation occurred for numerous, complex reasons related to disincentives for community placement and lack of an infrastructure to support integration. There were only the beginnings of federal and state agencies overseeing special education and adult-level services for individuals with disabilities, so very few standards or common expectations existed in service delivery.

Yes, things have changed. Today, the prospect of a young adult who has graduated from the special education system being able to hold a job, enroll in a postsecondary education program, or live independently is becoming increasingly common. But employment is, in many cases, less than 50% for former students up to 8 years out of high school. For those who do work, wages are low compared to their agemates. Total hours worked are less than full time, and few receive insurance or other benefits. Workshops and day programs serve increasing numbers of individuals with disabilities in segregated facilities. Although some employers have hired workers with disabilities, the majority are still hesitant. Postsecondary education institutions (meaning universities, colleges, adult education, etc.) are starting to "take hold" as options for young adults with disabilities. It is still unusual for college faculty to have been sufficiently trained in how to accommodate students with disabilities. Many high school special education teachers do not understand the concept of postsecondary education for young adults with disabilities, and they focus only on moving current students to the next grade level. Education budgets have been cut to the point that only essential, classroom-based academic services can be provided to students. Integrating classroom with community opportunities in real-world environments to reinforce academic skills and to teach functional skills are cost-prohibitive. Young adults with disabilities who have aspirations of determining and realizing their own career paths are, in some cases, told to "think more realistically." No, it is not nearly enough.

FINAL REFLECTIONS

Our interest in transition stems from years of working alongside youth and young adults as they seek their pathways to independence. We are captivated by their enthusiasm, motivation, and drive to determine their futures. Routinely, we are reminded of the exuberance of youth and feel privileged to experience it vicariously. And we ride the rollercoaster of emotion that comes with their successes, disappointments, and frustrations. Throughout the transition process, we have grown deeply respectful of parents, families, and teachers who catch the dream, learn the ropes, and defy the odds. Their hard work gives us hope for the future of the field of transition and the individuals with disabilities it serves. Collectively, the courage of youth and their stakeholders provides the motivation for this book. We are writing the book because we believe in the people, processes, and outcomes that are truly attainable with thoughtful planning and action.

Acknowledgments

Robert L. Morgan: I want to thank my dear family, Becky and Savanna, for their steadfast support. My daughter, Savanna, reminded me of the perseverance necessary to complete a project. Indeed, if you believe in your dream and remain steadfast, you will be guided in what you do every day.

Tim Riesen: I would like to acknowledge my family, Ashley, Zoe, and Audrey, for their continued support and patience. I would also like to acknowledge the individuals with disabilities with whom I've had the pleasure to work throughout my career.

Together, we would like to express appreciation to those who assisted in writing and researching material for the book, including Ms. Tashina Meaker (Teacher, Logan High School), Dr. Scott Kupferman (Assistant Professor, University of Colorado, Colorado Springs), Ms. Heather Weese (Clinical Instructor, Utah State University), and Dr. Jared Schultz (Associate Professor, Utah State University). Special thanks to the readers, Dr. David Test (University of North Carolina, Charlotte), Dr. Mary Morningstar (University of Kansas), Dr. Pattie Noonan (University of Kansas), Dr. Jim Martin (University of Oklahoma), Dr. Lori Peterson (University of Northern Colorado), Dr. David Ellerd (Humboldt State University), Dr. Shamby Polychronis (Westminster College), and Mr. Jeff Sheen (Utah State University). Next, we wish to express deep appreciation to Dr. Karen R. Harris (Arizona State University), Series Editor, and Rochelle Serwator, Senior Editor at The Guilford Press, for their guidance during the publication process. Finally, we are grateful to the students and families who participated in the Aggies Elevated Postsecondary Education Program at Utah State University, the young adults seeking employment through the EmployAbility Clinic, high school and post–high school students with whom we've worked, and the transition specialist teachers pursuing master's degrees in the Department of Special Education and Rehabilitation Master's Program at Utah State University. Collectively, they were the inspiration for this endeavor.

Contents

7. Student Involvement and Self-Determination to Guide Transition   132

8. Transition to Employment   152
with TASHINA MEAKER

9. Transition to Postsecondary Education   177
with SCOTT KUPFERMAN

CHAPTER 1

Transition to Adulthood

Creating a Pathway to Independence

This chapter addresses . . .

- The importance of successful transition to adulthood.
- Roles and responsibilities of various stakeholders from different disciplines.
- The relationship between transition and the Common Core curriculum.
- The critical role of self-determination.
- How students with disabilities can remain actively involved in their own transition process.
- Professionals from different fields and how they can contribute to the process.

WHAT DOES TRANSITION MEAN TO YOUTH?

Transition from school and special education services to adulthood is best understood by getting to know youth who are going through the process. Let us introduce you to three youth in transition. We refer to them as Demarius, Josefina, and Kenley. Each successive chapter will return to vignettes of these hypothetical youth as they make their transitions to adulthood.

Demarius is a 17-year-old student at Edison High School, an inner-city school in a large urban area. He returned to Edison after dropping out for a year and spending time in a juvenile facility due to an assault charge. The charge stemmed from an incident involving another 17-year-old youth who was hugging Demarius's girlfriend. Demarius reacted to the situation by physically assaulting the youth. His grandmother took Demarius in and insisted he return to school to get his diploma. Demarius describes his grandmother as the

1

"only constant thing" in his life. She thinks he knows right from wrong and can create a bright future despite his upbringing in poverty. His mom, whom Demarius describes as a "crackhead," disappeared years ago, and his dad left when he was 5.

Demarius receives special education services at Edison because of his classification of emotional disturbance. His high school resource teacher, Ms. Woolsey, describes Demarius as unmotivated. He reads and performs math at about the fifth- to sixth-grade level. His file describes a rebellious young man who lashes out at the world; terms such as *aggressive*, *defiant*, *oppositional*, and *noncompliant* appear in his file. Ms. Woolsey wants to help but feels like she has tried everything with Demarius. "He rejects everyone in authority as someone who is out to get him," she says. Demarius lives from day to day, seemingly waiting for the next crisis to "happen to him." He describes his future as "on the street." When asked about his hopes and dreams, he mutters "just surviving." When asked about what he needs, Demarius appears exasperated and walks away, saying "just need people to leave me alone." Conversation ended.

Josefina is a 18-year-old student at Ignacio High School. She has cerebral palsy, spastic type, which means she experiences loss of motor control such as slouching forward instead of sitting upright. She frequently has balance problems and hypertonicity (muscle stiffness) caused by inadequate oxygen during birth. Josefina uses a motorized, electric wheelchair to navigate Ignacio High School. She communicates with a slight articulation disorder, but her speech is understandable if she slows down to correctly position her tongue. She can feed herself and manage self-care tasks. Josefina scores in the normal range of intelligence on a non-language-based IQ test. She performs near grade level in math, language arts, and reading. Josefina is well liked by students at Ignacio and can often be found in the center of a group of students gathered in the hallway or cafeteria. Smiling widely, she often powers her wheelchair as she pulls her friends riding skateboards down the sidewalk, often drawing the vice principal to the front steps of the school shaking his head. "Gonna destroy the motor on that wheelchair," he says.

Josefina will soon graduate from Ignacio with a diploma and plans to join her class during the commencement ceremony. Because she has received special education services, particularly occupational and speech therapy, her special education teacher, Ms. Martin, developed an individual transition plan for her when she was 16 years old. Ms. Martin administered assessments and talked to Josefina about her career plans. At the annual individualized education program (IEP) meeting, Ms. Martin shared the assessment results and talked to Josefina's parents about the prospects of working toward a career in human services, perhaps as a paraprofessional in a classroom or as an assistant in a child care organization. Josefina felt she could assist a teacher with classroom tasks and deliver basic instruction to students. However, Josefina's parents, Raul and Mariana, responded cautiously at the IEP meeting. A career? Although they were appreciative of all the work Ms. Martin and others had done for Josefina, as well as grateful to the students for including Josefina in social activities, Raul and Mariana could not understand why a career was being considered. "We don't understand," Raul offered tentatively. "We see Josefina as needing to be home after high school, you know, taking care of her little sisters. Once she finishes at Ignacio, her responsibility is to serve her family."

Kenley is a 16-year-old student at Southridge High School who has autism spectrum disorder and moderate intellectual disability. Autism is characterized by limited communication and social skills as well as problem behaviors. A moderate intellectual disability means that Kenley does not process information readily and requires individualized lessons to learn basic self-care skills. Kenley does not initiate conversation, although he can express himself when prompted. He tends to hold back and remain quiet, and appears uneasy around classmates. His high school peer group has learned to accept Kenley, but it was a slow process and required a lot of help from Kenley's brother, Ashton. A senior and star player on the football team, Ashton has been Kenley's chief advocate and supporter. Since he will be graduating soon, however, Ashton worries about what will happen to Kenley. Reading has been the most difficult subject for Kenley. His special education teacher, Mr. White, tries to relate reading lessons to Kenley's physical world so the words take on relevance. Kenley's math skills are higher, but still below grade level. He understands basic arithmetic operations, number sense, and measurement.

Like some children with autism, Kenley's early years in school were extremely difficult and replete with tantrums. Kenley preferred to stare at the fluorescent lights on the classroom ceiling instead of listening to the teacher or playing games with classmates. When walking in the hallway, Kenley had to touch the wall at all times and screamed when unable to do so. In the school gym, Kenley wailed and screeched until allowed to leave. The expansive, wide-open facility seemed to frighten him. Ashton helped him acclimate by throwing and catching a ball and lifting weights in the gym.

Kenley had redefined the small community of Southridge, a farming hamlet in the Midwest. Consisting primarily of farmers, a grocery, grain mill, and farm implement business, Southridge residents had no understanding of autism and, at first, avoided Kenley and his family. Most of the community was quite reticent about involving the family in community activities. However, Ashton championed the cause for his brother, insisting that he be involved in inclusive classroom activities at school, community barbecues, and church events. With Ashton graduating from high school, his family is concerned that Kenley will be left at the high school with no clear plan for transition. The community has no system of support for Kenley. His parents, who both work at the grocery store, are unsure what to do. Kenley has not been taught vocational or social skills, and appears destined for an adulthood without direction.

Demarius, Josefina, and Kenley will soon enter adulthood. Like all of us, they will carry with them experiences, attitudes about those experiences, and uncertainty. They will bring hopes and aspirations. They will also bring fears and anxieties. Like many of us, they will find that adulthood is more complex than they imagined. The role of education is to provide knowledge and skills needed as an adult and to prepare individuals for life's complexities. For youth with disabilities, the importance of that preparation is heightened. Their skill sets and life circumstances present formidable challenges. These youth carry a heavy burden, and the transition process represents a steep climb. For them to succeed as contributing citizens in their communities, the transition process must be efficient, effective, and well coordinated.

HOW IMPORTANT IS SUCCESSFUL TRANSITION TO ADULTHOOD?

This question can be approached from several perspectives. For Demarius, Josefina, Kenley, and their families, successful transition is critical. But the probabilities of their success in adulthood are reduced by disability, poverty, and/or other factors. Yet each of them holds hope for success. Demarius is bright and athletic. Josefina is socially engaging. Kenley is meticulous. They each need well-coordinated assistance during transition to be successful.

Educators and parents have long understood the importance of successful transition. With the passage of the Education for All Handicapped Act in the mid-1970s (Public Law 94-142, 1975), these stakeholders prepared students with disabilities to enter an integrated community. Educators focused on procedural safeguards, entitlement for free and appropriate public education, and access to the least restrictive environments. About 10 years after passage of this law, researchers found that large percentages of young adults who had exited from special education after high school were unemployed or "underemployed" (i.e., working few hours and below minimum wage) (e.g., Hasazi, Gordon, & Roe, 1985). As described in Chapter 2, more recent surveys have shown only slight improvements in transition outcomes.

In 2012, the Government Accounting Office published a report detailing what its authors viewed as largely unsuccessful transition from school to adulthood for young adults with disabilities and called for better federal coordination in service delivery. The authors of the report noted that many young adults leave special education unemployed and without future educational opportunities. The Government Accounting Office report (2012) stated:

> Students with disabilities face several challenges accessing federally funded programs that can provide transition services as they leave high school for postsecondary education or the workforce. These include difficulty navigating multiple programs that are not always coordinated; possible delays in service as they wait to be served by adult programs; limited access to transition services; a lack of adequate information or awareness on the part of parents, students, and service providers of available programs that may provide transition services after high school; and a lack of preparedness for postsecondary education or employment. (p. 9)

The Government Accounting Office Report helped place the transition process in the national spotlight with new calls for cost-effectiveness in special education. Across government agencies, educators, and stakeholders supporting youth with disabilities, there is now general agreement that successful transition to adulthood is of paramount importance. And most important, we know that young adults with disabilities generally want to determine their own futures and make a difference in their lives, their families, and their communities. Successful postschool outcomes are vitally important to them. In Figure 1.1, we show the three primary areas of transition emphases.

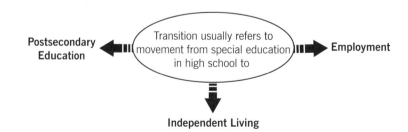

FIGURE 1.1. Three areas of transition emphasis for students with disabilities.

Respond to the following questions:

- For what additional reasons is successful transition important? What could successful transition prevent? Enhance? What could successful transition mean for young adults with disabilities? What could failed transition mean?
- What else should we investigate as desired outcomes for students in transition? What other outcomes should we anticipate? What outcomes should we seek to avoid by taking preventive measures in school activities?

WHAT CHANGES AWAIT A YOUTH WITH DISABILITIES IN ADULTHOOD?

Services in adulthood, particularly for individuals with developmental disabilities such as intellectual disability and autism (Westling, Fox, & Carter, 2015), are vastly different than school-based special education. Understanding the differences between the two is an important launching point for the reader. Throughout their school years, students with disabilities receive entitlements. In contrast, adulthood comes with major reductions or outright elimination of entitled services. In Table 1.1, we describe some of the differences between school-based entitlements and limited services in the adult world for individuals who have disabilities.

Throughout school, students and families expect special and general education teachers, along with related-services personnel (e.g., paraprofessionals, speech and language pathologists, occupational and physical therapists, school psychologists) to provide services if deemed necessary in the student's IEP. Annually, teachers and related-service personnel meet with the student, parents, and family to develop the IEP, based on the requirements set forth in the Individuals with Disabilities Education Act (IDEA, 2004; see Chapter 3 for a description of IDEA and related legislation). Special education services are available until a student graduates from high school at about age 18 with a diploma, or continue up to the 22nd birthday (called *post–high school*), if needed, for

TABLE 1.1. Differences between School-Based Services and the Adult World

Students with disabilities and their families are entitled to . . .	Adults with disabilities find that . . .
<ul><li>Free, appropriate public education in the least restrictive environment.</li><li>Preparation and implementation of an individualized education program (IEP).</li><li>Transition services starting at age 16 (in some states, age 14), as a part of the IEP.</li><li>Mandated protections of minority age.</li><li>A relatively predictable learning environment.</li></ul>	<ul><li>Entitlements are limited.</li><li>Adult services are available but limited to those who apply and are found eligible.</li><li>Number of applicants for services exceed number of slots, so waiting lists are common.</li><li>Employers hire the most qualified applicant.</li><li>Competition exists for jobs and postsecondary education (e.g., community college, 4-year college).</li><li>Colleges require a high grade-point average (GPA) and high scores on college entrance examinations.</li></ul>

the youth to complete requirements for a diploma or to become as independent as possible. Transition services designed to assist a student to prepare for adulthood must be included on the IEP by age 16 (in some states, age 14). Obviously, special education services should prepare the student for success in adulthood. However, most students with disabilities who leave special education services are likely to need additional services and supports going forward. As it currently stands, those adult services and supports are not guaranteed. Kochhar-Bryant, Bassett, and Webb (2009) stated:

> When students with disabilities exit secondary education, they must rely on adult service agencies to continue providing supportive services that may be needed in employment or postsecondary education. Services provided through adult agencies are not entitlements. These agencies have various eligibility requirements and, because of limited funding, cannot always immediately offer services to eligible citizens. Applicants for services are often placed on a waiting list. (p. 24)

Indeed, waiting lists for adult services are sometimes long and imperceptibly slow to change (see Chapter 10). One national organization sought to abolish waiting lists (National Organization to End the Waitlists, 2013). After years of entitlements, many young adults with disabilities and their families may be left without much-needed services.

For many young adults who do *not* have disabilities, the transition from high school to adulthood is a time of great expectations, although most who enter it are not fully equipped with the knowledge or skills to meet the challenge. Typical 18-year-olds find themselves looking to sort out various opportunities, such as entering college, getting a job, or living in an apartment. These opportunities come with heavy financial obligations and tremendous personal effort that can be overwhelming, but at least for some typical 18-year-olds, they are usually achievable given hard work, family support, tenacity, and luck.

For individuals who have developmental disabilities and their families, transition can be a time of shock, disillusionment, and discouragement. As a parent told one of us, "I felt like I was thrust into a foreign country where everyone spoke a different language." Another said, "I didn't have a clue what was happening. It was like we got [my young adult] ready for school and the bus didn't come . . . ever again."

The path from school to adulthood requires a thoughtful, systematic, calibrated, and well-planned transition process. Transition entails a team process involving the student, family, and other stakeholders actively engaged and clearly focused on the goal. In fact, students need to be the captains of the team, charting their futures according to their own vision. Transition also requires that all stakeholders understand their roles and responsibilities. Obviously, the best-laid plans in transition start early, long before the school bus does not come.

HOW DOES TRANSITION RELATE
TO THE STANDARDS-BASED EDUCATION?

The standards-based education movement represents an attempt to hold schools and educators accountable for student progress within a common framework of learning experiences (Nolet & McLaughlin, 2005). Some readers may be asking themselves "How can teachers competently carry out all the academic teaching requirements mandated by standards-based education and achieve successful transition outcomes as well?" At first blush, these appear to be competing priorities: meeting high standards of academic achievement while concurrently achieving successful postschool outcomes. Especially for educators at the secondary level, the sum of all responsibilities appears overwhelming and untenable. High academic standards require intensive teaching in science, technology, engineering, math, reading, language, and other subjects in classroom settings. On the other hand, transition to successful postschool outcomes requires working with students who have developmental disabilities in community sites, collaborating with agencies, and assisting families, little of which takes place in classroom settings. Indeed, this issue has been debated in many education circles from the nation's capital to faculty rooms in schools. Let's take a closer look.

In 1981, then Secretary of Education T. H. Bell created the National Commission on Excellence in Education to analyze the quality of education in the United States. Two years later, the commission published its report, *A Nation at Risk: The Imperative for Educational Reform* (National Commission on Excellence in Education, 1983). The commission found that the U.S. educational system was weakening as students received a substandard education compared to children from other countries. Educational reform became a force driving many subjects taught in the classroom. Since then, educators, parents, and legislators have sought to improve U.S. schools primarily by espousing higher standards based on high-stakes student testing (Vinovskis, 2009).

The 2001 reauthorization of the Elementary and Secondary Education Act, known popularly as the No Child Left Behind Act (2002), mandated that states create academic content and achievement standards in reading/language arts, math, and science. The achievement standards led to the development of assessment systems with proficiency requirements. All students were expected to meet the proficiency "cutoff" scores in periodic assessments, and, in turn, their schools were required to demonstrate adequate yearly progress toward achieving academic standards. In 2004, the reauthorization of IDEA attended closely to academic standards, requiring IEP teams to address how students participated in the general education curriculum.

Also, IDEA (2004) required that students with disabilities participate in the state's assessment system for all students or an alternative state assessment (Crockett & Hardman, 2010). The alternate assessments were modified versions of the state assessment that reduced the level of item difficulty but still required those items to be linked to goals in the state's achievement standards. However, alternate assessments could be taken only by 2% of all students in each grade assessed by the district and/or state, so many students with disabilities were not eligible. Students ineligible for the alternate assessment were required to take the same assessment as typical students. The rationale was to include students with disabilities and establish high expectations common to their peers without disabilities. Naturally, these requirements not only focused general educators on teaching to high academic standards but also galvanized special educators on the importance of holding students with disabilities to the same grade-level standards.

Concerns about weakened academic outcomes were based not only on comparisons to children from other countries, but also on readiness of U.S. students as they prepared for the transition to college and careers. In 2009, the National Governors Association and the Council of Chief State School Officers signed a memorandum to produce standards in the foundational subjects (English language arts and math) preparing high school graduates to succeed in college and careers (American Council on Education, 2011). This effort, which came to be known as the *Common Core State Standards Initiative*, resulted in most states adopting these standards in 2011–2012. The standards, according to the National Governors Association and the Council of Chief State School Officers, were designed to achieve the following outcomes:

- Align foundational subjects with college and work expectations.
- Include rigorous content and application of knowledge through higher-order skills.
- Build upon strengths and lessons of current state standards.
- Reflect expectations of top-performing countries so that all U.S. students are prepared to succeed in our global economy.
- Link to research and evidence-based practice (American Council on Education, 2011, p. 2).

More recently, the Common Core State Standards (CCSS) evolved into the College and Career Ready Standards (see the website at the end of this chapter). These standards were meant to articulate the expectations of higher education and the workplace. That is, education that is directed toward the standards should diminish and eventually eliminate the gap existing in the achievement level of a student exiting high school in comparison to the expectations of colleges and universities. With advent of the standards, state offices of education and institutions of higher education began working together to align curricula and instruction to increase the probability that high school graduates would pass entry-level college courses in language arts and math.

Career and Technical Education

At least for some students, attention to high academic standards may have obscured the importance of vocational education. Until the push for standards-based education, Flexer, Baer, Luft, and Simmons (2013) noted that vocational education, which is now called *career and technical education* (CTE), was the emphasis area for about 25% of secondary school students. These students received at least part of their education in career technical centers leading to occupational preparation and work experiences (Flexer et al., 2013, p. 156).

Even prior to the emphasis on standards-based education, educators and policymakers were concerned that many students were graduating from high school without requisite employment skills. The Secretary's Commission on Achieving Necessary Skills (SCANS) was organized to pinpoint knowledge and skills needed by high school graduates in the world of work (Flexer et al., 2013, p. 157). In 1991, SCANS published a report called *What Work Requires of Schools: A SCANS Report on America 2000* (U.S. Department of Labor, 1991). The SCANS Report called for secondary education to target basic skills, thinking skills, and personal qualities. SCANS also recommended five workplace competencies, including (1) identifying, organizing, planning, and allocating resources (e.g., time, money); (2) working with others (e.g., participating as a member of a team); (3) acquiring and using information; (4) understanding complex interrelationships (e.g., understanding systems); and (5) using technology.

SCANS suggested revamping traditional vocational education, which until that time had focused on specific trades and occupations. Occupation-specific courses in secondary vocational programs diminished, and instead, CTE emphasized broad technical preparation so that students could prepare for college. Some of the students who formerly sought occupational preparation and work experiences were now learning skills more broadly preparing them for college (Baer, Flexer, & Dennis, 2007). The push for standards-based education, fueled by the CCSS, was now having a profound effect on students taking CTE courses. While still focused on the trades, CTE courses are now designed to teach broad skills necessary to enter college.

Although the cumulative effect of these initiatives may be to substantially improve the educational experience for secondary students, we must now return to the question about standards-based education and transition of students with developmental disabilities. What has happened to students with disabilities and their teachers in an environment defined by standards-based education and diminished occupation-specific training? Students with disabilities and their families have long sought to be part of inclusive education, but were they being discarded in the push for higher standards? Was the race for higher test scores and college preparedness passing them by?

College and Career Readiness

The CCSS are meant to result in *college and career readiness*. This concept is described as follows:

> College and career readiness means that a high school graduate has the knowledge and skills in English and mathematics necessary to qualify for and succeed in entry-level, credit-bearing postsecondary coursework without the need for remediation—or put another way, a high school graduate has the English and math knowledge and skills needed to qualify for and succeed in the postsecondary job training and/or education necessary for their chosen career (i.e. community college, university, technical/vocational program, apprenticeship, or significant on-the-job training). To be college and career ready, high school graduates must have studied a rigorous and broad curriculum, grounded in the core academic disciplines, but also consisting of other subjects that are part of a well-rounded education. Academic preparation alone is not enough to ensure postsecondary readiness but it is clear that it is an essential part of readiness for college, careers, and life in the 21st century. Simply put, "college and career readiness" is the umbrella under which many education and workforce policies, programs and initiatives thrive. From high-quality early education and strong, foundational standards in elementary school to rigorous career and technical education programs and college completion goals, college and career readiness is the unifying agenda across the P-20 education pipeline. (*www.achieve.org/college-and-career-readiness*)

College and career readiness spans all years of formal education from preschool through college (sometimes referred to as *P–16*). Importantly, the term is applied to include students with developmental disabilities and to cover more than simply common-core academic skills. The expectation is that students with disabilities will receive the services and supports necessary so that they, too, may be ready for a college experience leading to a career pathway. The National Secondary Transition Technical Assistance Center (NSTTAC; 2012a) prepared a report titled *College and Career Ready Standards and Secondary Transition Planning for Students with Disabilities: 101.* The NSTTAC writes:

> The terms *Career Ready* and *College Ready* are often used interchangeably and most discussions focus on core academic skills. However, some suggest that Career Ready involves more than core academic skills. It also includes employability skills and technical, job-specific skills. . . . As states work to adopt and implement college and career ready standards for all students, the field must continue to consider the comprehensive secondary transition needs of students with disabilities. As suggested by Kochar-Bryant and Bassett (2002), the field may also consider this an opportunity to provide relevant, transition-focused education for all students within the standards. (pp. 14–19)

See the website at the end of this chapter more information.

HOW CAN TRANSITION COMPLEMENT RATHER THAN COMPETE WITH STANDARDS-BASED EDUCATION?

Instead of viewing transition to postschool outcomes and standards-based education as competing priorities, let's examine how they can be partners in the secondary educational system. What if both entities supplemented and reinforced each other? What if high-level academic and college preparation skills were mutually fortified through learning in virtual technology, community, and higher education settings?

What we sometimes see, especially when schools are under pressure to meet high standards, is that educators hunker down and work only with other educators. They are reluctant to reach out to bring in other interests for fear that they will lose focus on meeting high standards. Instead, at least for students at the secondary level and particularly for students with disabilities, we propose *interdisciplinary partnerships* to get students out of classrooms and into dynamic community work environments so that they can apply academic skills, learn new ones, and understand the relevance of what they are learning.

Some students complain that they do not see the applicability of academic skills taught in their classrooms. Where can students see the applications of academic skills? How can the relevance of academic skills be validated? What if secondary students could receive some of their education in community employment and/or university settings? We have worked with students who ask these questions. The first step is to take students in transition from school to adulthood outside the walls of the school and into the world of work or higher education where those skills are mandatory. Why not take students who complain of high math standards to work alongside engineers, architects, and computer programmers? Why not take students who complain of high language standards to shadow Web developers, newspaper journalists, and writers? Why not take students who complain about high reading standards to work with attorneys and medical professionals? But visiting community work sites is only the first step. Becoming invested in learning skills and carrying out assignments in real-world contexts is how careers are born. Teaching skills at construction sites, corporate offices, and university research labs may maximize the learning process by captivating the student's interest and unleashing motivation. When teaching in applied settings, at least in our experience, the learning process "sticks." Students who may have been reluctant or dubious usually understand the relevance of the skills to be learned and their potential to be contributing members of those environments. Parents begin to see their child's future as a competent adult.

Some students discover that standards-based education is like a fast-moving train leaving them behind. They drop out of school, complaining that they do not see the relevance of school when they can find entry-level employment on their own. In effect they ask, "Why finish school when I can find a job for myself?" As we examine in Chapter 2, youth who do not finish high school may find employment, but the wages of high school graduates quickly surpass them. Many students who leave school to take a job return at some future point to establish the credentials and knowledge base with which to create a career path. Why not catch them before they leave school to show them jobs that lead to real career opportunities?

At least in theoretical terms, we believe that transition educators and standards-based educators can work as partners. From general educators, special educators might learn that expectations for learning must be set extremely high and must continuously increase as learners "meet the bar." From special educators, general educators might learn that special education researchers have demonstrated that skills generalize, or transfer, when learning occurs in environments similar to the ones where the skills must be permanently exhibited (Stokes & Baer, 1977). The skills generalize because they serve a function, or a meaningful role, in that environment. As Crockett and Hardman (2010) state:

> The development of capacity is not simply demonstrating the mastery of curriculum content; it includes the ability to apply skills in real-life contexts and settings. Developing effective transition services will require schools to make a commitment to pedagogy that promotes the connection between skills learned in schools and performance in home and community settings. To achieve this, secondary programs will need to expand the typical instructional methods used by teachers to include the use of "situated" teaching models, community-based evaluation and instruction, and the integration of traditional "academic" and "vocational" curriculum through apprenticeship programs. (p. 49)

High academic standards can be taught and reinforced in virtual, community employment, and higher education settings. However, to achieve high standards under these circumstances, interdisciplinary collaboration is necessary. Professionals from different fields must work together. Business and labor must become partners in education, assisting in teaching secondary-age students with and without disabilities, and demonstrating their investment in the next generation of the U.S. workforce. Institutions of higher education should see the value of working with high school students in an effort to prepare them for college. Active collaboration should form among educators, business leaders, and higher education faculty. Most importantly, students must understand the relevance of the learning experience and become active learners. A shared investment in education across disciplines should focus on all students, including those with disabilities. See Chapter 12 for more information on interdisciplinary collaboration.

EXERCISE 1.2

Debates help us understand all sides of an issue. If you are in a transition class, take sides in a debate on standards-based versus vocationally focused, community-based training of functional skills for students with disabilities. Research both sides of the argument. If you are not in a class, consider both sides of the argument. What are the relevant arguments for and against each position? What is necessary to achieve the ideals represented by both sides of the debate?

WHO SHOULD PARTICIPATE IN TRANSITION AND WHAT IS THEIR ROLE?

A team approach is essential for successful transition. Potential transition team members are shown in Figure 1.2. Ideally, every youth with a disability needs a transition team of dedicated stakeholders who are competent to carry out their roles and responsibilities. The task is too formidable to rely on a single individual to get the job done. Transition has to involve a coordinated effort of multiple individuals playing distinct roles. This section examines transition participants and roles. In Chapter 12, we describe guidelines for creating and sustaining successful teams. For any given student, some professionals described below will not need to be represented, and for others, professionals not listed must become active members.

How Can Students Be Actively Involved in Determining Their Futures?

The most crucial member of a transition team is the student, who must determine the goal of his or her transition to adulthood. Self-determination involves far more than making choices about daily routine; it involves charting the course of one's future. It involves problem solving, decision making, setting and attaining goals, and advocating for oneself.

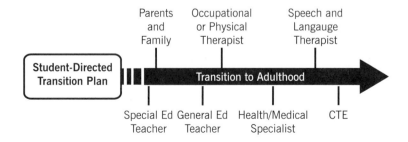

FIGURE 1.2. Graphic showing key transition team members. Depending on individual circumstances, not all members may participate, or additional members may play roles.

The extent to which students determine their own transition plans may have some degree of relationship to the characteristics of their disability or functioning level. Yet, we find that self-determination, like so many capacities, is more closely related to the student's and transition team's innovativeness. Researchers have shown that even students with multiple disabilities who require significant supports can develop extraordinary self-determination (e.g., Martin, Van Dycke, Greene, Gardner, & Christensen, 2006; Wehmeyer, Agran, & Hughes, 2000). Chapter 7 examines student involvement in guiding transition efforts.

What Can Parents and Families Do?

Much like students in transition, parents and families play critical roles in shaping the process. Because transition means the end of entitlements and predictable services, involvement of parents and families can bridge the gap and provide critical and necessary supports. Parents and families may become involved by encouraging self-determination for their transitioning youth with disabilities, contacting appropriate adult service providers (ASPs), coordinating supports (such as transportation), surveying extended family and neighbors to find supports, taking responsibility for appropriate goals in the individual transition plan, and advocating for their youth in transition. Researchers have shown that parent/family involvement is one of the most important factors in transition (e.g., Landmark, Ju, & Zhang, 2010). In fact, parents often report that they are desirous of training so that they can better help their youth navigate the transition process (e.g., Hetherington et al., 2010). Yet parents also report that they are not prepared and that educators do not provide sufficient information (Carter, Chambers, & Hughes, 2004; Tarleton & Ward, 2005). Chapter 11 provides an in-depth investigation of the value and barriers to parent/family involvement.

What Can Special Education Teachers Do?

Special education teachers, as we have mentioned, usually initiate the transition process and coordinate the activities of team members. They are responsible for organizing and coordinating the team to assure that activities are carried out. However, we argue that authority is often focused too strongly on the teacher and would be better distributed among the student, the family, and individual stakeholders. Teachers are primarily involved in transition assessment (Chapter 5); planning (Chapter 6); guiding student involvement (Chapter 7); teaching employment (Chapter 8), postsecondary preparation (Chapter 9), and independent living skills (Chapter 10); assisting families (Chapter 11); and collaborating with agencies (Chapter 12).

What Can General Education Teachers Do?

At least one general education teacher is required to participate if a student's IEP includes general education participation. According to IDEA (2004), the general educator must also (to the extent appropriate) determine which "supplementary aids and services, program modifications, and support for school personnel" are needed to help the child (1) progress toward attaining the annual goals; (2) be involved and make progress in the general education curriculum; (3) participate in extracurricular activities and other nonacademic activities; and (4) participate with other children with disabilities and those who are not disabled in the education process (§300.324[a][3][ii] and §300.320[a][4]). General education teachers are key players in acculturating students with disabilities into general education classrooms and school environments.

A teacher sets the tone for the entire classroom as to whether a student with a disability is socially accepted. Regarding academic achievement, teachers "set the bar" for students with disabilities much as they do for the rest of their students. As stated earlier, the bar should be set very high but achievable for students with disabilities. The teacher must convey that *all* students, including students with disabilities in transition from school to adulthood who participate in general education, can achieve at a high level, continuously set new marks, and take responsibility for their scholarship.

What Can Vocational Rehabilitation Counselors Do?

In each state, vocational rehabilitation (VR) is designed to assess, plan, develop, and provide rehabilitation services leading to employment for students with disabilities (Steere, Rose, & Cavaiuolo, 2007). Eligibility for VR services is described in Chapter 3. Given that a student is eligible, a VR counselor can be vital to the transition process. The focus of VR is to create and follow through with an individualized plan leading to employment (Wehman, 2011). Counselors often participate in IEP meetings when students are 16 years of age or older, describe VR services, and actively participate in providing services, especially when a student is preparing to exit from special education services. Special and general education teachers can communicate valuable data to a VR counselor on transition assessment results, academic achievement, and functional skill characteristics. Parents and family members can work with VR counselors to describe student strengths, preferences, interests, and abilities. CTE teachers can share with VR counselors their vocational assessment results and performance during work experiences.

Close collaboration between team members and VR counselors is pivotal to successful transition. It is important to note that VR services are short term, although exceptions exist. Longer-term services are provided by adult service agencies serving individuals with developmental disabilities. Names of these agencies vary from state to state. Chapter 12 provides information on collaboration with adult agencies, particularly VR.

What Can School Counselors Do?

School counselors assist students with academic, personal, and developmental support, including assessment of abilities and interests, application to college and for financial support, and determination of career path (Kochhar-Bryant et al., 2009). Although their job requires that they counsel all children needing services within a school, they can be particularly helpful in assisting students with disabilities by:

- Conveying information about career and personal competencies.
- Identifying the postschool opportunities and services to which students may have access.
- Working with students to develop their measurable postsecondary goals.
- Providing information to the IEP team on transition services that will help students realize measurable postsecondary goals.
- Conducting assessments across all life domains.
- Identifying the best curricular options and developing a course of study (*http://iris.peabody.vanderbilt.edu/module/cou2/cresource/what-is-the-school-counselors-responsibility-in-the-transition-planning-process/cou2_04/#content*).

What Can Career/Technical Educators Do?

As we mentioned earlier, CTE involves preparing students for careers in trades and technical fields. However, contemporary CTE has evolved to incorporate broader education goals involving academic and career-related education (Kochhar-Bryant et al., 2009). CTE specialists can be valuable members of a transition team because they understand occupational requirements, qualifications needed for jobs, job markets, and technical skills. Specifically, CTE specialists can assist with:

- Academic subject matter taught in relation to real-world contexts.
- Employability skills, such as job-related skills and workplace ethics.
- Career education and exploration of interests (Kochhar-Bryant et al., 2009, p. 73).

Much like school counselors, CTE specialists work in some, but not all, high schools. Small or rural districts may pool resources across schools, the entire district, or even across districts to amass CTE services. Some districts or rural cooperatives may have a career/technical center that serves multiple areas.

The participation of other team members depends on the needs of the individual in transition to adulthood. These team members are called *related-services staff* and may include paraeducators (i.e., paraprofessionals), speech and language therapists, occupational or physical therapists, health and medical specialists, and mental health specialists. The rationale for their inclusion and their roles are briefly described next.

What Can Paraeducators Do?

Paraeducators are direct service staff who work alongside teachers and other staff in special and general education. In relation to transition, paraeducators may teach skills on job sites, supervise in community or school settings, administer some assessments, describe careers, explore preferences with the student, assess performance by collecting data on work samples, develop task analyses (i.e., job tasks broken into component parts), and provide support. Training and supervision are imperative because a student's success depends largely on the paraeducator's being adequately trained to assist with instruction and assessment. Giangreco, Edelman, Luiselli, and MacFarland (1997) found that, without training and clear job descriptions, paraeducators interfered with instruction by "overprompting" (i.e., performing a task as opposed to waiting for the student to do the task), thus producing dependence on the part of the student.

What Can Speech and Language Therapists Do?

Researchers have shown risk of increased psychiatric difficulties associated with communication impairments for students in transition (e.g., Conti-Ramsden & Botting, 2008). For students who experience speech or language disorders, assistance of a speech and language therapist is critical in transition to adulthood. Speech–language pathologists provide a wide range of services to individual students with speech, language, or communication limitations. Speech services begin with initial screening for communication and continue with assessment and diagnosis, consultation for the provision of advice regarding management, intervention and treatment, or counseling. These professionals can assist with augmentative communication systems, assistive technology related to speech, accommodations in future environments, and referral to adult communicative services.

What Can Occupational or Physical Therapists Do?

Occupational therapists promote a student's functional skills and participation in daily routines, and can be especially useful in facilitating community mobility, identifying needed equipment for mobility, modifying equipment, and facilitating the acquisition of skills needed for employment (American Occupational Therapy Association, 2014; Pierangelo & Giuliani, 2004). Stewart, Law, and Willms (2002) conducted a qualitative study of 34 students with physical disabilities in transition from school to adulthood and recommended inclusion of occupational therapists to assist with person–environment fit and health promotion.

According to IDEA (1997), *physical therapy* refers to services that promote sensorimotor function through enhancement of musculoskeletal status, neurobehavioral organization, perceptual and motor development, cardiopulmonary status, and effective environmental adaptation. Services include (1) screening and assessment to identify dysfunction; (2) obtaining, interpreting, and integrating information appropriate to program planning to assist with movement; and (3) providing individual and group services or treatment (303.12[d][9]). Physical therapists promote sensory and muscular function through therapy and services. Specific to transition to adulthood, they can be instrumental in helping students who have sensorimotor problems (e.g., eye–hand coordination), limitations in muscular function or control, or restrictions in stamina or endurance (Palisano, Copeland, & Galuppi, 2007).

What Can Health and Medical Specialists Do?

Many students with disabilities experience various chronic health impairments and conditions that can significantly affect their transition from youth to adulthood. According to the Data Resource Center for Child and Adolescent Health (2012), 18.4% of students ages 12 through 17 had special health care needs. The Centers for Disease Control and Prevention (CDC) reported data from the National Health Interview Survey (2009) from

15,430 individuals, ages 18 through 29, in 2005 through 2007 and found that 12.9% of men and 17.4% of women reported one or more of the following conditions (in rank order): asthma, hypertension, arthritis, diabetes, cancer, and/or heart disease. Many disabilities result in additional (secondary) impairments, such as respiratory disorder and hypertension (Down syndrome) and eating disorders and obesity (Prader–Willi syndrome).

The overarching transition goal for students with chronic health impairments is to "maximize lifelong functioning and potential through the provision of high-quality, developmentally appropriate health care services that continue uninterrupted as the individual moves from adolescence to adulthood" (Joint Consensus Statement by the American Academy of Pediatrics, American Academy of Family Physicians, and American College of Physicians, as reported in the National Collaborative on Workforce and Disability for Youth, 2012, p. 4). Health care management involves monitoring medications, health status, insurance, medical appointments, hospital stays, and absence from school and work (National Collaborative on Workforce and Disability for Youth, 2012). However, only 16.4% of parents of transitioning youth with special health care needs discussed with their medical providers changing health insurance to adult providers (Scal & Ireland, 2005). Medical specialists, such as physicians, assistants, or nurses, can be important contributors to transition teams in cases where students experience chronic health impairments and conditions. Their areas of expertise usually do not overlap with other members of the transition team. Because of that, transition educators should be aware of the value of involving medical specialists.

What Can Mental Health Specialists Do?

One of the largest categories of disability listed in IDEA (2004) is that of emotional disturbance, accounting for 8.1% of all students served in special education (*www.education.com/reference/article/emotional-disturbance*). Large numbers of young adults in transition who experience emotional disturbance end up in mental health services or become incarcerated for legal offenses (Osgood, Foster, & Courtney, 2010). One study estimated that 46% of individuals fail to complete high school due to factors related to mental health problems (Vander Stoep, Weiss, Saldanha Kuo, Cheney, & Cohen, 2003). Only 14% of young adults with emotional disturbance who entered college graduated with degrees, which translated to approximately 4.29 million "dropouts" each year (Kessler, Foster, Saunders, & Stang, 2009). Mental health specialists could facilitate transition to adulthood by providing counseling and treatment services, working with families, or making referrals to appropriate mental health programs. Although school-based or center-based mental health services are available for adolescents, arranging ongoing and uninterrupted services is essential.

EXERCISE 1.3

The list of individuals described in this chapter who participate on a transition team is incomplete. For any given student, additional participants may play key roles. Who else might be involved in creating successful transition by participating on an individual's transition team? What roles might they play?

SUMMARY

In this chapter, we analyzed the current status of transition from school to adulthood for the purpose of understanding the magnitude of change confronting students, parents, families, educators, and other stakeholders. We made the case that successful transition to adulthood is critically important to the individuals involved, their families, educators, and other stakeholders. Successful transition begins with an educator who understands the significance of the challenge and possesses the competencies to address it. However, it also takes the efforts of all stakeholders. Transition has to involve a coordinated effort of multiple individuals playing different roles. The single most crucial member of transition teams is the student who must at least assist in determining transition goals. The student in transition should be enabled and respected as a causal agent.

Roles of other team members are briefly described in the chapter, including the parents and family, general and special education teachers, VR counselor, school counselor, and CTE. Where applicable, additional team members may include speech and language therapists, occupational or physical therapists, health and medical specialists, and/or mental health specialists. We compared and contrasted transition with standards-based education, stressing that transition educators and standards-based educators must work as partners. Special and general educators can learn from each other if they work together. Transition students with disabilities can be included in real work or postsecondary education (PSE) environments.

REVISITING DEMARIUS

The high school resource teacher, Ms. Woolsey, looked across the table at Demarius's grandmother, Elaine, and sighed. "I don't know, Elaine," started Ms. Woolsey, "I know Demarius has potential. I really want to help him. But he's got to get that chip off his shoulder."

"I know," muttered Elaine. "Not going to happen, though. He's stubborn."

Elaine had asked Demarius to attend their meeting. His absence sent a message—something like "I don't need your help." Ms. Woolsey knew Demarius was starting his junior year of high school and needed to earn credits to graduate. Plus, she had arranged for a work-based learning trial for Demarius at a local sports academy where he would be responsible for cleaning workout equipment and scheduling rooms at the gym for aerobics, yoga, and other classes. Ms. Woolsey had watched Demarius and knew he was interested in athletics and physical conditioning. She filled out the paper work and arranged a trial with the director of the sports academy. But again, Demarius did not show up for the interview.

"What really bothers me," Elaine began, "is that when you try to help him and he doesn't follow through, he turns it on you and makes you out to be the problem. You try to be part of the solution, and he acts like you are part of the problem. But he doesn't solve his problems. He says he can do it on his own, but he doesn't."

"I know what you mean. I wish I knew how to help without making it look like I'm helping," said Ms. Woolsey. "Make it like it was his idea, not mine."

Elaine sighed. "Yeah. Good luck. I've been at this a long time and I haven't found a way. I'm about to give up on him, tell you the truth."

"I know it's frustrating. But don't give up." Ms. Woolsey said. "Fact is, he respects you. You are the reason he's still in school. If it weren't for you, he'd be on the street. So try to keep him in school. Keep him coming to classes. He needs to be here. And keep in touch with me."

"I'll try."

(Case continued in future chapters.)

EXERCISE 1.4

Answer the following questions:

- What transitions were difficult for you?
- Why were they difficult?
- How did you get through them?
- What would have made them more tolerable?
- What would have enhanced the transition as a learning experience?
- Who might have participated more, and what role might they have played?
- How can your "lessons learned" be applied to students in transition from school to adulthood?

WEBSITES WITH ADDITIONAL INFORMATION

College and Career Ready Standards

www2.ed.gov/policy/elsec/leg/blueprint/faq/college-career.pdf

http://nsttac.org/sites/default/files/CCR101.updatedFall2012.pdf

National Secondary and Transition Technical Assistance Center

www.nsttac.org

CHAPTER 2

Establishing the Need for Successful Transition Outcomes

This chapter addresses . . .

- Desired outcomes for students in transition from school to adulthood.
- The status of postschool outcomes according to research on employment, PSE, and independent living.
- In-school predictors of successful postschool outcomes.
- Timelines of in-school transition activities across grade levels that lead to successful outcomes.

As we work with transition professionals, youth, and families, we ask that they start the transition process by conceptualizing successful outcomes they desire for the youth. When successful outcomes are envisioned, we can compare that to students' current transition status. With this comparison, we can ask, "What skills need to be taught to increase the chances of a successful transition?" "What supports need to be available?" and "What resources will be needed?" We can also examine research on factors found to predict successful postschool outcomes to see if schools can include these factors in transition planning or adjust curricula to better assist the student. Finally, we can decide how early in a student's educational experience to address transition-related activities.

WHAT ARE THE SOUGHT-AFTER TRANSITION OUTCOMES?

Halpern (1985) described employment, residential settings, and social and interpersonal networks as critical dimensions of postschool success for students with disabilities. Halpern's employment dimension consisted of a wide array of components, including "job finding networks, job search skills, minimum-wage levels, employer incentives, job discrimination and structural unemployment" (p. 481). The residential environment dimension was characterized by satisfactory home living, such as "the quality and safety of the neighborhood in which the home is located . . . [and] . . . availability of both community services and recreational opportunities" (p. 481). The social and interpersonal networks dimension consisted of "daily communications, self-esteem, family support, emotional maturity, friendship, and intimate relationships" (p. 481). These dimensions may be important when considering sought-after outcomes.

Many other researchers have envisioned transition outcomes. deFur and Patton (1999) described employment, PSE, maintaining a home, becoming involved in the community, and experiencing satisfactory personal and social relationships (p. 15). For Wehmeyer (2007), four essential characteristics of the dimension of self-determination were autonomy, self-regulation, psychological empowerment, and self-realization.

In summary, the sought-after outcomes for youth in transition from school to adulthood are similar to outcomes valued by most citizens in Western society:

- Having a job, establishing a career path, and maintaining employment to pay the bills and enjoy a relatively high quality of life.
- Getting involved, to some degree, in PSE, which can range widely from pursuing a degree at the college level to taking a course on a topic of interest in adult or community education.
- Becoming recognized as a valued, contributing citizen in integrated community activities.
- Participating in recreational and leisure activities.
- Acting in ways that enhance self-determination.

Although there may be differences or variations in these outcomes for individual youth, this list represents the target areas of educational efforts during the transition process. In any case, identifying desired outcomes provides the youth and his or her support team with a set of general goals with which to compare current skill levels, support systems, and resources. But before mobilizing the transition process, all stakeholders should carefully review the transition outcomes of individuals with disabilities who have already made the journey. Although the data are in some cases sobering, understanding the status of current transition outcomes will ensure that the youth and support team are fully informed and, hopefully, better prepared.

WHAT IS THE STATUS OF EMPLOYMENT OUTCOMES FOR ADULTS WITH DISABILITIES?

Before we examine the status of postschool outcomes for young adults with disabilities, we consider the status of employment outcomes for all adults with disabilities ages 18–65. The adult outcome data provide one perspective by which to compare data on young adults in transition. Also, adult outcomes provide a frame of reference for the world that transitioning students will soon enter.

From 1999 through 2012, the Administration on Intellectual and Developmental Disabilities commissioned a longitudinal survey to analyze service trends for adults with disabilities (cited in Butterworth et al., 2014). Adult agencies in all 50 states and the District of Columbia were asked to provide data on the employment status of adults with disabilities. Through 2012, data were received on an estimated 570,000 individuals in 45 states served by adult agencies through 2011. Overall, researchers estimated that 32.5% of working-age adults with disabilities were employed, compared to 71.4% of people without disabilities. For individuals with intellectual and developmental disabilities (IDD), 22.5% were employed. Of all adults with IDD receiving state-funded services, 14.7% were involved in "integrated employment," defined as services provided in a community setting involving paid employment such as competitive employment, group- or individual-supported employment, or self-employment (Butterworth et al., 2014, p. 15). The remaining 85.3% of adults with IDD receiving employment services were involved in "facility-based work or nonwork" activities or a segregated setting where the majority of employees had a disability (e.g., sheltered workshop) (Butterworth et al., 2014, p. 16). In Figure 2.1, we show the percentage trend in integrated employment from 1999 through 2011. Since 2001, the trend for integrated employment has decreased from 25 to

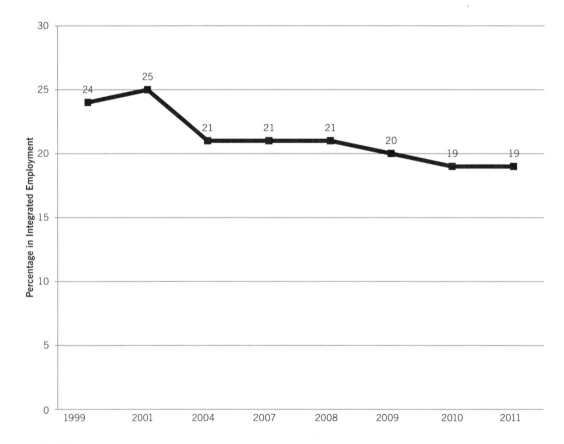

FIGURE 2.1. Percentage trend of adults with IDD in integrated employment in the United States, 1999 through 2011.

18.4%. Butterworth and colleagues (2014) stated that the decrease in integrated employment occurred because of systemic problems, such as state and federal policies that did not consistently prioritize employment, and ASPs (e.g., sheltered workshops or day programs) that did not allocate sufficient resources to community employment.

Butterworth and colleagues (2014) also reported data on average hours worked per week and wages of working adults with IDD in 2012. Overall, adults with IDD who had jobs worked an average of 23 hours per week (about half-time). Average wage was $8.13/hour (about $187 per week at 23 hours per week). For young adults with IDD who were working, the weekly wage placed them below the poverty line ($9,350 average annual wage for 50 weeks, compared to the poverty threshold of $11,945 in 2012; *www.census.gov/hhes/www/poverty/data/threshld*).

Butterworth and colleagues (2014) compared the data on individuals with IDD who were 2 years out of high school with same-age young adults who did *not* have disabilities. Sixty percent of young adults *without* disabilities were employed, compared to 22.5% of individuals with IDD. Researchers accounted for low employment data for post–high school adults with IDD by citing (1) lack of emphasis on integrated employment outcomes in state agencies, (2) inadequate collaboration between adult service agencies and transition educators, (3) limited vocational experiences in schools, (4) inadequate transition support related directly to community jobs, and (5) limited development of self-determination and career-related skills during the transition years in school. We should remember that the survey data reported above were for adults with IDD. No data were provided for adults with specific learning disabilities, emotional disturbance, physical disabilities acquired after childhood, or other types.

WHAT WERE OUTCOMES FOR STUDENTS WHO RECEIVED SPECIAL EDUCATION SERVICES?

As mentioned in Chapter 1, researchers in the 1980s conducted surveys of young adults who exited special education services and found that large percentages of them were unemployed or "underemployed." For example, Hasazi and colleagues (1985) surveyed 462 young adults with mostly mild disabilities 2 years after leaving high school and found that only 55% were employed, and most of those with jobs were in part-time, seasonal, or intermittent work.

The National Longitudinal Transition Study

In the 1990s, the U.S. Department of Education funded the National Longitudinal Transition Study (NLTS) to determine the employment, education, and independent living characteristics of young adults with disabilities who had exited high school. A follow-up study, the NLTS-2 (Newman et al., 2011), provided information over a 10-year period from a nationally representative sample of individuals with numerous types of disabilities. The NLTS-2 started by following youth ages 13–16 and ended 8 years after those youth had exited high school. The purpose of the NLTS-2 was to collect data on employment, PSE, productive engagement in the community, household circumstances, and social and community involvement in five "waves" (or successive surveys) beginning in 2001 and ending in 2009.

In Figure 2.2, we show the areas of emphases in the NLTS-2. Researchers used stratified random sampling (based on region, student enrollment, and community wealth) of 500 school districts and special schools in the United States. Students with disabilities or their parents/guardians were surveyed through telephone interviews and mailed questionnaires. The Wave 1 survey in 2001 started with 11,270 participants. Given attrition, the final Wave 5 survey in 2009 had about 4,810 participants. Comparison data were obtained from the 2009 U.S. Census Bureau survey of young adults ages 21–25 in the general population (i.e., young adults *without* disabilities). For a description of full methodology and statistical analysis of the NLTS-2, go to *www.nlts2.org.*

Employment Outcomes

Using the NLTS-2 data, researchers reported outcomes on:

- Employment outside the home.
- Employment according to type of disability.
- Employment according to parents' household income.
- Hours worked and wages per week.

The data reported in the NLTS-2 did not distinguish between competitive employment (i.e., hiring the most qualified applicant with no supports), supported or customized employment (i.e., levels or types of supports needed to maintain a job), or facilities-based employment (i.e., sheltered, segregated settings). That is, all types of employment were combined. In Chapter 8, we describe competitive, supported, and customized employment.

As shown in Table 2.1, 60% of young adults with disabilities reported that they were employed at the time of the 2009 interview. In comparison, 66% of young adults *without* disabilities reported employment, according to a U.S. Census Bureau survey. Thirty-one percent of young adults with disabilities reported employment after high school but were unemployed at the time of the interview. About 91% (i.e., 60% plus 31%)

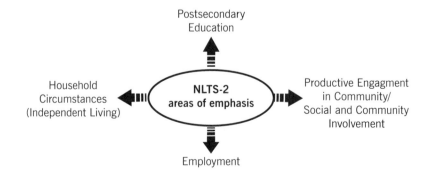

FIGURE 2.2. Areas of emphasis in NLTS-2 survey.

TABLE 2.1. Percentage of Young Adults with Disabilities Reporting Paid Employment Outside the Home

Employed at the time of the interview	60.2%
Employed after high school but unemployed at the time of the interview	31.0%
Employed at some point since leaving high school	About 91%

Note. From Newman et al. (2011). Reprinted with permission from SRI International.

reported employment at some point since leaving high school. These figures appear much higher than those from the Butterworth and colleagues (2014) survey, but the latter survey focused on more significant disabilities such as IDD, as opposed to all disability categories as in the NLTS-2.

In Table 2.2, we present employment status according to type of disability. Data are shown in two columns: (1) those who reported being employed at the time of the interview, and (2) those who reported being employed after high school but were unemployed at the time of the interview. The data showed that young adults with some types of disability, such as specific learning disability, other health impairment, and speech–language impairments, reported relatively high levels of employment (67.3%, 64.4%, and 63.9%, respectively). These levels were near those of young adults *without* disabilities

TABLE 2.2. Average Percentages of Paid Employment Outside the Home for Young Adults with Disabilities Up to 8 Years Post-High School, by Disability Category

Disability	Employed at the time of the interview	Employed since high school
Specific learning disability	67.3%	94.9%
Speech/language impairment	63.9%	94.0%
Intellectual disability	38.8%	76.2%
Emotional disturbance	49.6%	91.2%
Hearing impairment	57.2%	91.5%
Visual impairment	43.8%	78.0%
Orthopedic impairment	35.0%	67.7%
Other health impairment	64.4%	95.5%
Autism	37.2%	63.2%
Traumatic brain injury	51.6%	81.4%
Multiple disabilities	39.2%	62.5%
Deaf-blindness	30.1%	70.4%

Note. From Newman et al. (2011). Reprinted with permission from SRI International.

(i.e., 66%). Average percentages for other types of disability were much lower, such as deaf-blindness (30.1%), orthopedic impairment (35.0%), and autism (37.2%).

As you might surmise from reviewing data in Table 2.2, a category of disability does not describe a homogeneous set of characteristics. That is, abilities can vary widely even within a disability category. For example, we see that 38.8% of young adults with intellectual disability reported employment at the time of the interview, but we do not know if they experienced mild, moderate, severe, or profound intellectual disability. Furthermore, 37.2% of young adults with autism reported employment, but the autism spectrum includes functioning levels ranging from high to low. The percentages represent only average rates per disability category.

Also, the data in Table 2.2 do not show whether young adults worked in facility-based or integrated, community-based employment. Questions about these factors were not a part of the NLTS-2 interviews. For more information, see Newman and colleagues (2011) or *www.nlts2.org*.

In Table 2.3, we present percentages of young adults in paid employment outside the home according to household income of parents, race/ethnicity, and gender. Young adults with disabilities whose parents made more than $50,000 were employed at much higher percentages than young adults whose parents had less income. In addition, young adults of European (white) descent were employed more than African Americans or Hispanics. Males were employed slightly more than females. These findings remind us that advantages still exist for those of higher socioeconomic status, European descent, and male sex status. As might be expected, for young adults with disabilities, struggles of transition to adulthood are exacerbated by poverty, diversity-related characteristics, and gender. These data illustrate once again that equal access is an ongoing challenge requiring our steadfast efforts.

TABLE 2.3. Average Percentages of Young Adults in Paid Employment According to Household Income of Parents, Race/Ethnicity, and Gender

Factor	Employed at time of interview	Employed since high school
Parent income of $25,000 or less	44.4%	85.2%
Parent income of $25,001 to $50,000	65.2%	93.6%
Parent income of more than $50,000	70.7%	94.5%
Race/ethnicity: White	64.5%	93.6%
Race/ethnicity: African American	48.0%	86.4%
Race/ethnicity: Hispanic	53.6%	85.1%
Male	64.9%	91.6%
Female	52.1%	90.1%

Note. From Newman et al. (2011). Reprinted with permission from SRI International.

In Table 2.4, we present average hours worked per week among young adults according to disability category. As shown, young adults with specific learning disabilities, emotional disturbance, traumatic brain injury, other health impairment, and speech/language impairment all averaged more than 34 hours of work per week. Young adults within these categories worked significantly more hours than those with autism, deaf-blindness, multiple disabilities, orthopedic impairments, or intellectual disability, who worked between 24 and 28 hours per week. Young adults *without* disabilities reported working an average of 37.1 hours per week.

One positive finding from these data was that many young adults with disabilities were working full time or near full time when interviewed. It is unclear why young adults with some disabilities—particularly autism, deaf-blindness, multiple disabilities, orthopedic impairment, or intellectual disability—worked far fewer hours (only 24–28 hours per week), but these findings may be attributable to lower stamina or endurance, diminished productivity, behavior problems, or other factors (Frey, Buchanan, Rosser Sandt, & Taylor, 2005).

The average wage for young adults with disabilities who were employed full time was $11.10/hour. In comparison, the average wage for young adults with disabilities working part-time was $9.00. At the time of the 2009 survey, the minimum wage was $7.25/hour. In comparison, young adults *without* disabilities reported an average wage of $11.40/hour. These findings suggest that young adults with disabilities who were working at the time of the survey reported relatively high wages. Furthermore, these findings compare favorably to those of Butterworth and colleagues (2014), who reported average earnings of only $8.13/hour.

TABLE 2.4. Average Hours Worked per Week among Working Young Adults with Disabilities, According to Disability Category

Disability	Average hours worked per week
Specific learning disability	37.7
Speech/language impairment	34.2
Intellectual disability	27.6
Emotional disturbance	35.6
Hearing Impairment	31.3
Visual impairment	31.5
Orthopedic impairment	26.8
Other Health impairment	35.0
Autism	24.1
Traumatic brain injury	35.5
Multiple disabilities	24.8
Deaf-blindness	24.7
Young adults *without* disabilities	37.1

Note. From Newman et al. (2011). Reprinted with permission from SRI International.

Newman and colleagues (2011) described numerous other findings in the NLTS-2 report on the employment of young adults with disabilities. Key data included the following:

- Young adults with disabilities who completed high school averaged more hours worked per week than those who did not complete high school.
- The most common type of job worked for young adults of most disability categories was food preparation (13.1%), followed by sales (12.1%). Employment in these types of jobs diminished and other types of jobs increased the longer the time since leaving high school.
- The longer the amount of time since leaving high school, the more hours a young adult with disability worked per week.

EXERCISE 2.1

Answer the following questions:

- What, if any, NLTS-2 employment findings surprise you? What would you have expected the findings to be instead? Why?
- What NLTS-2 employment findings would you like to research further? Go to *www. nlts2.org/reports/2011_09_02/nlts2_report_2011_09_02_complete.pdf.*

Postsecondary Education

Newman and colleagues (2011) examined educational involvement for young adults with disabilities who were out of high school for up to 8 years. PSE programs included 2- or 4-year colleges; or vocational, business, and technical schools. Using the NLTS-2 data, researchers reported outcomes on:

- Percentages of young adults with disabilities enrolled in PSE programs.
- Enrollment according to type of program.
- Enrollment according to disability category.

In Table 2.5, we present data on PSE school enrollment of young adults with disabilities and a comparison sample of young adults *without* disabilities in the general population. Overall, 60.1% of survey respondents (or their children with disabilities) reported that they had enrolled in a PSE program at some point following high school. Over one-third indicated that they had enrolled in some type of PSE program in the past 2 years. At the time of the interview, 15.1% were enrolled. Higher percentages of young adults *without* disabilities in the general population sample indicated enrollment on all three measures.

Respondents were then asked to identify the type of PSE program in which they had enrolled. In Table 2.6, we find that young adults with disabilities had higher levels of enrollment in 2-year community colleges than in other types of schools, although few were currently enrolled at the time of the interview in any of the alternatives.

TABLE 2.5. Percentages of Enrollment of Young Adults with Disabilities and the General Population (i.e., Young Adults *without* Disabilities) in PSE Programs

	Young adults with disabilities	General population
Young adults who, since leaving high school, had enrolled in PSE	60.1%	67.4%
Young adults enrolled in past 2 years but not enrolled at the time of the interview	33.5%	51.2%
Young adults enrolled at the time of the interview	15.1%	28.3%

Note. From Newman et al. (2011). Reprinted with permission from SRI International.

TABLE 2.6. Percentages of Enrollment for Young Adults with Disabilities and Young Adults *without* Disabilities in the General Population in 2-Year, Vocational/Business/Technical, and 4-Year Colleges

	Young adults with disabilities	General population
Ever enrolled[a]		
Two-year community college	44.2%	20.6%
Vocational, business, or technical school	32.3%	20.3%
Four-year college	18.8%	40.2%
Enrolled at time of interview		
Two-year community college	9.0%	5.9%
Vocational, business, or technical school	2.2%	3.8%
Four-year college	5.2%	16.1%

Note. From Newman et al. (2011). Reprinted with permission from SRI International.
[a]Totals exceed 60.1% for students with disabilities because some respondents reported involvement in more than one type of PSE program.

In Table 2.7, we show percentages of PSE enrollment of young adults with disabilities who were ever enrolled by IDEA category. Data are divided into 2-year colleges; vocational, technical, or business colleges; and 4-year colleges. Enrollment varied widely by disability category. Across categories, respondents are shown in each type of PSE program. The 2-year college was the most common program for all categories. Respondents with intellectual and multiple disabilities were the least involved in PSE across all three types of programs.

Newman and colleagues (2011) described numerous other findings on PSE of young adults with disabilities. All findings were based on average or overall percentages. Key findings included the following:

- High school completers had significantly higher levels of enrollment in all types of PSE programs than noncompleters.
- Similar to employment, young adults with disabilities whose parents' household income was more than $50,000/year had significantly higher levels of enrollment in PSE programs than young adults of lower-income parents.
- Young adults with disabilities who were Hispanic or African American had slightly higher levels of enrollment in 2-year colleges and vocational, business, or technical schools than European Americans, who had higher enrollment in 4-year colleges.
- Females with disabilities had slightly higher levels of enrollment in 2-year colleges and 4-year colleges than males with disabilities. Males had slightly higher enrollment in vocational, business, or technical schools than females.
- Over 70% of young adults with disabilities who enrolled in any type of PSE program did not inform the school of their disability (or did not consider or know that they had a disability). Those most likely to inform the school of their disabilities were young adults with orthopedic (76.1%) and visual (73.0%) impairments. Those least likely to inform programs were young adults with speech–language impairment (16.6%) or with specific learning disabilities (24.2%).
- According to the survey of all respondents up to 8 years out of high school, over 40% of young adults with disabilities graduated from or completed a PSE program.

TABLE 2.7. Percentages of PSE Program Enrollment of Young Adults (Ever Enrolled), by Disability Category

Disability	Ever enrolled in:		
	2-year community college	Vocational/ technical/ business school	4-year college
Specific learning disability	49.9	35.8	21.2
Speech/language impairmentt	46.0	28.5	32.5
Intellectual disability	18.9	16.4	6.7
Emotional disturbance	37.7	33.3	10.8
Hearing impairment	51.5	42.9	33.8
Visual impairment	51.5	26.2	40.1
Orthopedic impairment	50.3	26.2	26.1
Other Health impairment	51.6	32.2	19.6
Autism	32.2	21.0	17.4
Traumatic brain injury	42.2	36.9	18.5
Multiple disabilities	21.7	17.5	7.4
Deaf-blindness	36.9	22.1	23.7

Note. From Newman et al. (2011). Reprinted with permission from SRI International.

EXERCISE 2.2

Answer the following questions:

- What, if any, NLTS-2 PSE findings surprise you? What would you have expected the findings to be instead? Why?
- What NLTS-2 PSE findings would you like to research further? Go to *www.nlts2.org/ reports/2011_09_02/nlts2_report_2011_09_02_complete.pdf.*

Household Circumstances

In the NLTS-2 report, Newman and colleagues (2011) described data on independence and living circumstances. A few highlights included the following:

- At the time of the interview, 45% of young adults with disabilities reported that they were living independently. This finding compares to 59% for young adults *without* disabilities. The highest percentages of young adults living on their own were those with specific learning disabilities (64.9%) and emotional disturbance (63.1%). The lowest percentages living on their own were young adults with multiple disabilities (16.4%) or autism (17%).
- At the time of the interview, 13.5% of young adults with disabilities reported that they were married, compared to 19.3% of young adults *without* disabilities. In terms of parenting status, 29.4% of young adults with disabilities reported they had a child or had fathered a child. This finding was slightly higher than young adults *without* disabilities (28.4%).
- Over half of young adults with disabilities who responded to the survey indicated they had both a savings and checking account, and 41.4% of respondents had a credit card.

Social and Community Involvement

The NLTS-2 researchers also examined involvement in social and community activities. A few noteworthy results included the following:

- In the preceding year, over half of young adults with disabilities reported involvement in community education lessons or classes, volunteer or community service activities, or community groups.
- Seventy-one percent of age-eligible young adults with disabilities reported being registered to vote.
- On a negative note, almost one-third (32.3%) of young adults with disabilities reported that they had been arrested by law enforcement authorities, as compared to 12.3% for young adults *without* disabilities. By far, the highest percentage of respondents with disabilities reporting arrest was young adults with emotional disturbance (60.5%). The next highest percentage was young adults with traumatic brain injury (35.0%).

EXERCISE 2.3

Answer the following questions:

- What NLTS-2 independent living or community/social involvement findings surprise you? What would you have expected the findings to be instead? Why?
- What NLTS-2 independent living or community/social involvement findings would you like to research further? Go to *www.nlts2.org/reports/2011_09_02/nlts2_ report_2011_09_02_complete.pdf.*

Analysis of NLTS-2 Findings

In Wave 5 findings of the NLTS-2, Newman and colleagues (2011) found generally high percentages of young adults with disabilities engaged in employment, PSE, independent living, and/or community involvement. These outcomes suggested that young adults with disabilities were getting involved in personal and community activities during their early adult years. Although outcomes varied widely across disability categories, parent income levels, and gender, the data provided a degree of optimism regarding transition efforts. Comparison of the NLTS-2 findings to surveys from the 1980s and 1990s is problematic because of differences in research methods. Any comparisons across studies should take into account a variety of contextual variables. For example, comparison of the NLTS-2 employment findings to the survey by the Administration on Intellectual and Developmental Disabilities (cited in Butterworth et al., 2014) showed far higher employment of young adults with disabilities. However, the NLTS-2 reported on all types of disabilities, whereas the Butterworth and colleagues (2014) survey focused on IDD. Researchers have pointed out that the measurement methods used in survey research on the employment of adults with disabilities can affect outcomes (Lengnick-Hall, Gaunt, & Brookes, 2001). Skeptics may note potential bias in survey methods (e.g., nonrespondents may have chosen not to respond because they were not employed or going to school). However, to their credit, NLTS-2 researchers anticipated bias problems by performing statistical "weighting" to adjust the reported data (Javitz, Wagner, & Newman, 2008). Clearly, vast improvement in transition outcomes is still possible, and major disparities still exist in data comparing young adults with and without disabilities.

WHAT FACTORS PREDICT SUCCESSFUL POSTSCHOOL OUTCOMES?

If we could identify factors, or *predictor variables* (i.e., knowledge, skills, and activities) relating to the future success of young adults with disabilities, then we could promote programs using those factors to improve transition practices. With knowledge of these predictor variables, we could examine a youth's desired outcomes, compare that to current skills, and recommend programs to bridge any gaps that existed.

The National Secondary Transition Technical Assistance Center (NSTTAC)[1] is a national center that provides technical assistance and information dissemination and

---

[1] NSTTAC has changed its name to the National Technical Assistance Center on Transition (NTACT). Individuals can still go to their website at *www.nsttac.org* or to *www.transitionta.org.*

is funded by the U.S. Department of Education's Office of Special Education Programs and Rehabilitation Services Administration. One of the NSTTAC's goals is to improve transition services leading to successful postschool outcomes for students with disabilities (NSTTAC, 2010, p. 3). For more information, see the website at the end of this chapter. The NSTTAC (2010) conducted a review of the secondary transition literature to identify in-school predictors of improved postschool outcomes. The researchers identified 22 studies meeting rigorous selection criteria that investigated the relationship between transition outcomes and predictor variables. We should note that existing research on predictor variables is correlational; there has been minimal intervention research to demonstrate cause and effect.

Across these studies, there were 26,480 transition-age participants. Based on the review, 16 in-school predictors correlated with improved postschool outcomes in PSE, employment, and/or independent living. These predictors are shown in Table 2.8, along with the outcomes each one predicted (designated by X).

Some variables predicted all three outcomes (PSE, employment, and independent living). These predictors were *inclusion in general education, paid employment/work experience during high school, self-care/independent living,* and *student support during transition.* Predictors of two outcomes (PSE and employment) were *career awareness, interagency collaboration, occupational courses, self-advocacy/self-determination, social skills, transition program,* and *vocational evaluation.*

TABLE 2.8. Predictor Categories and Associated Improvements in Postschool Outcomes

Predictors/outcomes	PSE	Employment	Independent living
Career awareness	X	X	
Community experiences		X	
Exit exam requirements/high school diploma status		X	
Inclusion in general education	X	X	X
Interagency collaboration	X	X	
Occupational courses	X	X	
Paid employment/work experience	X	X	X
Parental involvement/expectations		X	
Program of study		X	
Self-advocacy/self-determination	X	X	
Self-care/independent living	X	X	X
Social skills	X	X	
Student support	X	X	X
Transition program	X	X	
Vocational education	X	X	
Work study		X	

Note. From the National Secondary Transition Technical Assistance Center (2010).

Based on the statistical evidence, predictors were assigned *strong, moderate* or *potential* prediction for PSE, employment, or independent living. There were no strong predictors. The highest ranked predictor (moderate for all three outcomes) was *inclusion in general education,* followed by *vocational education, paid employment/work experience,* and *parent expectations.*

The presence of certain variables in predictor research was noteworthy. First, inclusion in general education emerged as the highest-ranked predictor. Earlier, we speculated that transition and standards-based education should work in partnership by providing learning opportunities in a range of learning environments from general education classrooms to community-based, real-life contexts. Transition research appears to support such a partnership. Second, self-advocacy and self-determination were predictive of successful employment and PSE outcomes. Students in transition should determine their own futures and advocate for themselves to the fullest extent possible.

The NSTTAC (2010) asserted that identification of these predictor variables provided information to practitioners on effective transition practices. As they evaluate their transition programs, state and local education agencies may want to determine whether these predictors are being implemented in schools. Rather than view predictors as "check-off" items for transition curricula, we propose more in-depth analysis. What matters most is how a school implements a predictor, how much time and effort are allocated, and how transition educators make decisions based on student data. For example, although it is important to know that involvement in inclusive classrooms predicts successful outcomes, we would speculate that it is the quality and intensity of involvement in inclusive classrooms that makes a difference.

The NSTTAC (2010) noted that data on predictors of successful outcomes were not "disaggregated" (i.e., divided into categories), so the strength of certain predictor variables for particular disabilities or characteristics (e.g., gender, ethnicity) is not clear. The authors also note that more research is needed. As more high-quality research is conducted, the list of predictor variables may grow or the strength of various predictors may change. Finally, although predictor variables were identified, the research does not provide guidance on when (i.e., at what age) various types of transition programs should be implemented. For example, transition educators might ask, "When should career awareness courses be taught in relation to graduation to be maximally effective?" In the next section, we examine these questions.

EXERCISE 2.4

Answer the following questions:

- What is your take on the NSTTAC findings regarding in-school predictors of postschool outcomes? What would you have expected as a predictor that was not present in the list of predictors. What was present in the list of predictors that surprised you?
- What would you recommend for future research on in-school predictors?
- Beyond PSE, employment, and independent living, what other categories should research consider for identifying predictor variables? Why?

TO ACHIEVE OUTCOMES, HOW EARLY SHOULD TRANSITION START? WHAT SHOULD BE TAUGHT?

In conversations about transition from school to adulthood, we often hear stakeholders say "Start early." The current thinking is to start several years prior to the student's departure from special education services. Although the IDEA requires that certain activities commence at age 16, many advocates recommend starting transition as early as sixth grade when students with disabilities begin middle school. But what exactly should be taught and when?

A *timeline*, in this context, is a list of skills and activities to be taught in a logical sequence across grades. Nielsen (2013) developed a sixth- to 12th-grade timeline for students with high-incidence disabilities (e.g., specific learning disabilities, emotional disturbance) based on perceptions of educators and parents. Although the timeline is for students with high-incidence disabilities, most items apply to students with all types of disabilities, including intellectual disabilities and autism.

Nielsen (2013) gathered information to produce the timeline from the existing transition literature. She examined the importance and age/grade-appropriateness of skills/activities on the timeline by collecting ratings from educators and parents in focus groups. Participants included eight secondary special educators with at least 10 years experience, and five parents of young adults with high-incidence disabilities who had graduated from both high school and PSE programs. These 13 individuals participated in focus groups to decide which items should be considered important and how items should be placed chronologically. Nielsen analyzed data based on median and range scores for each item, and rank-ordered items to produce a timeline of transition skills/activities. Only items rated highest (median = 4) are shown here. In Table 2.9, we present the highest-rated transition timeline items encompassing *all grades* (6th through 12th). In Table 2.10, we show a continuum reflecting the sequence of skills to be taught in grades 6–8, 9–10, 11, and 12.

TABLE 2.9. Highest Overall Ranked Items Encompassing All Grades 6–12

- Participates in core general education classes.
- Participates in general education math classes.
- Demonstrates appropriate social skills across settings.
- Learns self-advocacy strategy (e.g., asks teachers to clarify assignments).
- Attends meeting for IEP.
- Attends student educational occupational plan (SEOP).
- Comes prepared for each class (e.g., pencil, paper, text, completed assignments).
- Demonstrates good attendance and punctuality.
- Follows rules, routines, and procedures for each class.
- Takes core exams.
- Uses decision-making skills.
- Uses technology skills.

Note. From Nielsen (2013). Adapted with permission from the author.

TABLE 2.10. Highest Ranked Items within Grades 6–8, 9 and 10, 11, and 12

Grades 6–8 (top 12 items out of 16)

Demonstrates acceptable hygiene.

Follows one-step, two-step, and multistep directions.

Independently contacts teachers about missing work.

Memorizes class schedule, locker combination, student number, etc.

Writes assignments in a planner, uses an assignment calendar, and keeps a homework binder.

Understands safety skills (e.g., Internet safety).

Participates in IEP meeting by making introductions.

Understands assignment expectations.

Demonstrates respect for one's own property and property belonging to others.

Attends career and technical education classes (CTE) when beginning seventh grade.

Takes several assessments, including interest, learning style, etc.

Keeps work area and locker clean.

Grades 9 and 10 (top 12 items out of 27)

Participates in IEP meeting by making introductions and sharing career goals, strengths, weaknesses, accommodations, and how those accommodations affect performance.

Reviews credit history toward graduation at SEOP.

Identifies the remunerative, personal, and social benefits met through work.

Takes driver training if the state allows it or independently uses public transportation.

Obtains driver's permit.

Identifies factors that will affect retention and promotion on the job site.

Demonstrates understanding of time management.

Learns job-related social communication skills.

Demonstrates understanding of grade-point average (GPA) and American College Testing (ACT) scores required for admission to state colleges.

Identifies job requirements (e.g., gets food handlers' permit to work at a restaurant).

Begins development of career portfolio.

Demonstrates understanding of the level of education needed for various careers.

Grade 11 (top 10 items out of 15 items)

Reviews credit history toward graduation and ACT application during SEOP.

Identifies requirements for enrolling in college.

Participates in self-directed IEP meeting with VR counselor attending (student directs the IEP and the VR counselor participates).

Adds to career portfolio (resumé and reference list).

(continued)

TABLE 2.10. *(continued)*

Identifies how disability affects employment.

Identifies how accommodations affect employment.

Participates in career awareness class or work–study program.

Adapts to change in the work environment.

Demonstrates self-management in employment (e.g., initiates tasks).

Takes ACT preparation class.

Grade 12 (all 13 items considered important)

Obtains summary of performance documents.

Participates in college tour day at school, gets college applications.

Increases skills using assistive technology in preparation for college.

Retakes ACT test (if necessary).

Obtains necessary documentation for disability resource center at postsecondary settings.

Contacts agencies for support (PSE program disability resource centers, VR).

Completes applications for college admissions.

Self-directs IEP.

Enrolls in financial literacy and/or adult roles classes.

Participates in internship or apprenticeship.

Understands information on a pay stub.

Understands federal and state income tax.

Demonstrates how, when, and where to independently disclose one's disability, and when *not* to disclose a disability.

Note. From Nielsen (2013). Adapted with permission from the author.

Educators and parents commented that all of the 12 highest-rated items (see Table 2.9) should be priorities throughout secondary grades. The two highest-ranked items related to the active involvement of youth with disabilities in general education classes (i.e., core curriculum including math). Social and self-advocacy skills were next highest in importance. Many items ranked highest by educators and parents were similar to Test and colleagues' (2009) in-school predictors of postschool success (e.g., general education classes, social skills, self-advocacy).

Highest-ranked items for grades 6–8, 9–10, 11, and 12 in sequence are shown in Table 2.10. Placement of these items shows how educators and parents envisioned a sequence of transition teaching activities across grades.

Educators and parents rated multiple items as early as sixth through eighth grades as important in preparation for transition to employment, PSE, and independent living (e.g., acceptable hygiene, following directions). In ninth and 10th grades, highest-rated items were those reflecting more targeted, goal-directed skills (e.g., participating in one's IEP meeting, interview training for a job, building a resumé). Highest-rated items in 11th and 12th grades were more specific and reflected final preparations for future activities (e.g., college applications, self-management).

Nielsen's (2013) timeline showed that, according to a small sample of educators and parents, many transition skills and activities were considered important. Other important skills and activities may have been excluded because they were not identified in existing timelines in the literature. However, the study showed that educators and parents are able to set priorities on what must be taught, starting in the sixth grade.

EXERCISE 2.5

What skills or activities would you add to the timeline? At what grade(s) would you add them? Reflect on your own transition: What skills/activities would have helped? During which grade?

SUMMARY

For young adults with disabilities, sought-after outcomes in the transition from school to adulthood are similar to outcomes valued by most citizens in Western society: having a job, establishing a career path, and maintaining employment. Additional desired outcomes include PSE, which can range widely from pursuing a degree at the college level to taking a course on a topic of interest in adult or community education. Existing data on the extent to which young adults access these activities are variable. Although surveys of adults with IDD show relatively low levels of employment, low wages, and decreased jobs in integrated community settings (Butterworth et al., 2014), the NLTS-2 survey shows relatively high community engagement of young adults up to 8 years post–high school. The survey methods were vastly different, however, which accounts for differences in findings. In considering the NLTS-2 results, we reviewed data on employment, PSE, household circumstances (i.e., independent living), and social/community environments. With a better understanding of data on postschool outcomes, we examined factors in schools that predict the future success of young adults with disabilities. Test and colleagues (2009) systematically reviewed the secondary transition literature to identify in-school predictors of improved postschool outcomes for students with disabilities. Sixteen predictors were identified. Predictors of all three outcomes (PSE, employment, and independent living) were inclusion in general education, paid employment/work experience during high school, self-care/independent living, and student support during transition. If these activities predict postschool success, special educators should consider involving students with disabilities in them as early as possible, potentially starting in sixth grade (Nielsen (2013).

REVISITING JOSEFINA

Ms. Martin, Josefina's teacher, sat down to meet with Josefina's parents, Raul and Mariana. Josefina's senior year was a phenomenal success, Ms. Martin reported. In many respects, Josefina had changed the culture of Ignacio High School. She was elected to student council and was an active participant on the cheerleading squad. She was an integral part of the senior class and a rallying point for the entire school. Students with and without disabilities watched her as she worked relentlessly on assignments in the chemistry lab, a presentation in U.S. government class, and movements in the "Warrior Cheer" with the cheerleading squad. All seniors gathered in a circle to watch Josefina and her date dance at the senior prom. Her wheelchair was not an impediment; it was part of the dance routine! She had taught students at Ignacio something about motivation, persistence, and courage. Their comments in her yearbook reflected how Josefina became a model student that changed their way of thinking. "You made me understand how all people are capable of greatness," one student commented. Josefina, like many seniors at the center of the school's attention, was caught up in the process. After so many years dealing with her cerebral palsy, her hard work had paid off. She knew how vigorously she had to work to succeed. She knew about long hours working late at night on assignments. But now she was pleased as her senior year drew to a close. As Ms. Martin described Josefina's accomplishments, her parents felt pride and satisfaction. Josefina smiled broadly.

"Josefina has shown interest in working as a teacher's assistant. We call them paraprofessionals, or paraeducators. If you want, we could build on Josefina's success and think about job placement?" Ms. Martin asked.

Josefina's parents were silent.

Ms. Martin described what paraeducators do in classrooms to assist students. "If you wanted to consider this job, it would be an opportunity for Josefina."

"But Ms. Martin," Raul offered, "as we said before, we need Josefina at home. Her family needs her. Her responsibility is to serve her brothers and sisters, nieces and nephews. She can inspire them."

"I understand," said Ms. Martin. "You must be looking forward to having her at home to help out. And she will be a great helper. But she has had such success in school with all kinds of people. Shouldn't Josefina have the opportunity to inspire others?"

"We don't mean to be selfish," said Mariana. "But there is so much for her to do at home. We desperately need her now. I can't do it all anymore. I have some health problems. The last couple of years have been so hard. And I've been waiting for her to finish school. I need her help now. I respect what you are saying. I understand your wishes for Josefina. But we need her right now to help the little kids, especially nieces and nephews that I must take care of. Maybe someday she can get a job. But now is not the time."

Ms. Martin turned to Josefina. "What would you like to do?"

Josefina chose her words carefully and spoke slowly. "I know what you are saying, Ms. Martin. I've had a great year at school. I will never forget. I have many friends. I would love to have a job. But I know I need to help at home. That is what I want right now. I will be happy at home. Maybe later I will find a job. It's OK. Thank you."

(Case continued in future chapters.)

EXERCISE 2.6

- If you could craft an ideal transition timeline of all the necessary skills and activities to adequately prepare a student with a disability for the adult world, what would you include? Use information from the NLTS-2, the NSTTAC study on in-school predictors of postschool outcomes, the transition timeline, and the discussion about expectations of postschool environments.
- What advice would you provide to Josefina and her parents? Is there a way to fulfill her parents' wishes as well as Josefina's career aspirations?
- What about other outcomes for Josefina? How would you recommend supporting her in other transition outcomes?

WEBSITES WITH ADDITIONAL INFORMATION

National Longitudinal Transition Study–2

www.nlts2.org

National Secondary Transition Technical Assistance Center

www.nsttac.org or *www.transitionta.org*

Predictor Implementation School/District Self-Assessment

www.transitionta.org/download/PostsecondaryEducation/Predictor_Self-Assessment.final_07_02_13.pdf

Aligning Evidence-Based Practices and Predictors of Post-School Success

www.transitionta.org/download/PostsecondaryEducation/AlignEBPP_Resources_PSS_FINAL_2014.pdf

National Post-School Outcomes Center

www.psocenter.org

CHAPTER 3

Transition-Related Legislation and Policy

This chapter addresses . . .

- The transition mandate as outlined in the Individuals with Disabilities Education Act (IDEA).
- IDEA Indicators 13 and 14.
- The Rehabilitation Act as amended in the Workforce Innovation and Opportunity Act.
- The amended Americans with Disabilities Act.
- The Ticket to Work and Work Incentives Improvement Act.
- The Fair Labor Standards Act.

HOW CAN WE CATEGORIZE DISABILITY-RELATED LAWS?

Understanding the vast array of disability legislation and policy can be a daunting task for many professionals and families. Nonetheless, it is imperative that stakeholders have a basic understanding of the protections and opportunities that specific laws provide transition-age youth with disabilities. With a basic understanding, transition professionals can better advise youth and their families, work with representatives from other agencies, and develop transition plans taking advantage of the protections and opportunities.

Silverstein (2000) suggested that current laws affecting people with disabilities be divided into distinct categories, including *civil rights statutes, entitlement programs, discretionary grant-in-aid programs,* and *regulatory statutes*. These categories are illustrated in Figure 3.1.

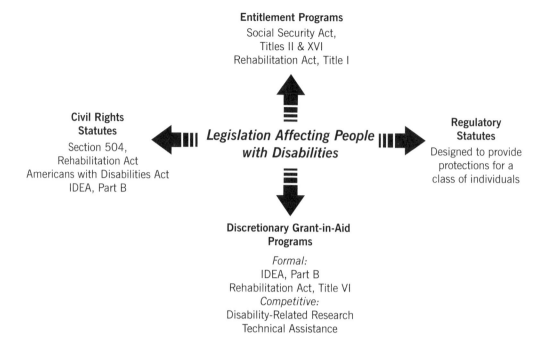

FIGURE 3.1. Categories of laws affecting individuals with disabilities (Silverstein, 2000).

Civil rights statutes prohibit discrimination based on a person's disability, sex, race, religion, and age. Section 504 of the Rehabilitation Act, the Americans with Disabilities Act (ADA), and Part B of the Individuals with Disabilities Education Act (IDEA) are examples of civil rights statutes.

Entitlement programs provide eligible individuals a certain level of benefit in the form of either monetary or program assistance. For example, Title II of the Social Security Act and Title XVI provide beneficiaries with federal financial assistance. Medicaid provides health care and long-term assistance to eligible individuals with low incomes. Title I of the Rehabilitation Act provides eligible individuals with disabilities with VR services.

Silverstein divided discretionary grant programs into two separate categories: formula grants and competitive grants. Formula grants, such as Part B of the IDEA and Title VI of the Rehabilitation Act, provide financial assistance to states to establish programs and supports for people with disabilities. Competitive grants are awarded to entities to conduct disability-related research, develop technical assistance programs, and develop training programs.

Finally, regulatory statutes were designed to provide certain protections for a class of individuals. Examples of regulatory statues include the National Voter Registration Act and the Family and Medical Leave Act (Silverstein, 2000).

WHAT IS THE IDEA?

The IDEA was preceded by the Education for All Handicapped Children Act, passed in 1975. This law, known as Public Law 94-142, was an important step in improving educational opportunities for students with disabilities. A number of court cases, most notably federal cases (*Mills v. Board of Education of the District of Columbia*, 1972; *Pennsylvania Association of Retarded Children v. Commonwealth of Pennsylvania et al.*, 1972), challenged how schools were educating students with disabilities. In the 1970s, education of students with disabilities was characterized by segregated schools and limited educational opportunities. These landmark cases prompted Congress to establish the "zero exclusion" principle and to provide a framework for due process outlined in Public Law 94-142.

In 1990, Congress reauthorized Public Law 94-142 and called it the IDEA. For the first time, Congress explicitly required school districts to assume more responsibilities in coordinating a student's transition from school to adult life. A child's IEP had to contain a statement of transition services.

In the 1997 reauthorization of the IDEA, Congress articulated that improving educational results for children was a national priority for ensuring "equality of opportunity, full participation, independent living, and economic self-sufficiency for individuals with disabilities" (20 U.S.C. § 1400 [c][1], 1997). Congress also added that children with disabilities were entitled to a free and appropriate education, emphasizing special education and related services designed to "prepare a student with disabilities for movement to post-school employment and independent living" (20 U.S.C § 1400 [d][1] [a], 1997).

The most recent reauthorization of the IDEA in 2004 included revisions to transition planning to strengthen it and improve outcomes for students with disabilities. Changes were made in response to the recommendations of the President's Commission on Excellence in Special Education report (U.S. Department of Education Office of Special Education and Rehabilitative Services, 2002). The report noted that the IDEA's requirements were too complex and needed better clarity for implementation. Also, the report recommended that the IDEA be changed to "clearly" link the long-range goals of a student with disabilities to the development of his or her annual IEP goals, objectives, and activities (p. 47).

EXERCISE 3.1

The President's Commission on Excellence in Special Education report recommended that the IDEA be changed to link a student's long-range goals to the development of his or her annual IEP goals, objectives, and activities. To the commission, long-range goals meant statements identifying a youth's aspirations after leaving school. How might a teacher find out what students and their parents want to identify as long-term goals?

The IDEA (2004) Transition Mandate

The IDEA (2004) defined transition services as a coordinated set of activities that are designed to facilitate movement of a child with a disability from school to employment, PSE, independent living, and/or participation in the community. According to the IDEA (2004), transition services should:

1. be designed as a results-oriented process focused on improving the academic and functional achievement of the child with a disability to facilitate the child's movement from school to post-school activities, including postsecondary education, vocational education, integrated employment (including supported employment), continuing and adult education, adult services, independent living, or community participation;
2. be based on the individual child's needs, taking into account the child's strengths, preferences, and interests; and
3. include instruction, related services, community experiences, the development of employment and other post-school adult living objectives, and, if appropriate, acquisition of daily living skills and functional vocational evaluation. (34 CFR 300.43 [a]] 20 U.S.C. 1401[34])

Four IDEA (2004) transition highlights are noteworthy:

1. The 2004 amendments establish a clear time frame to implement transition planning and instruction. IEP teams are required to develop a transition plan in the first IEP in effect when the child is 16 years of age, to be updated annually.
2. The transition plan must include measurable postsecondary goals based on age-appropriate transition assessments related to training, education, employment, and independent living.
3. The transition plan must outline the transition services, including course of study, to assist the child in reaching his or her transition goals.
4. Finally, 1 year prior to the child reaching the age of majority, the IEP should include a statement that the child was informed of any rights under Part B that would transfer to the child when he or she reaches the age of majority (20 U.S.C. § 1414). This means that the state needs to transfer all or some of the educational rights to the child when he or she reaches the age of 18, such as the student's right to consent to a change in placement, to receive notice of IEP meetings, and to consent to reevaluation.

ACCORDING TO THE IDEA (2004), WHO SHOULD ATTEND THE IEP TRANSITION MEETING?

The IDEA stipulates that the local education agency (LEA; e.g., a school district or charter school) must invite a child with a disability to attend the annual IEP team meeting "if a purpose of the meeting will be the consideration of the postsecondary goals for the child and the transition services needed to assist the child in reaching" (34 CFR 300.321[b][1]). If the student does not attend the IEP meeting, the LEA should take additional steps to ensure that the student's preferences and interests are being considered in the meeting. In addition, with the consent of the parent or student who has reached the age of majority, the LEA should invite a representative of a participating agency who is responsible for providing the services needed to assist the student in reaching specific postsecondary goals (34 CFR 300.321[b][3]). The most likely participating agency representatives are VR counselors, caseworkers from the state's developmental disabilities agency, or counselors from PSE disability service offices.

HOW ARE IDEA (2004) TRANSITION PERFORMANCE GOALS AND INDICATORS MEASURED?

The IDEA (2004) requires each state to develop performance plans that evaluate the effort to implement the IDEA's provisions (20 U.S.C. 1416[a][3][B]). Under the IDEA, states are required to submit an annual performance report (APR) based on IDEA indicators. The state's monitoring activities therefore have to be designed to improve the "education results and functional outcomes for all children with disabilities" (34 CFR 300.604 [a][1]). The Office of Special Education Programs (OSEP) regulates the IDEA and has developed 21 indicators to guide state educational agencies with implementation and reporting of progress on meeting state goals. The following four indicators are specific to the transition process:

- Indicator 1: percent of youth who graduate from high school.
- Indicator 2: percent of youth who drop out of school.
- Indicator 13: percent of youth with required transition components in the IEP.
- Indicator 14: percent of youth who achieve postschool outcomes outlined in the IDEA.

Indicators 13 and 14 are described below because they are central to the transition process. Indicators 1 and 2 are also critical to transition, but they are influenced by many factors not specifically related to transition (e.g., type of school attended, socioeconomic status).

Indicator 13

This indicator addresses the structure of written transition plans for students age 16 and above. Specifically, Indicator 13 addresses:

Percent of youth with IEPs age 16 and above with an IEP that includes appropriate measurable postsecondary goals that are annually updated and based upon an age-appropriate transition assessment, transition services, including courses of study, that will reasonably enable the student to meet those postsecondary goals, and annual IEP goals related to the student's transition services needs. There also must be evidence that the student was invited to the IEP Team meeting where transition services are to be discussed and evidence that a representative of any participating agency was invited to the IEP Team meeting with the prior consent of the parent or student who has reached the age of majority. (20 U.S.C. 1416(a)(3)(B))

Because Indicator 13 is a compliance indicator, states are required to show that 100% of all students who are age 16 and over have IEPs that include specific transition-related components. The NSTTAC (2012c) developed eight questions to determine compliance with each component (see website at the end of this chapter). The Indicator 13 checklist is presented along with information on how to write transition plans in Chapter 6.

Indicator 14

Indicator 14 is a results-based measure that addresses the percent of youth who are no longer in secondary school, have IEPs in effect at the time they left school, and are (1) enrolled in higher education within 1 year of leaving school; (2) enrolled in higher education or competitively employed within 1 year of leaving high school; and/or (3) enrolled in higher education or in some other postsecondary education or training program, or competitively employed or in some other employment within 1 year of leaving high school (20 U.S.C. §1416[a][3][B]).

The National Post-School Outcomes Center (NPSO) provided state education agencies with advice on how to develop a rigorous data collection system to measure the components of Indicator 14. (See website at the end of this chapter.) Table 3.1 provides definitions for each of the Indicator 14 categories as outlined by the NPSO. States are required to measure and report the percentages for these outcomes annually.

TABLE 3.1. NPSO Indicator 14 Definitions

Outcome	Definition
Enrolled in higher education	Youth have been enrolled on a full- or part-time basis in a community college (2-year program) or college/university (4-year or more program) for at least one complete term, at anytime in the year since leaving high school.
Competitive employment	Youth have worked for pay at or above minimum wage in a setting with others who do not have disabilities for a period of 20 hours a week for at least 90 days at any time in the year since leaving high school. This includes military employment.
Enrolled in other postsecondary education or training	Youth have been enrolled on a full- or part-time basis for at least 1 complete term any time in the year since leaving high school in an education or training program (e.g., Job Corps, adult education, workforce development program, vocational technical school which is less than a 2-year program).
Other employment	Youth have worked for pay or have been self-employed for a period of at least 90 days at any time in the year since leaving high school. This includes working in a family business (e.g., farm, store, fishing, ranching, catering services).

Note. From Falls and Unruh (2010). Reprinted with permission from the authors.

As readers may surmise from previous sections, the IDEA has placed greater emphasis on education results, courses of study, and functional outcomes, including measurable postsecondary goals. Through Indicators 13 and 14, the IDEA defines measurable outcomes and requires states to collect data on performance. Some scholars have commented that the IDEA has moved from a focus on process variables, such as services and supports, to outcomes as described above (e.g., Turnbull, Turnbull, Wehmeyer, & Park, 2003). But a focus on outcomes implies that processes are inherent and still in place (Browder & Spooner, 2011). The shift away from process variables, however, may mean that transition educators lose sight of effective, evidence-based teaching procedures that can lead to successful outcomes. Later chapters place considerable emphasis on "what works"—that is, on teaching procedures used in the process of reaching successful postschool outcomes.

EXERCISE 3.2

Given what you have read so far in this book, what is your view of the current status of the IDEA in regard to legislating transition from special education services to adulthood? Is the IDEA 2004 reauthorization on target by making schools more accountable for successful outcomes? Has it gone too far? Not far enough? What would you recommend for future reauthorizations of IDEA on transition?

WHAT IS THE REHABILITATION ACT?

The passage of the Rehabilitation Act of 1973 protected qualified individuals from discrimination in any program or activity that received federal funding. This Act also expanded the scope of rehabilitation to serve people with significant disabilities. The Rehabilitation Act, most recently reauthorized under the Workforce Innovation and Opportunity Act (2014), is divided into a preamble and seven separate titles. The preamble defines key terms such as *disability* and the intent of the Act. The term *disability* is defined as "a physical or mental impairment that constitutes or results in a substantial impediment to employment; or physical or mental impairment that substantially limits one or more life activities" (29 U.S.C § 705 [9][a][b]). The Act is designed:

1. To empower individuals with disabilities to maximize employment, economic self-sufficiency, independence, and inclusion and integration into society, through—
   a. Statewide workforce investment systems;
   b. Independent living centers and services;
   c. Research;
   d. Training;
   e. Demonstration projects; and
   f. The guarantee of equal opportunity; and
2. To ensure that the Federal Government plays a leadership role in promoting the employment of individuals with disabilities, especially individuals with significant disabilities, and in assisting States and providers of services in fulfilling the aspirations of such

individuals with disabilities for meaningful and gainful employment and independent living. (29 U.S.C § 701 (b)(1))

The seven titles serve as a framework for the Act. Table 3.2 describes each of the titles.

WHO IS ELIGIBLE FOR VR SERVICES?

To be eligible for VR services, a person must (1) have a physical or mental impairment that constitutes or results in a substantial impediment to employment, and (2) require VR services to prepare for, secure, retain, or regain employment. In addition, Title II (Social Security Disability Insurance [SSDI]) and Title XVI (Supplemental Security Income [SSI]) beneficiaries are automatically presumed to be eligible for VR services given that the individuals intend to achieve an employment outcome.

Additionally, the Act requires that states develop a plan outlining how they will implement an "order of selection" if there are insufficient resources to serve all eligible individuals (Section 101[a][5][A]). Under an order of selection, individuals with the most significant disabilities are selected first for VR services. A person with a significant disability is defined as an individual:

- who has a severe physical or mental impairment which seriously limits one or more functional capabilities (such as mobility, communication, self-care, self-direction, interpersonal skills, work tolerance, or work skills) in terms of an employment outcome;
- whose VR can be expected to require multiple VR services over an extended period of time; and
- who has one or more physical or mental disabilities. (29 USC § 705 [21] [A])

WHAT SERVICES DOES VR PROVIDE?

Once an individual is determined eligible for VR services, an individualized plan for employment (IPE) is developed. (The IPE should not be confused with the individualized education program for students with disabilities, referred to as the *IEP*.) At a minimum, the IPE must include (1) a description of a specific employment outcome, (2) a description of the specific services needed to achieve the employment outcome, (3) a description of the entity that will provide the VR services, (4) a description of evaluation criteria used to measure progress toward achieve the employment outcome, (5) the terms and conditions of the IPE, and (6) if supported employment is an outcome, the IPE must identify the extended services. Title 1, Section 103 of the Rehabilitation Act describes the types of services used to assist an individual with a disability in preparing for and securing an employment outcome. Table 3.3 lists VR services as outlined by the Act.

TABLE 3.2. Titles of the Rehabilitation Act

Title	Description
Title I. VR Services	• Describes basic structure, framework, and principles of VR and provides formal grants to designated state VR agencies. • Establishes client assistance programs (CAPs) that are designed to inform and assist people in accessing programs authorized by the Act. • Establishes state rehabilitation councils (SRCs) comprised of at least one member of the Statewide Independent Living Council, one representative of a parent training and information program, one representative of the CAP, one qualified VR counselor, one representative of a community rehabilitation service provider (CRP), four representatives of business, representatives from a cross-section of disability groups, one representative from the state education agency responsible for education of students with disabilities, and one representative of the state workforce investment board.
Title II. Research and Training	• Provides for research, demonstration projects, training, and related activities to maximize the full inclusion and integration of individuals with disabilities. • Establishes the National Institute on Disability and Rehabilitation Research, which is designed to promote, coordinate, and provide for research, demonstration projects, and related activities.
Title III. Special Projects and Demonstrations	• Provides funding for personnel preparation and training programs to ensure that rehabilitation professionals provide services to people with disabilities. Provides funds for training programs such as parent and Braille training. • Establishes regional rehabilitation continuing education programs.
Title IV. National Council on Disability	• Establishes the National Council on Disability, which is comprised of 15 members who are appointed by the president. • The purpose of the National Council is to promote policies, programs, and practices that guarantee opportunity and empower people with disabilities to achieve economic self-sufficiency, independent living, and inclusion in all aspects of society.
Title V. Rights and Advocacy	• Title V is the civil rights component of the act. Title V is comprised of nine sections that address the rights and advocacy of people with disabilities. o Section 501. Employment of Individuals with Disabilities. o Section 502. Architectural and Transportation Barriers Compliance Board. o Section 503. Employment under Federal Contracts. o Section 504. Nondiscrimination under Federal Contracts. o Section 505. Remedies and Attorney Fees. o Section 506. Secretarial Responsibilities. o Section 507. Interagency Disability Coordinating Council. o Section 508. Electronic and Information Technology. o Section 509. Protection and Advocacy.

(continued)

TABLE 3.2. (continued)

Title	Description
Title VI. Employment Opportunities for Individuals with Disabilities	• Strategies to promote employment of people with disabilities: Projects with Industry and Supported Employment. • Projects with Industry is a program that expands job and career opportunities for people with disabilities by encouraging business involvement in rehabilitation and hiring people with disabilities. • Supported Employment is designed to assist people with the most significant disabilities to obtain and maintain employment.
Title VII. Independent Living Services and Centers for Independent Living	• Provides funds to assist states in helping people with live independently. • Establishes a national system of centers for independent living. • Establishes independent services for older individuals who are blind. • Establishes state independent living councils.

WHAT IS THE ROLE OF VR IN PROVIDING TRANSITION SERVICES TO STUDENTS WITH DISABILITIES?

The 2014 Workforce Innovation and Opportunity Act (WIOA) contains a number of amendments to the Rehabilitation Act and places considerable emphasis on transition-age students with disabilities. Specifically, the amendments require state vocational agencies to set aside at least 15% of federal funds for pre-employment transition services. These services include (1) job exploration counseling, (2) work-based learning experiences (school or after-school experiences) provided in the most integrated setting, (3) counseling opportunities for enrollment in PSE programs at institutions of higher education, (4) workplace readiness training to develop social skills, and (5) instruction in self-advocacy (Workforce Innovation and Opportunity Act, Public Law 113-128 § 422, 4069, 2014). Another important provision in the 2014 WIOA relates to subminimum wage. The Act specifies how an entity cannot employ an individual with a disability at wages below minimum wages unless the individual first receives pre-employment transition services, applies for VR services, makes attempts to gain competitive integrated employment, and receives information about alternatives to subminimum wages (Workforce Innovation and Opportunity Act, Public Law 113-128 § 458, 2014).

VR services are important in transition because the Rehabilitation Act emphasizes collaboration between state VR programs and state education agencies. Under Title I, states are required to submit a plan of rehabilitation services that outlines how the state will meet the provisions outlined in the Act. One of these provisions is related to transition. Specifically, the state plan must contain policies and procedures for cooperation, collaboration, and coordination between the state rehabilitation and state education agencies developed to facilitate transition students from educational services to rehabilitation services. According to the Act, states are required to develop formal interagency agreements that provide for:

TABLE 3.3. VR Services (29 USC § 723)

Types of VR services that must be described in the IPE

- An assessment for determining eligibility and VR needs by qualified personnel, including, if appropriate, an assessment by personnel skilled in rehabilitation technology.
- Counseling and guidance, including information and support services to assist an individual in exercising informed choice consistent with the provisions of section 722(d).
- Referral and other services to secure needed services from other agencies.
- Job-related services, including job search and placement assistance, job retention services, follow-up services, and follow-along services.
- Vocational and other training services, including the provision of personal and vocational adjustment services, books, tools, and other training materials, except that no training services provided at an institution of higher education shall be paid for with funds under this title unless maximum efforts have been made by the designated state unit and the individual to secure grant assistance, in whole or in part, from other sources to pay for such training.
- To the extent that financial support is not readily available from a source (such as through health insurance of the individual or through comparable services and benefits consistent with section 721 [a][8] [A] of this title) other than the designated state unit, diagnosis and treatment of physical and mental impairments, including:
  o Corrective surgery or therapeutic treatment necessary to correct or substantially modify a physical or mental condition that constitutes a substantial impediment to employment, but is of such a nature that such correction or modification may reasonably be expected to eliminate or reduce such impediment to employment within a reasonable length of time.
  o Necessary hospitalization in connection with surgery or treatment.
  o Prosthetic and orthotic devices.
  o Eyeglasses and visual services as prescribed by qualified personnel who meet state licensure laws and who are selected by the individual.
  o Special services (including transplantation and dialysis), artificial kidneys, and supplies necessary for the treatment of individuals with end-stage renal disease.
  o Diagnosis and treatment for mental and emotional disorders by qualified personnel who meet state licensure laws.
- Maintenance for additional costs incurred while participating in an assessment for determining eligibility and VR needs or while receiving services under an individualized plan for employment.
- Transportation, including adequate training in the use of public transportation vehicles and systems, that is provided in connection with the provision of any other service described in this section and needed by the individual to achieve an employment outcome.
- On-the-job or other related personal assistance services provided while an individual is receiving other services described in this section.
- Interpreter services provided by qualified personnel for individuals who are deaf or hard of hearing, and reader services for individuals who are determined to be blind, after an examination by qualified personnel who meet state licensure laws.
- Rehabilitation teaching services, and orientation and mobility services, for individuals who are blind.
- Occupational licenses, tools, equipment, and initial stocks and supplies.

(continued)

TABLE 3.3. *(continued)*

- Technical assistance and other consultation services to conduct market analyses, develop business plans, and otherwise provide resources, to the extent such resources are authorized to be provided through the statewide workforce investment system, to eligible individuals who are pursuing self-employment or telecommuting or establishing a small business operation as an employment outcome.
- Rehabilitation technology, including telecommunications, sensory, and other technological aids and devices.
- Transition services for students with disabilities to facilitate the achievement of the employment outcome identified in the IPE.
- Supported employment services.
- Services to the family of an individual with a disability necessary to assist the individual to achieve an employment outcome.
- Specific postemployment services necessary to assist an individual with a disability to retain, regain, or advance in employment.

1. Consultation and technical assistance to education agencies in planning for the transition of students with disabilities for school to post-school activities, including VR.
2. Transition planning by personnel of the State agency for students with disabilities that facilitates the development and completion of their IEP under IDEA.
3. The roles and responsibilities, including financial responsibilities, of each agency, including provisions for determining State lead agencies and qualified personnel responsible for transition services.
4. Procedures for outreach to and identification of students with disabilities who need the transition services. (Rehabilitation Act, Title 1 Section [a] [11] [D])

Once a student in special education reaches age 16 and thus requires a statement of transition services in the IEP, a VR counselor may be invited to participate on the IEP team. VR services can be instrumental in achieving successful postschool outcomes. VR counselors can describe eligibility requirements and services that enable successful transition, facilitate employment placement, and provide access to reasonable accommodations. In future chapters, we describe the integral role of the VR counselor in facilitating the transition process.

EXERCISE 3.3

Based on your knowledge, describe ways in which your state rehabilitation and education agency are collaborating to facilitate the transition of students with disabilities. Are there any areas that you see that need improvement? If you are not sure, look on your state websites for VR and special education. Are there agreements or other information that suggests collaboration between VR and special education agencies?

WHAT IS THE ADA?

The ADA was signed into law in 1990 and amended in 2008. This legislation extended the civil rights, nondiscrimination mandate of Section 504 of the Rehabilitation Act to private employers and organizations that did not receive financial assistance. The broader protections outlined in the ADA prohibit discrimination against people with disabilities in employment, public services, public accommodations, transportation, and telecommunications. The definition of a disability under the ADA ensures that individuals with a broad range of disabilities are protected from discrimination. An individual is considered to have a disability under the ADA if he or she has a physical or mental impairment that substantially limits one or more major life activities, has a record of such impairment, or is regarded as having an impairment (42 U.S.C § 12102).

WHY DO TRANSITION PROFESSIONALS NEED TO UNDERSTAND THE ADA?

As shown in Figure 3.2, the amended ADA is divided into separate titles, including Employment (Title I), Public Services (Title II), Public Accommodation (Title III), Telecommunications (Title IV), and Miscellaneous (Title V). Each of these titles is designed to ensure that people with disabilities participate in all aspects of society. From a transition perspective, we believe that professionals should understand the basic provisions

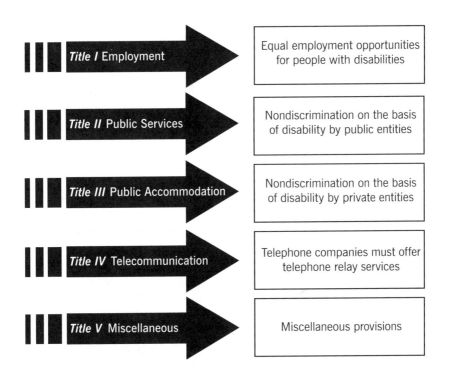

FIGURE 3.2. Titles of the ADA.

outlined in Titles I, II, and III to ensure that students with disabilities participate, to the maximum extent, in employment, education, and community activities.

Employment (Title I)

Title I prohibits employers with 15 or more employees from discriminating against a qualified individual with a disability in all aspects of employment. This means that employers cannot discriminate against qualified individuals in relation to the application procedures, hiring, advancing or discharging, compensating, job training, or any other privilege of employment (42 U.S.C § 12112). ADA defines a *qualified individual* as "an individual who, with or without reasonable accommodation, can perform the essential functions of the employment position that such individual holds or desires" (42 U.S.C § 12112 [8]). Essential functions are fundamental duties of the job outlined in written job descriptions or determined by observing workers in similar positions.

Employers are obligated to provide a reasonable accommodation regardless of the hours the employee works or if the employee is considered probationary (U.S. Equal Opportunity Commission, 2002). Accommodations are generally provided upon the request by the employee with a disability and with disclosure of that disability. Reasonable accommodations may include:

- Making facilities accessible.
- Modifying work schedules.
- Restructuring jobs.
- Changing test or training material.
- Providing qualified readers or interpreters.
- Reassignment to vacant positions.

It is critical to understand that employers are not required to eliminate essential functions of a job or lower performance standards. Reasonable accommodations do not mean changing the essential functions or standards of a job. The Job Accommodation Network (see website at the end of this chapter) is a resource for exploring accommodations in the workplace.

The employment provisions of the ADA may be important to transition teachers seeking job placements. Teachers should keep these provisions in mind as they work with employers. Also, we find that employers will occasionally ask transition teachers for help in interpreting the ADA. So in this way, transition teachers can become valuable assets to employers.

Public Services (Title II)

Title II of the ADA prohibits public entities such as state and local governments, including colleges and universities, from discriminating against a "qualified" individual with a disability. Under Title II, qualified individuals with disabilities cannot be excluded from participation or be denied benefits of services, programs, or activities of a public entity.

Public entities must ensure that people with disabilities have access to services and that buildings are accessible. In addition, Title II stipulates that public entities furnish auxiliary aids and services to ensure effective participation by students with disabilities (35.CFR. § 35.160[b][1]). These auxiliary aids and services may include note takers, qualified interpreters, captioning, audio recordings, taped texts, texts in Braille, large-print material, talking calculators, etc. In addition, public entities such as colleges and universities are required to make reasonable accommodations when a student with a disability discloses the disability. Public colleges and universities are required to provide auxiliary aids and services to both matriculating degree-seeking students and to non-degree-seeking students (U.S. Department of Education Office of Civil Rights, 1998).

Title II of the ADA contains an integration mandate stating that "a public entity shall administer services, programs, and activities in the most integrated setting appropriate to the needs of qualified individuals with disabilities" (28 C.F.R. § 35.130[d]). This mandate influences the way programs and services are provided to people with disabilities. For example, many cities have recreation programs, such as adapted basketball, that are designed for individuals with disabilities. Creating these separate programs is not a violation of the integration mandate. However, the city would violate the integration mandate if it only allowed youth with disabilities to participate in adapted programs and would not allow them to participate in its other recreational programs.

The ADA integration mandate influenced the Supreme Court in its decision involving *Olmstead v L.C.* (1999). The Court held that unjustified segregation of people with disabilities was a clear violation of the Title II integration mandate. The Court concluded that states were required to provide community-based treatment for people with disabilities when (1) such services were appropriate; (2) the person with a disability did not oppose the services; and (3) community-based placements provided reasonable accommodations, taking into account the resources of the state and the needs of other people with disabilities receiving services (*Olmstead v. L.C.*, 527 U.S. 607). *Olmstead* and the Title II integration mandates have been the catalysts for changing the way states deliver services to individuals with disabilities. For example, advocates successfully challenged the placement of individuals with disabilities in sheltered workshops (*U.S. v. Rhode Island and City of Providence*, 2013). Also, the Department of Justice intervened to assist states in complying with the integration mandate (U.S. Department of Justice, 2012). Finally, Massachusetts unveiled a plan to no longer place people with disabilities in sheltered workshops by 2014 and to close all workshops by 2015 (Massachusetts Department of Developmental Services, 2013).

EXERCISE 3.4

Here's a hypothetical situation: Let's say that during a transition planning meeting, a parent states that he would like to see his youth with intellectual/developmental disability transition to a sheltered workshop. How would you respond to the parent while also explaining postschool employment options for students with more significant support needs in integrated, community settings? How would you find out your state's position on sheltered workshops?

The public services provisions of the ADA are important to transition teachers because they protect students who wish to enroll in public PSE, such as colleges and universities. In addition, the integration mandate creates and expands more community-based employment options for individuals with significant disabilities. Transition teachers should explain these changes and advise both parents and students about integrated postschool options.

Public Accommodation (Title III)

The ADA defines a public accommodation as a facility, operated by a private entity, whose operations affect commerce and fall within at least one of the following categories: (1) an inn, hotel, or place of lodging; (2) a restaurant or bar; (3) a place of exhibition or entertainment (e.g., theater, auditorium, convention hall); (4) a sales or rental establishment (e.g., bakery, grocery store, clothing store, shopping center); (5) a service establishment (e.g., laundromat, professional office, hospital, pharmacy); (6) areas used for public transportation; (7) places of recreation (e.g., zoos, parks); places of education (e.g., nursery, elementary, secondary, undergraduate, and graduate school); (8) social service centers (e.g., homeless shelter, food bank); and (9) places of exercise and recreation (e.g., bowling alley, golf course) (28 C.F.R. § 36.104). Title III covers public accommodations, commercial facilities, and private entities. The ADA requires removal of architectural barriers in existing facilities when removal is achievable without difficulty and expense. Removal of barriers could mean installing ramps, making curb cuts, widening doorways, installing grab bars on toilets, etc. All new construction occupied after January 1993 is required to be accessible to individuals with disabilities.

Title III also requires that courses and examinations related to professional, educational, or trade-related applications, licensing, certifications, or credentialing be provided in a place and manner accessible to people with disabilities, or offer alternative accessible arrangements for qualified individuals with disabilities (28 C.F.R. § 36.309). Accommodations include auxiliary aids and services outlined in the previous section. Title III applies to both public and private colleges and universities. The public accommodations provisions of the ADA may be important to transition teachers because they provide protection for students who wish to enroll in public and private colleges and universities. In addition, Title III calls for removing architectural barriers. Transition teachers should understand how private entities, such as community businesses, are required to make their facilities accessible.

EXERCISE 3.5

Let's say that during a transition planning meeting, one of your students with a specific learning disability indicates the she would like to attend a community college to pursue an associates of applied science degree (A.A.S.) in culinary arts. The parents of the youth ask, "Who conducts the IEP meeting at the college so that we can get needed accommodations?" How would you reply?

WHAT IS THE TICKET TO WORK AND WORK INCENTIVES IMPROVEMENT ACT?

The Ticket to Work and Work Incentives Improvement Act is designed to remove barriers to work for SSI and SSDI beneficiaries. One of the primary purposes of the Act is to "establish a return to work ticket program that will allow individuals with disabilities to seek the services necessary to obtain and retain employment and reduce their dependency on cash benefit programs" (Public Law 106-170 sec 2 [b]). The Act also provides grants to states for Work Incentives Planning and Assistance (WIPA). The WIPA program is designed to assist SSI or SSDI beneficiaries to make informed choices about work. The program stipulates that trained professionals provide counseling that describes how working would impact an individual's benefits. In addition, the Act created Medicaid "buy-in" programs to cover working individuals with disabilities who meet the income and resource limits set by each state. The buy-in allows working beneficiaries to share some of the cost of their coverage. The Ticket to Work and Work Incentives Improvement Act was amended in 2008. This amendment, among other things, was designed to improve the outcome milestone payment system. This system provides financial payments to approved service providers who assist individuals with disabilities in reaching specific employment-related milestones.

Ticket to Work Program

The ticket program is a voluntary one designed for individuals between the ages of 18 and 64 who are blind or receive SSI or SSDI benefits. The program offers expanded choice for individuals seeking supports to enter or maintain employment. Beneficiaries can redeem a "ticket" to an employment network (EN) or state VR agency. An EN contracts with Social Security to provide employment supports and services to ticket holders. Either the EN or VR will provide appropriate services to help the beneficiary find and maintain employment. Services may include training, career counseling, VR, job placement, and ongoing supports to achieve a work goal. ENs are reimbursed by Social Security using an outcome payment system established by the Social Security Administration. For example, in 2015 an approved EN may receive milestone payments totaling $24,919 for SSDI beneficiaries and $24,072 for SSI. The Social Security Administration provides a list of approved ENs for each state at *www.choosework.net/resource/jsp/searchByState.jsp.*

Transition teachers should be aware of the Ticket to Work Program because it is one of many benefits available to transition-age students who are either SSDI or SSI beneficiaries. The ticket program can be a valuable tool in helping a student attain an employment goal. For example, a school can apply to be an EN that provides supplemental supports to help transition-age students obtain meaningful employment. It is not uncommon for parents and students to express concerns about working because they mistakenly assume that a job means loss of SSI or SSDI benefits. This assumption is incorrect. Therefore, transition teachers need to be aware of their states' WIPA program so that referral to a VR benefits counselor can be made. Once a referral is made, a WIPA staff will conduct a benefits analysis and answer questions about how working would impact an individual's benefits.

WHAT IS THE FAIR LABOR STANDARDS ACT?

Transition professionals should understand certain provisions of the Fair Labor Standards Act (FLSA) because it can impact youth with disabilities who are placed in community work settings to learn employment skills. Youth with disabilities often participate in various types of work-based career exploration programs, assessment, and training. The FLSA sets basic minimum wage and overtime pay standards, provides standards for youth employment, and provides guidance on individual rehabilitation programs for youth with disabilities. Employees are entitled to the established minimum wage and hour and overtime pay of at least time and a half for nonexempt workers. The Department of Labor, Wage and Hour Division, administers and enforces the provisions of this Act.

HOW DOES THE FLSA APPLY TO YOUTH IN TRANSITION?

The U.S. Department of Labor recognizes the importance of providing valuable community-based work experiences to students with disabilities. Section 64c08—Students with Disabilities and Workers with Disabilities Who Are Enrolled in Individual Rehabilitation Programs—of the *Wage and Hour Field Operations Handbook* provides specific guidelines for students with disabilities who participate in vocational programs. In 1993, the Wage and Hour (WH) Division issued a statement that reflects the commitment to supporting transition programs:

> The U.S. Departments of Labor and Education are committed to the continued development and implementation of individual education programs, in accordance with the Individuals with Disabilities Education Act (IDEA) that will facilitate the transition of students with disabilities from school to employment within their communities. This transition must take place under conditions that will not jeopardize the protections afforded by the Fair Labor Standards Act to program participants, employees, employers, or programs providing rehabilitation services to individuals with disabilities. (U.S. Department of Labor, n.d.)

The Department of Labor created specific guidelines to determine if an employment relationship exists between an employer and an employee (see Table 3.4). Based on these guidelines, students with disabilities can participate in unpaid vocational exploration, vocational assessment, and vocational training as long as there is not a clear employment relationship. If all criteria are met, the Department of Labor will not assert that an employment relationship exists and the student, under the supervision of the teacher, can participate in unpaid job training. If however, there is an employer relationship, the employer is responsible for compliance with FLSA.

TABLE 3.4. 64c08 Guidelines for Students with Disabilities Who Are Enrolled in Vocational Programs

1. Participants are individuals with physical and/or mental disabilities for whom competitive employment at or above the minimum wage level is not immediately obtainable and who, because of their disability, will need intensive ongoing support to perform in a work setting.

2. Participation is for vocational exploration, assessment or training in a community-based work site under the general supervision of rehabilitation organization personnel, or in the case of a student with a disability, public school personnel.

3. Community-based placements must be clearly defined components of individual rehabilitation programs developed and designed for the benefit of each individual.
   - Each student with a disability shall have an IEP that lists the needed transition services established for the exploration, assessment, training, or cooperative vocational education components.

4. Documentation will be provided to WH upon request that reflects that the individual is enrolled in the community-based placement program, that this enrollment is voluntary and that there is no expectation of remuneration. However, the information contained in the IEP or IPE does not have to be disclosed to WH. The individual with a disability and, when appropriate, the parent or guardian of each individual must be fully informed of the IEP or IPE and of the community-based placement component of the plan.

5. The activities of the individuals with disabilities (participants) at the community-based placement site do not result in an immediate advantage to the business. Factors that would indicate the business is advantaged by activities of the individual include:
   - Displacement of regular employees.
   - Vacant positions have been filled with participants rather than regular employees.
   - Regular employees have been relieved of assigned duties.
   - Participants are performing services that, although not ordinarily performed by employees, clearly are of benefit to the business.
   - Participants are under continued and direct supervision of employees of the business rather than representatives of the rehabilitation facility or school.
   - Placements are made to accommodate the labor needs of the business rather than according to the requirements of the individual's IEP or IPE.
   - The IEP or IPE does not specifically limit the time spent by the participant at any one site, or in any clearly distinguishable job classification.

6. While the existence of an employment relationship will not be determined exclusively on the basis of the number of hours spent in each activity, as a general rule, an employment relationship is presumed not to exist when each of the three components does not exceed the following limitations:
   - Vocational explorations—5 hours per job experienced
   - Vocational assessment—90 hours per job experienced
   - Vocational training—120 hours per job experienced
   - In the case of students, these limitations apply during any one school year.

7. Individuals are not entitled to employment at the business at the conclusion of the IEP or IPE. However, if an individual becomes an employee, he or she cannot be considered a trainee at that particular community-based placement unless in a different, clearly distinguishable occupation.

CAN STUDENTS WITH DISABILITIES BE UNPAID VOLUNTEERS?

In our work, we occasionally hear teachers state that students are "volunteering" at a local business. It is important that transition teachers understand that volunteering and job training are completely different concepts. Specifically, *volunteering* typically occurs in religious, charitable, or nonprofit organizations and is designed so that an individual freely offers a service to the community. *Job training*, on the other hand, occurs in a local business and is designed to teach a student necessary skills for employment. Students with disabilities may participate in unpaid volunteer work as long as the minimum requirements of Section 64c04 of the *Field Operations Handbook* are met. According to the WH Division, volunteer work can occur on a part-time basis if there is no expectation of payment or employment. Students with disabilities may volunteer their time as long as criteria outlined in Section 64c04 are met. These criteria include:

1. The worker with a disability must be legally competent to freely volunteer his or her services. A worker with a disability who is at least 18 years of age is often his or her own guardian, but if not, the parent or guardian must have approved such volunteer work.
2. The work performed must be substantially different from the work performed during duty hours. (*Duty hours* refers to time on the clock for paid employment.).
3. The work must be of the type normally classified as "volunteer" work described in the *Field Operations Handbook* 10b03(c) (e.g., religious, charitable, and nonprofit organizations).
4. The work must be performed outside normal duty hours.

SUMMARY

Legislation is designed so that individuals with disabilities can fully engage in inclusive education and community environments and opportunities. Although there are additional laws related to education and employment that are *not* described here (e.g., Carl D. Perkins Vocational and Technical Education Act, Higher Education Opportunity Act, Social Security Act), we chose to highlight what we believe are the major pieces of legislation impacting transition-age youth and young adults with disabilities.

The IDEA and its transition mandate provide clear direction on assisting students to achieve valued transition outcomes. The Rehabilitation Act is designed as civil rights legislation to prohibit discrimination against people with disabilities who are in programs and activities that receive federal dollars. The Act also provides funds for research, technical assistance, and training and services to maximize employment opportunities for people with disabilities. The ADA extends the civil rights protection of the Rehabilitation Act to the private sector and contains provisions to ensure that individuals receive services and supports in integrated settings. The Ticket to Work and Work Incentives Improvement Act provides SSI and SSDI beneficiaries with specific incentives and supports to actively pursue employment. Finally, the FLSA ensures that transition-related work-based learning programs for students with disabilities follow specific guidelines to guarantee that no employer relationship exists.

REVISITING KENLEY

Kenley's special education teacher, Mr. White, cleaned the white board in his classroom after school. Another day was in the books. Today, Kenley, a 16-year-old with autism, learned to orally read the sentence "I see the ball." Putting words together to form a sentence was exceedingly difficult for Kenley, so today's event was a major accomplishment. As Mr. White thought about Kenley's success, he also considered how far Kenley had to go to achieve functional reading skill. "What is Kenley going to do in this little farming town when he becomes an adult?" he thought.

"Hey, Mr. White, can I interrupt?" Kenley's brother, Ashton, was at the classroom door.

"Oh, Ashton, how are you? Hey, I was just thinking about Kenley."

"Yeah, me too," Ashton responded. "Do you have a couple of minutes? I won't be long."

Mr. White had known Ashton as a football player on the Southridge team. They started by talking football, then talk returned to Kenley.

"I'm worried about him, Mr. White," Ashley started. "He's going to be done with school in 2 years. What will happen to him?"

"Yeah, I understand your concern. We've been working so much on getting his behavior under control. But his reading is so low. I mean, it's coming along and we've had some successes. But still."

"Does he have any possibility of working someday? I mean, I know he has to read and write. But I wonder if he can do anything around town. You know?"

Ashton and Mr. White continued to discuss Kenley's situation and his future. Southridge was a farming community with a small group of close-knit families and a few businesses. Mr. White was the only special education teacher at the high school that served surrounding communities. He was really the only expert in how to work with youth who experienced disabilities, but he hadn't focused on Kenley's transition to adult life.

"I don't know of any jobs that Kenley could do around town," said Mr. White. "We haven't really been teaching him job skills because of other priorities. Any ideas, Ashton?"

"Not really. I just want to see him do well. I'm going to graduate this year. I'll probably just work out at Reicker's—you know, the farm implement place. But I'm thinking about college, too. If I go to college, I'd have to move away. I just don't want to leave him in a lurch."

"Well, Ashton, you know your mom and dad will take good care of him. You should join us when we have a meeting to review your brother's IEP and plan his transition. You know, maybe if we all put our heads together. Hmm." Mr. White paused. "There's Teresa Schmidt. She's a voc rehab counselor from Garden City. She doesn't get out here often, but maybe I could call her and see if she can join us for the review meeting. She might be able to tell us whether Kenley would be eligible for VR services or Ticket to Work. Do you know if Kenley receives SSI benefits?

"I think so," said Ashton. "Could she get Ashton a job?"

"I don't think so, but she could tell us what services might be available if Kenley qualifies for VR and how to plan for his future. I could call her and see if she can join us."

"Thanks, Mr. White."

WEBSITES WITH ADDITIONAL INFORMATION

National Secondary Transition Technical Assistance Center

www.nsttac.org or *www.transitionta.org*

Job Accommodation Network

http://askjan.org/index.html

National Post-School Outcome Center

www.psocenter.org

Social Security Administration Employment Networks

www.choosework.net/resource/jsp/searchByState.jsp

CHAPTER 4

Overview of Transition Models and Practices

This chapter addresses . . .

- Early transition model programs and their influence on policy and practice.
- Evidence-based practices that promote successful transition outcomes.
- Practices that promote integrated employment outcomes and PSE.
- Practices identifiable across transition models.

WHAT IS THE HISTORY OF TRANSITION PROGRAMS?

Researchers and policymakers have long recognized how complex and intricate the transition process can be for youth with disabilities. Starting years ago, professionals from various disciplines discussed how to make a youth's transition a smoother process. For example, in 1968, the Western Interstate Commission for Higher Education held a conference on developing cooperative agreements between special education and rehabilitation services. The conference recognized the importance "of planning toward an effective and comprehensive program between special education and VR during the transitional period of the child's life from the more formal training of the classroom to work activities in the labor community" (Hensley & Buck, 1968, p. 33). One of the goals of the conference was to develop innovative strategies for special education and VR during the critical transition years. This type of dialogue about improving the vocational process and outcomes for youth with disabilities provided a platform for later transition models.

It may appear ironic that models of transition services have been proposed for about a half-century when outcome data indicate that today's youth with disabilities still struggle. This lag between discussion and positive outcomes raises questions about the history of model transition programs. Are the models effective? Are they not being adopted in practice? If not, why not? Investigating model transition programs may guide us in understanding the complexity of the issues.

WHAT WERE THE EARLY TRANSITION MODELS?

In the 1980s, researchers (e.g., Hasazi et al., 1985) conducted survey studies and found that high percentages of students with disabilities were unemployed after leaving special education services. Policymakers took notice and expressed concerns. In 1984, the U.S. Department of Education's Office of Special Education and Rehabilitation Services issued a position paper referring to bridging the gap between school and working life. Will (1984) defined transition from school to working life as

> an outcome-oriented process encompassing a broad array of services and experiences that lead to employment. Transition is a period that includes high school, the point of graduation, additional PSE or adult services, and the initial years of employment. Transition is a bridge between the security and structure offered by the school and the opportunities and risks of adult life. (p. 2)

Will (1984) established a national priority for improving the transition from school to working life for students with disabilities. She described the *bridges model* as a way to improve employment outcomes for youth with disabilities (see Figure 4.1). Three "bridges" from school to employment were conceptualized as ways to support a student's transition to employment: (1) no special services, (2) time-limited services, and (3) ongoing services. *No special services* referred to trade schools, community colleges, and other services available to anyone living in the community. *Time-limited services* were specific services, such as VR, for eligible individuals with a disability. These were designed to be short-term services and were configured to assist an individual in finding employment. *Ongoing services* were designed to provide longer-term support to an individual over a lifespan (e.g., state IDD agencies).

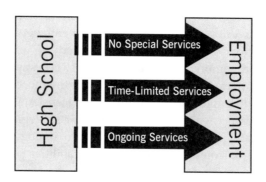

FIGURE 4.1. The bridges model (Will, 1984).

Will (1984) reinforced the importance of employment as an outcome for students with disabilities. Shortly after its introduction, Halpern (1985) suggested the model needed modification because there were other nonvocational transition outcomes considered to be equally important for students with disabilities. He proposed a revised model that viewed community adjustment as the ultimate goal of transition services, consisting of a residential environment, employment, and social and interpersonal networks. Community adjustment involved examining the quality of all three factors. Halpern developed a conceptual diagram depicting community adjustment as supported by three pillars: residential, employment, and social and interpersonal networks, stating that "if any of the three pillars are inadequate and do not carry their own weight, then the entire structure is in danger of collapse, and a person's ability to live in the community is threatened" (pp. 480–481).

The 1990 IDEA took into account these formative transition models and helped set the stage for rigorous research and model development. Models continued to evolve after the 1990 IDEA transition mandate as researchers and practitioners recognized the importance of coordinated services.

In order to present a comprehensive, conceptual understanding of effective transition practices, Kohler (1996) developed a *taxonomy for transition programming* using an iterative process that included literature reviews, evaluation studies, and model project outcomes. She organized the taxonomy into five categories: (1) student-focused planning, (2) student development, (3) interagency collaboration, (4) family involvement, and (5) program structure. The five taxonomy areas interact and collectively impact the effectiveness of transition processes. Transition professionals can use the taxonomy as a framework for designing comprehensive transition education. The categories are described in the following sections.

Student-Focused Planning

Student-focused planning uses assessment information to develop specific measurable postsecondary goals in education and training, vocation, community-related/residential living, and recreation and leisure. Part of the planning process includes addressing personal needs such as financial, medical, and guardianship issues.

Student Development

Student development emphasizes coordinated instruction across several domains, including social skills, self-determination and self-advocacy skills, independent living skills, and employment skills. Career and vocational curricula may be included, such as structured work experiences (e.g., apprenticeships, paid work experience, work–study, and job placement services).

Interagency Collaboration

Interagency collaboration encourages involvement of various adult service agencies, community businesses, and organizations through collaborative service delivery and frameworks. Collaboration requires shared delivery of transition services and shared funding, staffing, coordination of information, and consultation.

Family Involvement

Kohler (1996) listed three core components in this category: (1) family involvement, (2) family empowerment, and (3) family training. Family involvement includes family members' participation in program policy development, service delivery, assessment, and evaluation of a student's program. Family empowerment includes implementing pre-IEP planning activities, identifying family support networks, and developing structured methods to identify family needs. In family training, members learn how to assist with self-determination, self-advocacy, natural forms of support, empowerment, and accessing agency services.

Program Structure

Program structure relates to how the delivery of transition-related education and supports are viewed across programs and organizations. This category covers program philosophy, program evaluation, strategic planning, program policy, human resource development, and resource allocation as key elements.

EXERCISE 4.1

Respond to the following questions:

- Based on what you have read so far, how have models of transition evolved since 1968? That is, what changes are apparent?
- What elements in transition models have remained relatively unchanged since 1968?
- As you review these historical models and compare them to what you know about transition today, what, if any, elements are still missing? What would you add to a current transition model?

WHAT ARE EVIDENCE-BASED PRACTICES?

Most of the early model programs in transition provided research evidence to support them. However, the NCLB Act of 2001, particularly its insistence on "scientifically based research," galvanized the entire field of education. The NCLB Act requires that educators implement instructional programs and practices that "involve the application or rigorous, systematic, and objective procedures to obtain reliable and valid knowledge relevant to education activities and programs" (20 USC § 7801 [37]). Congress believed that special education "has been impeded by low expectations, and an insufficient focus on applying replicable research on proven methods of teaching and learning for children with disabilities" (20 USC §1400[c][4]). Consequently, the 2004 amendments to IDEA require that a student's IEP, including the individual transition plan, contain "a statement of the special education and related services and supplementary aids and services, based on peer-reviewed research to the extent practicable" (20 USC §1414 [D] [1][A][i][IV]).

Several federal policy initiatives were developed to support the implementation of research-based practices, including the U.S. Department of Education's *What Works Clearinghouse* (see website at the end of this chapter). Developers of the Clearinghouse, created in 2002, stated that educational practice needs to be evaluated using scientifically based research to determine if it is evidence-based. The purpose of the clearinghouse was to review research studies to find evidence of the effects of specific practices. The rationale was that states, districts, and local schools would only use practices with evidence-based data to support them.

Cook, Smith, and Tankersley (2012) claimed that educators have been unaware, or at least desensitized to, the importance of research evidence to support educational practice. The gap between educational practice and research on what works may be the primary reason for disappointing school outcomes. They called on educators to insist on *evidence-based practice*, defined as a systematic approach to determining those practices that are

> supported by a sufficient number of research studies that (a) are of high methodological quality, (b) use appropriate research designs that allow for assessment of effectiveness, and (c) demonstrate meaningful effect sizes such that they merit educators' trust that the practice works. (p. 497)

HOW DO EVIDENCE-BASED PRACTICES RELATE TO TRANSITION?

The Office of Special Education Programs funded the NSTTAC (see website at the end of this chapter) to provide technical assistance and information on evidence-based practices in transition. The NSTTAC defined four levels of evidence-supported practices: as *evidence-based*, *research-based*, *promising*, or *unestablished* practices, as shown in Figure 4.2.

To determine the evidence base for secondary transition practices, the NSTTAC conducted a two-part analysis of transition research: the first examined evidence-based practices using group and single-subject designs, and the second examined correlation research to determine predictor variables. Chapter 2 describes predictor variables.

Evidence-Based Practices	Research-Based Practices	Promising Practices	Unestablished Practices
Evidence-based practices are based on rigorous research designs, have demonstrated a record for improving outcomes, and have been through a systematic review process that uses quality indicators to evaluate level of evidence.	Research-based practices are also based on rigorous research designs and have demonstrated a record for improving student outcomes.	Promising practices are based on research, have limited success, and have weak research designs.	Unestablished practices are not based on research, have no data to support their effectiveness, and are based on anecdotal evidence.

FIGURE 4.2. NSTTAC (2014) definitions of types of practices.

To examine evidence-based practices, the NSTTAC reviewed research that (1) involved students with disabilities who were participating in middle or high school programs; (2) included an independent variable, predictor variable, or discussion point that centered on transition; (3) included a dependent variable that centered on students' in-school or postschool outcomes; (4) reported results; and (5) included a discussion of in-school or postschool outcomes. Information was organized in broad areas of the transition taxonomy (e.g., student-focused planning, student development, interagency collaboration, family involvement, and program structure; Kohler, 1996). The research was coded and categorized based on evidence of causal inference (i.e., the extent to which a cause–effect relationship could be inferred, which was rated as *strong, moderate, potential,* or *weak*). Based on this review, the NSTTAC identified 64 evidence-based practices used to teach 26 different skills. In Table 4.1, we list these evidence-based practices organized by taxonomy area.

EXERCISE 4.2

The NSTTAC noted that evidence-based transition practices were limited by the existing research, and that the list could be expanded if more high-quality experimental research were conducted. Based on what you know about transition practices at this stage, what additional transition practices should be researched? What else would you suggest as a potential evidence-based practice?

These findings compel transition professionals to consider developing secondary transition programs with a strong evidence basis. Programs containing these components, if implemented as prescribed, have higher probabilities of successful transition outcomes for the youth with disabilities they serve.

National Collaborative on Workforce and Disability for Youth Guideposts for Success

The National Collaborative on Workforce and Disability for Youth (NCWD/Y, n.d.) recognized that transition from school to adulthood presents many challenges for students with disabilities and identified guideposts for success. Each guidepost is based on a number of principles, including:

1. High expectations for youth with disabilities.
2. Individualization, inclusion, and integration for all youth with disabilities.
3. Full participation supported by self-determination, informed choice, and decision making.
4. Independent living, including the development of long-term supports and services.
5. Competitive employment.
6. Individualized, person-centered, and culturally and linguistically appropriate transition planning (NCWD/Y, n.d.).

TABLE 4.1. Evidence-Based Transition Practices

Taxonomy	Practice	Skill/knowledge	Potential	Moderate	Strong
Student-focused planning (6) Includes practices in the areas of IEP development, student participation in planning, and planning strategies	1. Using *Whose Future Is It Anyway?* to teach....	Student knowledge of transition planning		✓	
	2. Using *Check and Connect* to teach....	Student participation in the IEP meeting	✓		
	3. Using computer-assisted instruction to teach....	Student participation in the IEP meeting	✓	✓	
	4. Using self-advocacy strategy to teach....	Student participation in the IEP meeting		✓	
	5. Using self-directed IEP to teach....	Student participation in the IEP meeting		✓	
	6. Using published curricula to teach....	Student participation in the IEP meeting			✓
Student development (57) Includes strategies in the areas of life skills instruction, career and vocational curricula, structured work experiences, assessment, and support services.	1. Using mnemonics to teach ...	Academic skills			✓
	2. Using peer-assisted instruction to teach....	Academic skills			✓
	3. Using self-management instruction to teach....	Academic skills			✓
	4. Using technology to teach ...	Academic skills			✓
	5. Using visual displays to teach....	Academic skills			✓
	6. Using backward chaining to teach....	Functional life skills		✓	
	7. Using constant time delay to teach....	Functional life skills		✓	
	8. Using forward chaining to teach....	Functional life skills		✓	
	9. Using progressive time delay to teach ...	Functional life skills		✓	
	10. Using self-monitoring instruction to teach....	Functional life skills	✓		
	11. Using simultaneous prompting to teach ...	Functional life skills		✓	
	12. Using systems of least-to-most prompts to teach...	Functional life skills		✓	
	13. Using systems of most-to-least prompts to teach....	Functional life skills		✓	
	14. Using total task chaining to teach....	Functional life skills		✓	
	15. Using community-based instruction to teach....	Safety skills		✓	
	16. Using progressive time delay to teach....	Safety skills		✓	
	17. Using systems of least-to-most prompts to teach...	Safety skills	✓		
	18. Using the "one more" strategy to teach ...	How to count money	✓		

(continued)

TABLE 4.1. (continued)

Taxonomy	Practice	Skill/knowledge	Potential	Moderate	Strong
	19. Using extension of career planning services after graduation to teach. . .	Increased finance skills	✓		
	20. Using community-based instruction to teach. . .	Purchasing skills	✓		
	21. Using one more strategy to teach. . .	Purchasing skills	✓		
	22. Using progressive time delay to teach. . .	Purchasing skills	✓		
	23. Using response prompting to teach. . .	Purchasing skills		✓	
	24. Using simulations to teach. . .	Purchasing skills		✓	
	25. Using systems of least-to-most prompts to teach. . .	Purchasing skills	✓		
	26. Using *Whose Future Is It Anyway?* to teach. . .	Self-determination skills		✓	
	27. Using self-determined learning model of instruction to teach. . .	Goal attainment		✓	
	28. Using response prompting to teach. . .	Social skills		✓	
	29. Using self-management to teach. . .	Social skills		✓	
	30. Using simulations to teach. . .	Social skills		✓	
	31. Using systems of least-to-most prompt to teach. . .	Communication skills	✓		
	32. Using community-based instruction to teach. . .	Communication skills	✓		
	33. Using computer-assisted instruction to teach. . .	Job-specific skills	✓		
	34. Using constant time delay to teach. . .	Job-specific skills		✓	
	35. Using self-management skills to teach. . .	Job-specific skills		✓	
	36. Using system of least-to-most prompts to teach. . .	Job-specific skills	✓		
	37. Using mnemonics to teach. . .	How to complete a job application	✓		
	38. Using community-based instruction to teach. . .	Employment skills		✓	
	39. Using response prompting to teach. . .	Employment skills		✓	
	40. Using community-based instruction to teach. . .	Banking skills	✓		
	41. Using constant time delay to teach. . .	Banking skills	✓		
	42. Using simulations to teach. . .	Banking skills	✓		

#	Teaching practice	Skill	
43.	Using community-based instruction to teach...	Community integration skills	✓
44.	Using community-assisted instruction to teach...	Food preparation and cooking skills	✓
45.	Using constant time delay to teach...	Food preparation and cooking skills	✓
46.	Using response prompting to teach...	Food preparation and cooking skills	✓
47.	Using video modeling to teach...	Food preparation and cooking skills	✓
48.	Using systems of least-to-most to teach...	Food preparation and cooking skills	✓
49.	Using community assisted instruction to teach...	Food preparation and cooking skills	✓
50.	Using community-based instruction to teach...	Grocery shopping skills	✓
51.	Using response prompting to teach...	Grocery shopping skills	✓
52.	Using systems of least-to-most prompts to teach...	Grocery shopping skills	✓
53.	Using response prompting to teach...	Grocery shopping skills	✓
54.	Using video modeling to teach...	Home maintenance skills	✓
55.	Using response prompting to teach...	Home maintenance skills	✓
56.	Using response prompting to teach...	Laundry tasks	✓
57.	Using constant time delay to teach...	Leisure skills	✓
		Leisure skills	✓

Family involvement (1)

Includes practices in family training, family involvement, and family empowerment.

#	Teaching practice	Skill	
1.	Using training modules to teach...	Parent involvement in the transition process	✓

Program structure (3)

Includes practices in program philosophy, policy and evaluation, strategic planning, resource allocation, and human resource development.

#	Teaching practice	Skill	
1.	Using check and connect to teach...	Student engagement	✓
2.	Using community-based instruction to teach...	Banking skills	✓
		Grocery shopping skills	✓
		Community integration skills	✓
		Purchasing skills	✓
		Safety skills	✓
3.	Using extension of career planning services after gradation to teach...	Communication skills	✓
		Increased finance skills	✓

Interagency collaboration (0)

No evidence-based practices identified.

Note. From the National Secondary Transition Technical Assistance Center (2010). *Evidence-based practices and predictors in secondary transition: What we know and what we still need to know.* Charlotte, NC: Author. *www.nsttac.org.*

71

Each guidepost is an evidence-based practice. The guideposts provide a statement of principles, information about how to produce better outcomes for all young people, and information about how to organize policy and practice. The NCWD/Y recommended that guideposts be used as a "strategic organizational framework" at multiple levels, such as (1) state policy, (2) local administration policy, (3) youth service, and (4) youth and family (NCWD/Y, n.d.). In Table 4.2, we provide details on these guideposts and the specific recommendations for youth with disabilities.

TRANSITION TO EMPLOYMENT: WHAT RESEARCH AND PROMISING PRACTICES EXIST?

Project SEARCH; the transition service integration model; Project Summer; and Achieving Rehabilitation, Individualized Education, and Employment Success (ARIES) are four model programs with research demonstrating employment outcomes. These models are reviewed below.

Project SEARCH

Project SEARCH was designed to provide students with significant disabilities with meaningful work experience during transition (Ruthowski, Datson, Van Kuiken, & Riehle, 2006). Originally developed at the Cincinnati Children's Hospital, Project SEARCH was expanded to include a high school transition program providing students the opportunity to spend their entire day in the workplace for 1 year. The project primarily focused on the health care industry but has application to other employment sectors such as banks, universities, and county park systems.

To be eligible for Project SEARCH, a student had to be age 18–22 and in the last year of high school. In addition, the student had to possess basic communication skills; independent toileting and feeding skills; appropriate social, grooming, and hygiene skills; and a desire to work in the community. Students attended the program for an entire academic year in the host business or hospital location. The host provided an on-site classroom and was staffed by transition educators and job coaches. Students received job skills instruction and unpaid internship experience and rotated through a series of internships throughout the year. The SEARCH model established a series of unique programmatic features distinguishing it from other transition-related employment programs. Ruthowski and colleagues (2006) outlined these critical features:

1. A customized career exploration package with three to four work experiences
2. Instruction and support provided by a job coach during work experiences
3. Assessment of adaptive skills
4. Identification of community services and agencies (e.g., case management, health care, interpreters, behavioral counseling, job coaching, follow-along employment, and/or residential)
5. Development of functional curricula (e.g., money management, social skills, and adult living)

TABLE 4.2. The National Collaborative on Workforce and Disability Guideposts for Success

Guidepost	Recommendations for Youth with Disabilities
1. School-based preparatory experiences	1. Use their individual transition plans to drive their personal instruction, and use strategies to continue the transition process after leaving school. 2. Have access to specific and individual learning accommodations while they are in school. 3. Develop knowledge of reasonable accommodations that they can request and control in educational settings, including assessment accommodations. 4. Be supported by highly qualified transitional support staff who may or may not be school staff.
2. Career preparation and work-based learning	1. Understand the relationships between benefits planning and career choices. 2. Learn to communicate their disability-related work support and accommodation needs. 3. Learn to find, formally request, and secure appropriate supports and reasonable accommodations in education, training, and employment settings.
3. Youth development and leadership	1. Mentors and role models, including persons with and without disabilities. 2. An understanding of disability history, culture, and disability public policy issues as well as their rights and responsibilities.
4. Connecting activities	1. Acquisition of appropriate assistive technologies. 2. Community orientation and mobility training (e.g., accessible transportation, bus routes, housing, health clinics). 3. Exposure to postprogram supports such as independent living centers and other consumer-driven community-based support service agencies. 4. Personal assistance services, including attendants, readers, interpreters, or other such services. 5. Benefits-planning counseling, including information regarding the myriad of benefits available and their interrelationships so that youth may maximize those benefits in transitioning from public assistance to self-sufficiency.
5. Family supports and involvement	1. An understanding of the youth's disability and how it may affect his or her education, employment, and daily living options. 2. Knowledge of rights and responsibilities under various disability-related legislation. 3. Knowledge of and access to programs, services, supports, and accommodations available for young people with disabilities. 4. An understanding of how individualized planning tools can assist youth in achieving transition goals and objectives.

From the National Collaborative on Workforce and Disability for Youth (n.d). Reprinted by permission.

6. Development of a work portfolio
7. Provision of additional support as necessary

Researchers (Ruthowski et al., 2006) provided evidence of successful outcomes noting that Project SEARCH placed 78.3% of its participants in paid, inclusive employment with a mean wage of $7.89/hour.

Wehman and colleagues (2012) adapted the SEARCH model for transition-age students with autism seeking competitive employment. The authors embedded additional levels of support to the SEARCH model for employees with autism. They added (1) weekly meetings with a behavior analyst to develop positive behavioral support; (2) consistent structure and schedules for internship experiences; (3) definitions of idioms, social skills, and work expectations to meet employer expectations; (4) visual supports such as task lists, social skills cue sheets, and behavior checklists; (5) self-monitoring checklists and reinforcement programs; (6) role playing and practice for social skills; and (7) intensive instruction and monitoring procedures. Wehman and colleagues implemented the "problem-solving" model in a single-subject research design with two students with autism. Both students met training criteria and obtained inclusive employment working 20 hours a week for $9.14/hour.

Transition Service Integration Model

The service integration model was created in response to the unemployment of individuals with significant disabilities. Certo, Pumpian, Fisher, Storey, and Smalley (1997) found systemic problems impeding transition to inclusive employment for students with significant disabilities. The first problem was that when community-training sites were developed, they were based on proximity to the school and not proximity to student residences. Without proximity to home, students could not get to and from training sites. The second problem was that schools often did not have staff or resources to independently support transition-age students seeking employment. Schools needed help with staffing and paying for job training. The third problem was the discrepancy between entitlement, support, and services. Many adult service programs were neither fully funded nor equipped to support individuals with more significant needs because of the time required to place them in inclusive employment. The model recognized that without a high level of support and service coordination, students with more significant disabilities were at risk of transitioning to adulthood without employment. The service integration approach attempted to address these problems by focusing on the transition from school to employment as an integrated process. Rather than developing individual supports in isolation, the model provided coordinated supports from the school and adult agencies during the student's last year of school. These supports continued after the student exited from school.

Certo and colleagues (2003) outlined the programmatic components of the transition service integration model. During the student's last year of school, the local education agency enters into a formal service agreement with a hybrid adult service agency comprised of VR and developmental disability systems. The goal of the agreement is to provide the resources and supports that would facilitate the immersion of students with disabilities in integrated employment and community activities prior to leaving school. Instruction and support are provided by the school system and the hybrid agency. Typically, a transition educator is assigned to a group of students in the community setting, and the district subcontracts funds to the hybrid agency to provide instructional aides or job coaches. Regular meetings are held between representatives from the school, VR, and developmental disability systems to discuss student progress in both work and community activities. Information obtained from these regular meetings is used to establish continued services with the hybrid agency *after* a student exits school. The researchers found that a critical feature of the service integration model was authorization from both the VR and the developmental disability system to concurrently fund and support a student.

Certo and colleagues (2008) piloted the service integration model in 14 urban, suburban, and rural school districts with 293 students. Of these students, 269 (92%) exited school with support from a hybrid agency. Furthermore, 177 (60%) exited school with a paid job averaging $6.62/hour (the minimum wage was $6.55/hour in 2008) for 14 hours a week. Three-year maintenance data indicated that 90% of students were still supported by the same hybrid agency and 71% were still employed.

Project Summer

In a 3-year development project funded by the Institute of Educational Sciences, Carter and colleagues (2010) developed a summer employment intervention strategy for transition-age students with emotional disturbance, intellectual disability, autism, and multiple disabilities. Project Summer consisted of community conversations, resource mapping, summer-focused planning, community connectors, and employer liaisons. These components are described here.

- *Community conversations.* Interagency meetings were designed to facilitate conversations about ways that schools, businesses, organizations, families, and youth could collaborate to expand employment options. During 2-hour events, the researcher asked two primary questions: "What can we as a community do to increase summer employment for youth with disabilities?" and "What would I be willing to do to facilitate summer employment opportunities for youth with disabilities?" Information was synthesized into a report.

- *Resource mapping.* The researchers compiled information about informal and formal resources used to improve employment outcomes. Specific resources were organized by domains (e.g., transportation, employment, recreation and leisure) and distributed to school staff.

- *Summer focus planning.* The researchers developed a two-page planning template to structure conversation among stakeholders. Short- and long-term goals, supports, and resources were also identified. The planning session was held during students' spring semester.

- *Community connectors.* The connector's role was to attend community conversations, facilitate the planning process for youth with disabilities, collaborate with employer liaisons, and serve as a link between parents and school staff. Follow-up contacts were made with parents, students, and employers during the summer months.

- *Employer liaisons.* The researchers identified a person to serve as an employer liaison in local communities to work with chambers of commerce, local employers, and employees from nonprofit organizations. The role of the liaison was to attend community conversations, expand networks, collaborate with community connectors, and attend planning meetings when appropriate.

Carter and colleagues (2010) piloted Project Summer with 67 youth with disabilities. Thirty-eight were placed in the intervention group and 29 in a control group. Researchers found that youth in the intervention group were 3.5 times more likely to have paid or unpaid summer work experiences than youth in the control group. Of students in the intervention group, 44.7% had paid competitive employment, 21.1% held unpaid jobs, 7.9% had sheltered work, and only 26.3% did not work in the summer. These results compared favorably to those of the control group.

Achieving Rehabilitation, Individualized Education, and Employment Success (ARIES)

As a 4-year multicomponent program designed for youth with emotional disturbance (Bullis, Moran, Benz, Todis, & Johnson, 2002), ARIES was staffed by three certified special education teachers who each maintained a caseload of 12–15 students. The program was comprised of (1) functional skills assessment (see Chapter 5), (2) person-centered planning (see Chapter 6), (3) individual education placement and support, (4) competitive job placement, (5) service coordination, and (6) multiple opportunities for success. According to Bullis and colleagues (2002), the project served 85 students with a mean age of 17.4 years. Sixty-one percent of the ARIES participants completed an educational program and 55% of participants worked in some capacity during the project. Moreover, the authors reported that students were successfully engaged in project activities.

TRANSITION TO PSE:
WHAT RESEARCH AND PROMISING PRACTICES EXIST?

The need for appropriate PSE for students with developmental disabilities has received considerable attention in recent years. Increasing numbers of youth with disabilities, including those with significant disabilities such as intellectual disability and/or autism, are involved in PSE. Most seek involvement in 2- and 4-year colleges, but others become involved in vocational, technical, or business schools. See Chapter 9 for more information on PSE. Because of this growth, PSE models have emerged.

Transition Programs for Students with Intellectual Disabilities

In 2010, the Office of Postsecondary Education awarded grants to 27 institutions of higher education to fund model transition programs for students with intellectual disabilities (TPSIDs). TPSIDs were designed to support students with intellectual disabilities so they could fully participate in inclusive higher education leading to an employment outcome (Grigal, Hart, Smith, Domin, & Sulewski, 2013). In 2012, there were 27 model demonstration projects on 43 campuses in 23 states working with 792 students with intellectual disability, autism, and/or developmental delays. Of those, 24% were dually enrolled in postsecondary and K–12 transition programs (Grigal et al., 2013).

The Think College National Coordinating Center issued an annual report (Grigal et al., 2013) on 2011–2012 TPSID activities, providing information on the structure and outcomes of TPSIDs. One of the primary functions of TPSIDs was to provide students with intellectual disabilities access to credit, noncredit, and/or audited college courses. These courses were either inclusive ones (47%) attended by both students with disabilities and typical college students, or specialized ones (53%) designed for students with disabilities. Examples of courses ran the gamut from art appreciation, automotive assistant, and English, to tai chi, study skills, career exploration, and introduction to business. Accommodations were provided by colleges and extra support was provided by paid TPSID staff. Additionally, TPSIDs were required to offer some type of meaningful credential for students upon completion, the most common being a certificate of completion.

In addition to academics, students in TPSIDs participated in career development and employment activities, including paid employment and unpaid career development. Employment options included individual paid jobs, paid internships, group work, sheltered work, and federal work–study. Students in paid positions used natural supports and job coaching. Grigal and colleagues (2013) noted that paid competitive employment was a critical outcome for TPSIDs. Unpaid career development activities included volunteer and/or community service, internships, and service learning.

TPSIDs also promoted self-determination. According to Grigal and colleagues (2013), all TPSIDs were required to incorporate person-centered planning (see Chapter 6). These programs provided supports to students so they could participate in extracurricular activities and all other college campus services. Finally, some students enrolled in TPSIDs had access to college residential living. According to Grigal and colleagues, in 2012, 16% lived in residences provided by the college, 20% lived in other residences, and 64% lived with family.

Weir, Grigal, Hart, and Boyle (2013) described the background and structure of five postsecondary programs receiving TPSID funding. Each of the profiles provided information on academic access, career development and employment, self-determination, and community membership. Western Carolina University's *University Participant Program* was one of these. Started in 2007, the program led to a 2-year "certificate of accomplishment," with students participating in academic course work, career development, self-determination activities, and all aspects of campus living. Students were not eligible to earn college credit or a degree. To obtain the certificate of accomplishment, students were required to:

- Complete 1,800 hours of learning activities over a four-semester period.
- Achieve a minimum of 80% of the objectives per semester.
- Obtain a recommendation for a University Participant Certification of Accomplishment.

The program, which involved eight student participants, used unpaid volunteers to facilitate student class attendance, engagement in social and recreational activities, and social skills. Each student was required to have an on-campus job, most of which were unpaid. However, the program strived to develop paid employment during the student's final semester. A career development coordinator helped facilitate on-campus job rotations and job development activities.

Evaluation of TPSIDs is ongoing. The effects on knowledge and skills, social and psychological impacts, and long-term impacts should become clearer with additional research. For more information, see the website at the end of this chapter.

SELF-DETERMINATION: WHAT RESEARCH AND PROMISING PRACTICES EXIST?

Researchers (e.g., Martin, Marshall, & De Pry, 2005; McGlashing-Johnson, Agran, Sitlington, Cavin, & Wehmeyer, 2003; Wehmeyer & Palmer, 2003) demonstrated that individuals with disabilities who exhibit self-determined behaviors were more successful in employment settings. Self-determination programs consisted of (1) setting goals and solving problems, (2) making appropriate choices based on personal preferences, (3) advocating for oneself, and (4) regulating and managing one's day-to-day behavior. Additional skills included teaching students to recognize their strengths and weakness, establish goals based on this information, recognize different sources of support, and self-monitor progress toward meeting employment goals and objectives. Model self-determination programs were described by Wehmeyer, Garner, Yeager, Lawrence, and Davis (2006). See Chapter 7 for details.

WHAT COMMON PRACTICES EXIST ACROSS EVIDENCE-BASED TRANSITION MODEL PROGRAMS?

We presented evidence-based transition model programs focusing on employment, PSE, and self-determination. These programs were evaluated using various research methodologies to determine their efficacy in improving outcomes.

Comparing across programs, we found common features and processes, many of which harken back to the recommendations of "early" transition models. Common components included (1) goal directedness, (2) multiple components, (3) active interdisciplinary and interagency collaboration, (4) self-determination, (5) student development, and (6) individualized focus. Let's take a closer look:

- *Goal directedness.* All models had clear goals for the overall program and for individual participants. Both program and individual participant goals were specific and measurable.

- *Multiple components.* All model programs were multifaceted to meet the various needs of individual participants. In this respect, all programs recognized individual differences and needs.

- *Interdisciplinary and interagency collaboration.* All model programs stressed how different disciplines and agencies needed to work together. Collaboration was active, with frequent interactions designed to achieve individual participant goals. For example, Project SEARCH, the transition service integration model, and Project Summer described collaboration, roles, and responsibilities of various professionals.

- *Self-determination.* Most model programs included active student involvement such as determination of goals and direction of the program by the individual participant. In particular, the ARIES, TPSID, and self-determination models emphasized that programs were driven and directed by the individual participant.

- *Student development.* Most programs emphasized the need for students to develop new skills as active participants. For example, Project SEARCH, Project Summer, ARIES, and TPSID models focused on increasing skills of individual participants.

- *Individualized focus.* Most model programs described how plans were individualized for each participant.

At least in a broad sense, the components necessary for a transition program to result in successful postschool outcomes are well established. Additionally, for different transition outcomes (e.g., employment vs. PSE) and for different types of disabilities, models are available for states, districts, and schools to emulate. At the outset of this section, we speculated about ongoing low rates of employment and other transition outcomes and asked questions about whether model programs were ineffective or not being adopted. Researchers have shown the model programs to be effective. The question about adoption remains open. So the question moving forward, to be considered in future chapters, is "What facilitates or hinders adoption of model programs?"

SUMMARY

With early model programs, such as Will's (1984) bridges model, Halpern's (1985) community adjustment model, and Kohler's (1996) taxonomy of transition programming, transition experts sought to increase employment and community integration outcomes for youth with disabilities. Although these model programs were evidence-based, the NCLB Act of 2001 insisting that all educational programs be based squarely on "scientifically-based research" strengthened the need for evidence underlying model programs in all areas. The What Works Clearinghouse required educational or instructional practice to be evaluated using scientifically based research to determine if the practice was evidence-based. The OSEP funded the NSTTAC to guide secondary and transition programs by providing technical assistance and information on evidence-based practices in transition. Project SEARCH, the transition service integration model, Project Summer, ARIES, TPSIDs, and self-determination programs are models with research demonstrating successful outcomes. Common practices across model programs are described.

Margaret Mead once said, "Never doubt that a small group of thoughtful, committed citizens can change the world; indeed it's the only thing that ever has" (*www.values. com/inspirational-quotes/6694-Never-Doubt-That-A-Small-Gr-*). Like Mead, we believe it is small groups of individuals that can make big changes. The challenge for transition educators is to learn how to incorporate elements of research and model projects into day-to-day classroom practices to promote effective postschool outcomes.

EXERCISE 4.3

Answer the following questions individually or in a discussion group.

- To what extent could each model transition program be adopted in your school or district? What changes may need to be made? What barriers would need to be overcome?
- Model programs require that all participants (administrators, transition educators, parents, youth, community members) "buy in" to a new set of approaches and commit to those approaches for a periodv of several years. What barriers might be encountered in implementing a model transition program in your school or district? How could you reduce those barriers?

REVISITING DEMARIUS

"I told you, I need people to just leave me alone," Demarius said.

"I'm not going to leave you alone until you try to get a job," Elaine responded. The tone of Demarius's grandmother's voice made it clear she was frustrated. "You're not going to turn out like your mother!"

Demarius looked at the floor.

"Demarius," Ms. Woolsey started, "We're on your side. We're not the bad guys. We want you to succeed by working and bringing home a paycheck. We want you to work with us because we believe in you."

Demarius looked up briefly from his shoes. "What do I have to do?"

Ms. Woolsey chose her words carefully. "I want to find out what you're good at. I want to find out what you would like to do—what career would work best for you."

"I ain't got no career!"

"Demarius, you stop that!" Elaine was not in the mood for hearing self-doubt.

"Like I said, we believe in you. Just try it. OK?"

Ms. Woolsey first explained to Demarius that career assessments were not tests in the traditional sense. He was not being scored or graded. Instead, he was identifying preferences for potential work and career. She then administered a career preference assessment (see Chapter 5 for details). Results confirmed what Ms. Woolsey had suspected: Demarius enjoyed working around athletic activity, such as a sports center or gymnasium. But she knew that he had "no-showed" previously when she arranged a work-based learning trial at a local sports academy. Although she wanted to set up another community opportunity, Ms. Woolsey knew she needed someone to offer support, perhaps someone who represented a role model. But who would Demarius look up to? Over the years, Ms. Woolsey had learned that neighborhood youth who turned their lives around sometimes became valuable role models for youth who were still struggling. She kept a "mental file" of such young adults. Recently, she had talked to Gabriel, a former drug addict who had cleaned up and played football on the junior college level. Gabriel had worked for the past year as a personal trainer at a local sports academy.

"Will Gabriel be up to the challenge of dealing with Demarius?" Ms. Woolsey pondered.

WEBSITES WITH ADDITIONAL INFORMATION

What Works Clearinghouse

http://ies.ed.gov/ncee/wwc/default.aspx

National Secondary and Transition Technical Assistance Center

www.nsttac.org or www.transitionta.org

National Collaborative on Workforce and Disability

www.ncwd-youth.info/guideposts

Project SEARCH

www.projectsearch.us

Transition Services Integration Model

https://interwork.sdsu.edu/web_programs/potsip.html

Project Summer

www.waisman.wisc.edu/cedd/projectsummer/Welcome.html

TPSID

www.thinkcollege.net

CHAPTER 5

Transition Assessment

This chapter addresses . . .

- The purpose of transition assessment.
- Characteristics and roles of transition assessment.
- Formal and informal assessments.
- The process for selecting transition assessments.
- The summary of performance document and processes.

WHAT IS THE PURPOSE OF TRANSITION ASSESSMENT?

Transition assessment is used for gathering and analyzing information on knowledge, skills, needs, preferences, and interests so that a student and the transition team can plan, implement, and evaluate transition activities. The data collected from transition assessment should be used to make decisions that better adapt and tailor transition planning. Once implemented, transition assessment should continue so that changes are made "on the fly" based on the changing needs of the youth. Following implementation, transition assessment should determine the effectiveness of planning and implementation activities.

WHAT ARE THE GOALS OF TRANSITION ASSESSMENT?

Test, Aspel, and Everson (2006, p. 64) identified three goals of transition assessment:

1. *To help students make informed choices that will enhance their postschool lives.* Some assessments provide various types of information about a student's performance

in potential future work, social, school, and community environments. This assessment information clarifies how students perform on job tasks so they can make informed choices (Sitlington, Neubert, & Laconte, 1997). Later in this chapter, we examine some of these assessment instruments.

2. *To help students take charge of the process.* Results of assessments should allow "students to assume the responsibility of coordinating their own . . . transition process" (Sitlington et al., 1997, pp. 70–71). As youth with disabilities make informed choices about their transition to adulthood, the assumption is that they will become more invested in managing, monitoring, and directing efforts in the process of realizing their goals. This assumption is supported by research on self-determination (e.g., Wehmeyer & Palmer, 2003). See Chapter 7 for more information.

3. *To help students understand the skills they need for postschool environments.* This goal draws attention to the importance of examining not only the skills of the student but how those skills interface with the requirements of postschool employment and PSE settings.

These goals reflect the importance of assessment in providing practical data and useful information to assist in the transition process. As Flexer and colleagues (2013) noted, "Transition assessment involves more than administering, scoring, and reporting tests and results. It involves careful analysis of the assessment results and provides functional, relevant, appropriate recommendations and decisions" (p. 99).

Transition assessment emphasizes gathering information about a student's strengths and skill characteristics. By assessing strengths, students can build on their strong points, determine their futures, and market their skills.

Unlike standardized, norm-referenced assessments for academic skills, the selection of a particular transition assessment depends on the individual student. Because transition is so wide-ranging and diverse, choice of transition assessment varies according to individual strengths, preferences, and needs, as well as the environments the individual seeks to access during or after transition (e.g., job setting, apartment, college campus).

To illustrate, Linda and Brenda are two 16-year-old students in a classroom who take the same standardized, norm-referenced test to assess their reading skills. They are presented the same set of reading items on the test and their responses are scored according to a preestablished protocol that produces *grade-equivalence scores,* that is, scores that describe estimates of their reading performance in relation to average grade-level scores. But the same two students, even though similar in their level of reading skill, may participate in very different transition assessments based on their interests and future directions. Linda, who has mild intellectual disabilities, is interested in a food service career, so her teacher uses an assessment for students entering culinary arts school. Also, her teacher has Linda fill out an assessment on the extent to which she is ready to determine and be responsible for her own future. The results of Linda's assessments are used to set her transition goals. In contrast, Brenda, a youth with cerebral palsy who uses a wheelchair, wants to work in a library because she loves reading literature. Her teacher assesses Brenda's reading, language, and computer skills. The teacher talks to a librarian and takes Brenda to the library to assess her ability to move about the reference desk area and perform work samples in a "situational assessment." The results of Brenda's assessments are used to set her transition goals.

WHAT ARE THE CHARACTERISTICS OF TRANSITION ASSESSMENTS?

Seven characteristics of assessments are described below. Note how these characteristics align with the models of transition discussed in the previous chapter.

Transition Assessment Must Be Student-Centered

Choice of assessment depends on what the individual student wants to do in the future. Therefore, selection of assessments depends on the student's vision of career, educational, and independent living aspirations. A student interested in a career as a welder would be given a different assessment than a student who wants to become a floral designer. A student interested in entering a 4-year college to pursue a degree in exercise science would use an assessment on college preparedness. Many students enter the transition process without preferences for the future. In this case, during the transition years (ages 14–18), these students should be exposed to numerous careers through job shadowing and job training experiences (see Chapter 8). With exposure, they can better make informed decisions using preference assessments described later in this chapter.

Transition Assessment Should Involve Several Stakeholders

Relevant members of the IEP team should provide input into assessment, including the youth; parents; special, general, and vocational educators; related-services personnel (e.g., speech therapists), and others. Although the student should drive the process and the decision making, the perspectives from several stakeholders can be very useful.

Transition Assessment Must Be Ongoing

Because transition assessment should provide the information necessary for making practical decisions at various points in time, ongoing assessment is recommended (Test et al., 2006). Unlike some assessments that are administered every 1–3 years, transition assessments should be administered on a frequent basis (at least once per year) because adolescents experience rapid and dramatic changes in development, skills, and interests.

Transition Assessment Should Occur in Many Environments

Unlike a reading assessment, most transition assessments that measure performance are closely tied to given environments, whether employment, community, residential, or school settings. For example, some transition programs in high schools arrange for students to rotate through numerous employment samples in effort to diversify and strengthen their employment skills and allow them to develop preferences (and dislikes). These provide occasions for assessing skills, environmental characteristics, and preferences. Transition educators can then compare the results of assessments across job sites.

The Selected Transition Assessment May Change as the Youth Gets Older

Neubert (2003) described transition assessments for students in middle school, high school, and at the "exit point" from school services (pp. 68–70). In middle school, assessment should help students identify interests and preferences, increase awareness of jobs and postsecondary academic alternatives (e.g., vocational/technical courses), determine needed accommodations and supports, and develop tentative postsecondary goals. Assessment methods can include interviews and interest inventories (described later). In high school, the focus turns to environments and job/educational requirements identified in assessments of interests and preferences. The youth and educator ask, "To what extent is there a match between requirements [of a certain job or a college course, for example] and current skills?" The answer to the question may target skills to be taught or strengths to be emphasized in the transition plan.

Transition Assessment Should Take into Account Academic Preparedness for College or Technical Schools

Young adults with disabilities, even those with significant challenges, are becoming increasingly involved in PSE (e.g., 2-year, 4-year, or business college) or vocational/technical schools (Grigal & Hart, 2010; Kochhar-Bryant et al., 2009; Neubert, 2003). This trend heightens the importance of preparing youth academically during middle and high school years. In fact, deficits in required academic skills can be a major blow to career aspirations of some youth with postsecondary goals of pursuing college careers. The trend should compel transition educators to identify interests in pursuing PSE early through interviews with the youth and parents, then gear transition planning to the needs of a college-bound learner. Although it is not realistic to target *specific* aspirations of a college-bound student at an early age, transition educators should at least identify students who see college in their future. In any event, the transition educator can be certain that academic standards will be high priority and should arrange transition assessment and planning accordingly.

Transition Assessment Must Consider Family Interests and Characteristics and Be Particularly Sensitive to Cultural Diversity

Transition assessment should tap into expectations, perceptions, and values of youth and their families, including those who come from culturally diverse backgrounds.

Greene (2011) noted the importance of using multiple and culturally responsive transition assessments for these youth. Additionally, he recommended the youth's family be involved in the assessment process from the outset and continuously throughout the transition years so that information gathered can reflect the expectations, perceptions, and values of the family. In transition from school to adulthood, many youth seek to retain the values coveted by their families and use them as strengths to define and represent their movement to adulthood. Educators and all stakeholders must acknowledge and adopt these values. We explore these issues more closely in Chapter 11.

WHAT ARE FORMAL ASSESSMENTS?

The first phase in categorizing transition assessment is to divide them into formal and informal types. Formal assessment strategies are structured assessment procedures with specific guidelines for administration, scoring, and interpretation of results (McLoughlin & Lewis, 2008). In some cases, formal assessments are norm-referenced. That is, they are based comparison of one person's score to scores of others with similar characteristics. Also, formal assessments are based on standardized procedures. That is, the examiner must follow a strict protocol to administer and score the test (Salvia, Ysseldyke, & Bolt, 2007). Only when the examiner follows the strict protocol can scores be compared across individuals or across subject matter with validity.

Formal assessments have undergone extensive test development, including evaluations of validity and reliability (Salvia et al., 2007). Examples of formal assessments are tests of intelligence, achievement, adaptive behavior, vocational and career aptitude, and occupational skill (Flexer et al., 2013). Test results are usually expressed as standard scores and percentile ranks. Standard scores typically have a mean (arithmetic average) score of 100. A score of 85 would correspond with a percentile rank of 16, which means that the student's score ranked 16th out of 100 students the same age who took the same test. These results can be used for various purposes, often as documentation for eligibility for special education (McLoughlin & Lewis, 2008).

Formal Assessments Used in Special Education

In Table 5.1, we list a sample of formal educational assessments. All listed assessments have been researched and found to have high levels of reliability and validity. Assessments shown in Table 5.1 are a very small sample of all formal tests. For a more comprehensive review, see McLoughlin and Lewis (2008). Only a brief synopsis of assessments is provided here.

Although formal assessments can yield scores that compare a student's performance to others or compare performance to a criterion, they provide little information about an individual's functional skills or progress over time. Nonetheless, there are formal assessments used in transition from school to adulthood that provide information on eligibility, predictors of performance, and characteristics that are important in transition planning. Here, we describe specific assessment instruments.

TABLE 5.1. A Sample of Formal Assessments Often Used in Special Education

Formal assessment	Characteristics
Wechsler Intelligence Scale for Children—Fourth Edition (WISC-IV; Wechsler, 2003)	Norm-referenced test of general intelligence. Yields scores for verbal and performance intelligence, as well as composite scores in subareas (e.g., verbal comprehension, perceptual reasoning). Mean score = 100; standard deviation = 15. Ages 6–16.
Woodcock–Johnson Tests of Achievement (WJ-III; Woodcock, McGrew, & Mather, 2001)	Norm-referenced test of student achievement. Yields scores in reading, oral language, mathematics, written language, and academic knowledge. Scores are expressed as "grade" or "age equivalents," as well as standard scores (mean score = 100; standard deviation = 15) and percentile ranks. Ages 2–adulthood.
Brigance Diagnostic Comprehensive Inventory of Basic Skills—Revised (CIB-R; Brigance, 1999)	Criterion-referenced test. That is, scores are compared to a criterion. Useful for pinpointing skills for instruction. Major areas: readiness, oral language, reading, writing, and mathematics. Early childhood through secondary grades.
Vineland Adaptive Behavior Scale (Vineland–II; Sparrow, Cicchetti, & Balla, 2005)	Adaptive behavior scale that measures student's level of functioning in areas of communication, daily living, socialization, and motor skills. Subdomains exist within each area. There is also a maladaptive behavior index. Scores are expressed as standard scores (mean score = 100; standard deviation = 15) and percentile ranks. Ages 3–18.

Formal Assessments Used in Transition from School to Adulthood

Before examining specific assessments, we divide them into a usable taxonomy. IDEA (2004) included three transition domains: education, employment, and independent living. Also, IDEA described the importance of an individual's strengths, preferences, interests, and needs (SPIN). In Figure 5.1, we illustrate this taxonomy using these four subareas to examine formal transition assessments.

Education

Many of us can relate to taking formal assessments for purposes of determining eligibility for college. The American College Testing college readiness assessment (ACT) and Scholastic Aptitude Test (SAT) are the most popular college entrance examinations. One of these two standardized, norm-referenced assessments will probably be taken by some youth in transition from school to college if they plan to take courses for credit. The ACT yields scores in English, math, reading, and science. Composite scores range from 1 to 36. The SAT yields scores in math, critical reading, and writing. Each subtest is worth 800 points; the overall score can range from 600 to 2400. Minimum scores on these tests are established for entry into most colleges if students plan to take credit-bearing

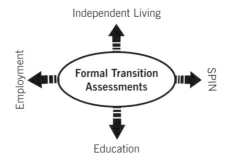

FIGURE 5.1. Types of formal transition assessment.

courses. Testing accommodations can be arranged for any college-entry test, including extended time, alternative format or location, and adaptive equipment.

Formal assessments are administered for many reasons beyond determining eligibility for PSE. With increasing frequency, students with disabilities are being held to CCSS, as mentioned in Chapter 1. With the Common Core comes standards-based assessment—that is, tests administered at periodic intervals for most children receiving public education, including those with disabilities. Standards-based assessment usually involves taking a formal instrument called a *criterion-referenced test* (CRT). A CRT determines whether students have mastered specific skills by comparing "performance to a curricular goal rather than performance of other students" (McLoughlin & Lewis, 2008, p. 59). Transition students with disabilities participate in CRTs to assess their mastery of curricular goals or determine progress over time (i.e., trends in curricular areas from unmastered to mastered material).

Employment

Formal assessments predicting employment skills usually focus on various occupational and vocational skills, including work behaviors, decision making, socialization, and information processing (Niles & Harris-Bowlsbey, 2005; Szymanski & Hershenson, 2005), among many others. There are numerous tests for assessment of skills in specific vocations and occupations. Interested readers should refer to *A Guide to Vocational Assessment* (Power, 2013).

One of the most popular vocational assessment instruments is the *Career Ability Placement Survey* (CAPS; *www.edits.net/products/copsystem.html*), a comprehensive, multidimensional battery designed to measure vocationally relevant abilities. There are eight ability dimensions: (1) mechanical reasoning, (2) spatial relations, (3) verbal reasoning, (4) numerical ability, (5) language usage, (6) word knowledge, (7) perceptual speed and accuracy, and (8) manual speed and dexterity. This test takes 5 minutes for each of the eight dimension tests and yields standard scores. Data on reliability and validity were reported by Knapp-Lee (1995). The CAPS is appropriate for individuals with mild disabilities. It is part of a three-component assessment consisting of CAPS, *Career Occupational Preference System* (COPS: assessment of interests), and *Career*

Orientation Placement and Evaluation Survey (COPES: assessment of work values). The system is available online as a package (*www.edits.net*).

Other recently published formal assessments for employment include *Bennett's Mechanical Comprehension Test* (Bennett, 2006), *Life-Centered Career Education Program* (LCE; Wandry, Wehmeyer, & Glor-Scheib, 2013), and *O*NET Ability Profiler* (U.S. Department of Labor, 2002).

Independent Living

Assessment in independent living relates to functional skill development in health and hygiene, home care, safety and community survival, community transportation, shopping, cooking, house cleaning, and money management (Flexer et al., 2013). As youth approach adulthood, assessment of independent living skills becomes crucial. Formal assessments are usually checklists or rating scales estimating performance of activities required for personal and social sufficiency (Sparrow, Cicchetti, & Balla, 2005). One particular instrument for measuring independent living skills is the *Ansell–Casey Life Skills Assessment–III* (Nollan, Horn, Downs, Pecora, & Bressani, 2002). This assessment measures a youth's independent living skills and is completed by the student and his/her caregivers. The authors claim the assessment is culturally sensitive and is appropriate for all students regardless of their living circumstances. Life skill areas addressed include: career planning, communication, daily living, home life, housing and money management, self-care, social relationships, work life, and work and study skills. The Ansell–Casey Life Skills Assessment–III is appropriate for youth with mild to significant disabilities. No research was found assessing reliability or validity.

The *Enderle–Severson Transition Rating Scales* (ESTR-J and ESTR-III; Enderle & Severson, 2003) are scales for identifying skills of students with disabilities from mild to those requiring significant supports. The informant scores each response as "Yes," "No," or "Yes, with supports." Subscales cover jobs and job training, recreation and leisure, home living, and postsecondary training and learning opportunities. No research was found assessing reliability or validity.

SPIN Assessments

We develop interests at an early age and they are often wide-ranging. Interests are usually related to personal strengths. Either we identify interests in areas we have strengths, or we spend time in areas of interests and, because of the time commitment, develop strengths. When we are presented with different interests and asked to select one, the response is called a *choice*. When choice responses are reliably repeated, we call them *preferences* (Lohrman-O'Rourke & Gomez, 2001). Considerable research exists on preferences, especially in relation to persons with significant disabilities (e.g., Tullis et al., 2011). Based on preference research, educators and practitioners have emphasized the importance of providing choice opportunities so that students, including those with disabilities, can identify their preferences.

SPIN instruments are consistent with the values inherent in self-determination and self-direction. The *Arc Self-Determination Scale* (Wehmeyer & Kelchner, 1995) allows students to rate themselves on 72 items according to four characteristics of self-determination: autonomy, self-regulation, self-realization, and psychological empowerment. An overall score is determined as well as scores in each of the four categories. A student profile is generated that provides data on each student's degree of self-determination skills. The instrument is appropriate for students with mild to significant disabilities. The authors (Wehmeyer & Kelchner, 1995) described data on the instrument's high levels of reliability and validity. The language on some items may be too complex for youth with significant reading limitations, so a reader may need to assist.

The *AIR Self-Determination Scale* (Wolman, Campeau, Dubois, Mithaug, & Stolarski, 1994) offers a profile of the student's level of self-determination, identifies areas of strength and needs, and suggests educational goals for a youth's IEP. Versions are provided for the student, educator, and parent. Scales consist of 30 questions providing measures on capacity and opportunity for self-determination. Items are arranged in a 5-point rating scale. The AIR self-determination scale is appropriate for students with mild to significant disabilities. Researchers (e.g., Carter, Lane, Pierson, & Glaeser, 2006) report high levels of reliability and validity.

A popular career preference assessment for individuals with and without disabilities is the *Self-Directed Search* (SDS; Holland, Powell, & Fritzsche, 1997). The SDS is based on Holland's personality theory, which describes the relationship between an individual's characteristics and the career selected. Career dimensions are categorized as *Realistic, Investigative, Artistic, Social, Enterprising,* and *Conventional* (abbreviated *RIASEC*). As Holland and colleagues (1997) stated,

> cultural and personal forces—parents, social class, culture, and the physical environment—shape people in different ways. Out of these experiences, a person learns first to prefer some activities over others. Later, the preferred activities become strong interests, which tend to lead to a special group of competencies. (p. 5)

The user self-directs the search by checking statements related to *Jobs You Have Thought About, Activities* (you might like), *Skills* (you have), and *Jobs* (you think you might like/dislike). The user then sums the number of checked items for each of the six types (RIASEC) and goes to a jobs finder to identify jobs that correspond with the highest numbers. There is an "easy" form of the SDS (Form E) for adults and high school students who have limited reading skills. Considerable research exists on reliability and validity of the SDS, including studies with users who have specific learning disabilities or intellectual disability (e.g., Mattie, 2000).

WHAT ARE INFORMAL TRANSITION ASSESSMENT PROCEDURES?

Informal assessments are used to determine current levels of performance and to document student progress (McLoughlin & Lewis, 2008). Compared to formal assessments, the procedures involved in informal assessments are less structured. Although most informal assessments are subjective, require interpretation by an individual, and do not yield scores that are comparable across different tests, they nevertheless

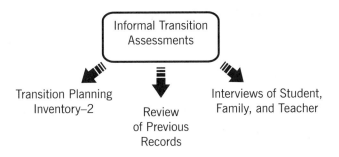

FIGURE 5.2. Types of informal transition assessment.

provide pertinent and very specific information about an individual. In this section, we describe informal assessments relevant to transition, including the *Transition Planning Inventory—Second Edition* (TPI-2; Gaumer Erickson, Clark, & Patton, 2013); a review of previous records; and interviews of the student, family, and teacher (see Figure 5.2).

Transition Planning Inventory—Second Edition

The TPI-2 (Gaumer Erickson et al., 2013) was designed to provide an assessment of a youth's capabilities in 11 transition areas, including career choice and planning, employment knowledge and skills, further education/training, functional communication, self-determination, independent living, personal money management, community involvement and usage, leisure activities, health, and interpersonal relationships. It requests information from the student, parents/guardians, and school personnel in order to identify areas of need that allow the transition team to develop services. Components include student, home, and school forms. The TPI-2 consists of 57 items (e.g., names occupations he or he prefers over all others, knows job requirements and demands for preferred occupations). Each of these items is broken into subcompetencies (e.g., identifies various jobs performed by family or friends). The instrument was developed for individuals with mild disabilities, although a modified form for students with significant support needs is provided. Data on high levels of reliability and validity were reported on the original TPI instrument (Kohler, 1998). The TPI-2 is available at *www.proedinc.com/customer/ProductView.aspx?ID=6063*.

Review of Previous Records

An individual's records may contain observations of previous educators, past IEPs, previous assessments, living situation, employment experiences, and health-related information (Sitlington & Clark, 2007). Generally, a record review is a good starting point in gathering informal assessment data because it answers some questions and sets up additional ones to be addressed in an interview. For example, an educator might review a student's records and discover a history of problem behavior according to a teacher's report and the teacher's behavior intervention plan. However, there may be no indication whether problem behaviors still occur, which sets up questions to ask in an interview.

Interviews of Student, Family, or Educator

Interviews can be useful for gathering a wide range of information (Sitlington & Clark, 2007). For example, an interview with a student can yield information on goals, preferences, interests, attitudes toward school and work, fears/anxieties, barriers encountered, and perspectives on various topics. In a survey of transition goals and experiences, researchers (Hogansen, Powers, Geenen, Gil-Kashiwabara, & Powers, 2008) asked female young adults with disabilities questions such as:

"What are your goals?"
"What are you doing to accomplish these goals?"
"What have other people done to help you work towards your goals?" (p. 219)

A discussion with family members can produce information on history, experience, and shared values. For example, Lindstrom, Doren, Metheny, Johnson, and Zane (2007, p. 353) sought to identify the role of the family in career development and asked parents questions such as:

"In what ways did you say that you [or other family members] were involved in helping [child's name] decide or prepare for a job after high school?"
"Did [child's name] have any role models that he/she could look up to that influenced his/her career choices or other life decisions?"

As noted by Sitlington and Clark (2007), interviews allowed "the assessor to clarify any responses that are not understood, pursue answers to incomplete responses, and verify or validate information collected through other methods" (p. 136).

EXERCISE 5.1

Write three questions you think would reveal important information if asked in an interview of:

- Youth with disabilities in transition from school to adulthood.
- Parents of youth with disabilities in transition from school to adulthood.
- Educators of youth with disabilities in transition from school to adulthood.

WHAT OTHER ASSESSMENT PROCEDURES AID IN TRANSITION DECISION MAKING?

Other assessment procedures combine formal and informal methods and include curriculum-based assessment (CBA), direct observation, ecological assessment, situational assessment, task analysis, portfolio assessment, assessment of PSE readiness, and competency-based assessment of skills of students with significant/multiple disabilities (see Figure 5.3).

- Curriculum-based assessment
- Direct observation
- Ecological assessment
- Situational assessment
- Task analysis

- Portfolio assessment
- Postsecondary rfeadiness
- Competency-based assessment:
  Students with significant/
  multiple disabilities

FIGURE 5.3. Other types of transition assessment.

Curriculum-Based Assessment

CBA refers to an approach designed to pinpoint a student's performance within a particular curriculum (Deno, 2003). It involves taking samples from a curriculum in a particular content area, presenting them to a student in sequence, and scoring his or her performance. The purposes of CBA are to pinpoint current student performance within a curriculum and develop specific lesson plans (Test et al., 2006). CBA can increase the effectiveness of instruction by precisely identifying a student's performance within a curriculum, as well as his or her strengths, weaknesses, and learning style (Deno, 2003). As related to transition, CBA may be instrumental in assessing the vocational skills a student needs for an employment task or measuring a student's academic skills in preparation for PSE.

Direct Observation

Much like CBA, direct observation involves collecting samples of a student's performance on a particular task by watching his or her behavior in a particular setting and collecting data. Although direct observation can be time-consuming and laborious—the observer must make frequent or continuous observations—the outcome can be an objective and specific record of performance. A starting point is to define the behavior being observed in operational terms, that is, in terms of what the observer is likely to see and hear. For example, an operational definition of street crossing with a pedestrian light might be:

1. Stands on the curb and waits until the light indicates "Walk."
2. When the light indicates "Walk," looks both ways and then begins walking.
3. Walks across the entire street staying within white lines (Page, Iwata, & Neef, 1976).

Second, the observer identifies a recording system that lends itself to the behavior being observed. For example, an observer may define following job-related instructions as "performing all actions requested by a supervisor by saying 'OK,' starting the first action within 5 seconds of the instruction, completing all actions within 1 minute, and returning to the supervisor to report actions completed." The recording system for observing instruction following may be to mark "+" or "−" at the end of 1 minute if all component parts of the behavior were completed. Over time and after several instructions, the recording system would yield pluses and minus, which could be compiled to show the percentage of total instructions (or components) followed. With teaching, the observer could examine for trends in increased instruction following.

Because behaviors vary along dimensions of time, movement, quality, and work (Johnston & Pennypacker, 1993), several observational methods may be necessary. Ellerd and Morgan (2013) described various observational methods related to the performance of behaviors in employment, independent living, or postsecondary settings, including (1) frequency, (2) rate, (3) percent of opportunities, (4) percent correct, (5) level of prompt required, and (6) quality rating. In Table 5.2, we describe some of the key elements of observation.

Some behaviors can be recorded using multiple observation methods. Observers should select one method that best addresses the accuracy of the observation process and the learning needs of the student. According to Sitlington and Clark (2007), behavior observation requires that the educator (1) clearly define the behavior to be observed, (2) select the observation method that most accurately reflects the occurrence of behavior, (3) determine the amount of time each day for observation, (4) decide who should conduct the observation, and (5) share results with the student. In some cases, interobserver agreement, or reliability of behavior observation, can be established by having two observers independently observe the same behavior from different vantage points (Kratochwill et al., 2013).

Ecological Assessment

Ecological assessment examines all aspects of a physical and/or social environment (people, places, things) and the relationships among those aspects and a student's performance (Flexer et al., 2013). McLoughlin and Lewis (2008) referred to ecological assessment as the measure of the degree of match or mismatch between a student's performance and the constraints of an environment. All relevant aspects of an environment can be assessed: number of people, noise levels, temperature, physical dimensions, lighting, furniture/equipment, pace of work and movement of people, social interactions, etc. These aspects are considered for their degree of match (interrelationship) with the student's performance and needs. Clearly, these relationships are not reducible to a single measure, but instead may yield either multiple measures or qualitative information that helps a transition educator develop an environment to accommodate a student's needs.

Situational Assessment

A *situational assessment* is a type of ecological assessment involving the collection of direct observation data on a student's job performance. Its purpose is to observe and record a student's work performance and adaptation needs in a specific work or community setting (Flexer et al., 2013). Ideally, a student is placed in a series of situational assessments for purposes of generating comparison data to identify the most compatible job.

TABLE 5.2. Observation Methods Used in Transition Settings

Method	Description	Examples
Frequency recording	A count of the number of occurrences of a behavior. To be counted, the behavior must have a clear beginning and end, and cannot occur at an extremely high rate.	Number of parts assembled; number of math problems correct.
Rate	Number of occurrences of a behavior divided by elapsed time. This is usually expressed as the rate per minute or hour.	Rate of parts assembled per hour; rate of correct math problems per minute.
Percent of opportunities	Number of times an individual's behavior occurred in relation to total opportunities. Total correct divided by total opportunities times 100 = percent correct.	Percent of instructions followed; percent of work days attended.
Percent correct	Percent of actions scored correct (+) divided by total actions scored correct (+) plus incorrect (−) times 100.	Steps correct in bed-making; steps correct in making coffee.
Duration of time	The amount of time (seconds, minutes, or hours) that elapses while an individual sustains work on a task.	Time to complete an assignment; time worked before requesting a break.
Level of prompt required	The minimum level of prompt necessary to successfully perform a task. Example: no prompt, verbal, gesture, touch, tap, hand-guided, multiple prompts.	Selecting the correct city bus at a bus terminal; cleaning a window using soap, water, and pad.
Quality rating	Comparison of an individual's performance to a standard or criterion. Example: low quality (multiple problems), moderate quality, good quality, excellent quality (no problems observed).	Making a pizza; using a drill press to drill holes.

Steere and colleagues (2007) noted that situational assessments provide functional and practical ways to determine individual strengths and weaknesses on a job. Assessment of individual characteristics is closely tied to the work environment and job requirements. For example, one of the authors recently consulted with a teacher who supervised a 21-year-old post–high school student (Randall) whose preferred job was as a farm equipment mechanic. Randall was completing his final year of special education service eligibility and wanted to be competitively employed. He had significant intellectual disability and communicated in single words. Randall followed instructions and evidenced good hearing and vision. His teacher, Ms. Alvarez, found a temporary job training opportunity at a local farm implement repair shop. The shop repaired tractors with mechanical problems, and the boss thought it would be a good idea to clean the tractor cabs before they were returned to farmers. Randall agreed to participate in the temporary training opportunity.

A situational assessment by Ms. Alvarez revealed that Randall was well liked by the supervisor and coworkers. His job training involved vacuuming the cab areas of tractors and washing interior and exterior windows surrounding cabs. Ms. Alvarez conducted a situational assessment to determine whether Randall's performance in this particular situation could lead to employment. Early in the situational assessment, barriers were noted. Randall was small in stature (less than 5 feet tall) and possessed underdeveloped physical strength and endurance. Many tractor tires were 7 feet or larger in diameter. The foot- and handholds built into the tractors were beyond Randall's reach, so Ms. Alvarez found a sturdy stepladder that made it possible for him to access the cab area. Although Randall vacuumed and cleaned the dashboard area of the cab, the interior windows were challenging. They rose high above his outstretched arms, even when he stood on the seat in the cab. Ms. Alvarez provided a squeegee with a long handle, which allowed Randall to reach the top edges of interior windows with soap and water. However, the exterior windows produced a new challenge. Randall could not safely stand on the tops of tractor tires and maneuver around the exterior to access windows. Also, he did not possess the strength and flexibility to reach the upper extremes of the windows while pressing and dragging the squeegee down the window surface. He realized there was a mismatch between his performance and the characteristics of the environment, and he turned his attention to auto detailing.

Task Analysis

A *task analysis* involves breaking down, or dividing up, a task into specific component skills (Flexer et al., 2013) for purposes of systematically delivering instruction to a learner. A task analysis should arrange component skills in sequence from beginning to end to facilitate teaching. A good way to start analyzing a task is to ask someone proficient in the skill (a model) to perform and "talk through" each step, noting aspects of the task that are important. Observing the model perform the task allows the educator and learner to see the entire sequence and take notes. Eventually, the model should perform the task at the speed typically required so the educator and student can note the allotted time for each step. The sequencing process allows both the learner and the educator to understand as clearly as possible what is necessary to successfully complete the task (Storey & Montgomery, 2013).

Each task analysis should specify (1) the name of the task; (2) the data to be collected on the performance of each task; (3) criteria for successful completion of the entire task; (4) stimuli, or cues, that serve as the "occasion" for beginning and performing each step of a task; (5) the response that must be performed; (6) speed, quality, or accuracy criteria for each task; (7) reinforcement for satisfactory learner performance; and (8) error correction procedures in case the learner makes a mistake. For example, Storey and Montgomery (2013) described a task analysis for bussing tables (e.g., pick up dishes, take dishes to cleaning area, return to unwashed table, use cleaning cloth to wipe down table). For each response, a stimulus should be identified that serves as the occasion for performing that response. The reason for identifying naturally occurring stimuli that serve as the occasion for performing a response is to assure that a learner is responding to the environment, not to a prompt from a transition educator. For example, the stimulus that sets the occasion for the first step is an unoccupied dirty table with used dishes. In response to this stimulus, the employee begins picking up dishes.

Performance on each of these steps can be scored "+" or "−" according to speed, quality, or accuracy criteria. The transition educator also records reinforcement and error correction procedures. Assuming the educator is using reinforcement and correcting errors so the learners do not practice inaccurate responses, their performance should improve over time. An example of a task analysis for boarding and riding a city bus appears in Figure 5.4.

Task analysis is often conceptualized as a procedure for basic self-help or domestic tasks. However, many complex tasks can be divided into component parts, such as following steps in a computer program, carrying out high school biology experiments, filling out college application forms, or assembling an automobile engine.

Advantages of Task Analysis

As an informal assessment strategy, task analysis is useful because (1) stimuli and responses are specified in sequence, (2) it facilitates data collection on each task, (3) the educator can identify steps that are troublesome for the learner and "isolate" them for further instruction, and (4) the learner can use it as a self-management strategy by "checking off" tasks performed in sequence.

How Many Steps?

A frequently asked question is "How many steps should be included to analyze a task?" The answer depends on the learning needs of the student (Flexer et al., 2013). For example, the task of washing a delivery truck at a parcel company may be one step in a larger task analysis for a learner with high-level skills. The entire task analysis may appear as follows: Wash vehicle, fill with gas, note odometer mileage, check oil, check window wash fluid, vacuum interior, and drive to loading dock. Yet, for a learner with more significant training needs, the task of washing the vehicle may need to be broken down (e.g., obtain bucket, fill with soap and water, obtain water brush, turn on water, spray with water all surfaces of truck, rub all surfaces of truck with water brush using soapy water, spray with water all surfaces to rinse).

Analyzing Different Kinds of Tasks

McLoughlin and Lewis (2008) reminded us that not all tasks follow a time-based sequence of subtasks performed from beginning to end. First, some tasks must be analyzed according to *developmental sequence* (Affleck, Lowenbraun, & Archer, 1980, p. 87). That is, there may be a progression of steps built on previously acquired skills, such as in arithmetic skills. Addition and subtraction must be learned to mastery before introducing multiplication and division, which must be learned before introducing rules about the order of operations. In this case, the sequence is developmental, not time-based. Second, some tasks must be analyzed according to *difficulty level* of subskills. Affleck and colleagues (1980) used the example of letter writing: straight-line letters ("*l, t, i*") are

Student Alias: _Jared_   Date: 10/24

Measurable Objective: _Jared will increase independent travel by boarding and riding the city bus from school to a predetermined location_
on two consecutive trials at 100% accuracy and independence.

Settings: _School, bus, 12th St. and Washington Blvd._   Materials: _Bus token, warm clothing (if needed)_

Step #	Stimulus	Task/Response	Speed/Quality/Accuracy
1	Receive bus token from secretary.	Say "Thank you." Walk to bus stop in front of the school.	2 minutes
2	See bus stop sign.	Stand near the bus stop sign and watch for bus.	4–10 minutes
3	See the bus approaching.	Remain standing by the sign until the bus comes to a complete stop.	30 seconds
4	The bus comes to a stop.	Wait for the bus door to open.	20 seconds
5	The bus door opens.	Step into the bus and walk up the stairs.	5 seconds
6	See token box at top of stairs.	Deposit the bus token into the slot on the token box.	10 seconds
7	See the driver.	Ask the driver for a transfer slip.	10 seconds
8	Receive transfer slip.	Say "Thank you" to the driver and place the transfer slip in your pocket.	10 seconds
9	See an open seat on the bus.	Walk to the open seat and be seated.	10 seconds
10	The bus starts to move.	Watch out the window for the bus stop on 12th and Washington.	15–20 minutes
11	See the bus stop on 12th and Washington.	Pull the cord to notify the bus driver to stop.	10 seconds
12	The bus stops.	Exit the bus and step away from it.	10 seconds

Teaching Procedures: Teach the whole task. Use least-to-most prompts (i.e., no prompt, open-ended verbal prompt such as "What next?", specific verbal prompt, verbal prompt + gesture, and if none of these is sufficient, demonstrate the task).

Data Collection: Educator marks data sheet with I for independent, O for open-ended verbal prompt, S for specific verbal prompt, and G for gesture. Data are collected for each step across five trials. Educator stays within close proximity, observes, and prompts student using the prompt hierarchy throughout task. When student obtains 80% or above in overall independence on the task analysis, educator then fades observation to indirect observation—that is, following the student from a distance and following the bus from another vehicle. When the student successfully completes the task analysis with 100% independence on indirect observation for one trial, the educator can terminate the indirect observation. The student then completes the task independently, with no observation, for two trials to demonstrate task mastery, with the educator meeting the student at the bus stop (end of the route).

Reinforcement: In the initial teaching phase, verbal praise is offered for each step of the task analysis independently completed. In the second phase, verbal praise is offered after every four correct tasks/responses completed independently. When the student demonstrates mastery by completing the entire task independently, the educator should take the student to his or her favorite fast-food restaurant that is at the bus stop for a chocolate frosty.

FIGURE 5.4. Example of a task analysis for boarding and riding a bus.

less difficult than straight line and slant letters (*"v, x, w, y, z"*), which are less difficult than circle and curve letters (*"o, c, s"*), and so forth. Letter writing progresses by writing simple letters first and then letters with increasing difficulty. Learning machine trades (e.g., operating a lathe), actions in sports (e.g., a backhand return in tennis, parallel turns in skiing), and decision making in organizational management may be viewed as possessing different levels of difficulty. Transition educators must understand whether tasks should be learned based on time sequences, developmental sequences, or degree of difficulty.

EXERCISE 5.2

Analyze one of the following time-based tasks. Follow the steps described in this chapter in conducting the task analysis. Specify (1) the name of the task; (2) data to be collected on performance of each task; (3) criteria for successful completion of the entire task; (4) stimuli that serve as the "occasion" for performing each step of a task; (5) the response that the learner must make to the stimulus for each task; (6) speed, quality, or accuracy criteria for each task; (7) reinforcement for satisfactory learner performance; and (8) error correction procedures in case the learner makes a mistake.

- Changing a fluorescent light bulb in a large machine shop
- Using a microwave to heat a TV dinner
- Withdrawing $40 from one's personal checking account at an ATM

Portfolio Assessment

Collecting samples of one's best performance in various content areas is called *portfolio assessment* (Sitlington & Clark, 2007, p. 137). To develop the portfolio, a transition educator and student collect materials from personal and medical information, educational assessments, employment training, work samples, and so forth (Demchak & Greenfield, 2003). A popular way to develop a portfolio is to record video to communicate one's accomplishments (Graph Paper Press, 2014). A video of the student's performance in work samples may be an effective way to show pace, accuracy, and quality of job skills to VR counselors or potential employers. To promote self-determination, the student should be involved as much as possible in developing and updating the portfolio. A portfolio can be configured in such a way as to fulfill federal requirements for the summary of performance document (discussed later in this chapter).

EXERCISE 5.3

If you could develop your own transition assessment, what would you assess? What areas would be included? How would you address strengths, preferences, and interests? How would you address skill limitations? Select the context for your assessment (e.g., employment, PSE, independent living) and the level, age, and characteristics of your student. Then design your own assessment. (Obviously, if you were actually developing an assessment, before administering your assessment you would evaluate its reliability and validity for specific purposes.)

HOW DOES ONE SELECT ASSESSMENTS FOR A STUDENT?

With the variety of assessment instruments and procedures available, and with such diversity among youth in transition, the process of selecting assessments can be daunting. We offer the following decision rules to guide selection of assessments. Although these rules attempt to isolate the relevant variables in decision making, they still leave considerable latitude regarding specific assessments to choose.

1. Pay particular attention to assessments designed to assess strengths, preferences, and interests (see the section "SPIN Assessments" earlier in this chapter) because their approach is positive, goal-directed, and consistent with self-determination. The results they yield are designed to guide personal decision making by allowing the youth and the transition team to weigh options.

2. Select assessments whose results can be easily interpreted to the youth and family. Because the youth should self-determine his or her transition, assessment results should be straightforward, understandable, and meaningful. Because the goal of transition assessment is to help the youth make informed decisions about his or her direction in adulthood (Test et al., 2006), test results should facilitate, not confuse, decision making.

3. According to the NSTTAC (2014), the assessor should select instruments that are appropriate for students. Key considerations include the nature of each student's disability (e.g., reading level and general intelligence), his or her postschool ambitions (e.g., college vs. other training options or immediate employment), and community opportunities (e.g., local training options, employers and ASPs). For more information, see the website at the end of this chapter.

4. If an assessment does not yield data that seem to target the needs of the youth, select another. Transition assessment should be ongoing and focused on the youth's unique needs.

5. Select assessments with demonstrated reliability and validity. Note that the validity of an assessment instrument is based on a specific purpose (e.g., characteristics of a student, prediction of performance in a specific environment). Empirical research on reliability and validity should be considered when selecting an assessment instrument.

WHAT IS THE SUMMARY OF PERFORMANCE?

The reauthorization of IDEA (2004) required a document called the *Summary of Performance* (SOP) to be developed before students exit from special education. As a mechanism for sharing relevant information with ASPs, the purpose of the SOP was to provide "a summary of the child's academic and functional performance which shall include recommendations on how to assist the child in meeting post-secondary goals" (IDEA, 2004, Section 614 [c] 5ii). According to Richter and Mazzotti (2011), a well-developed SOP provides adult service agencies, PSE, students, families, and others with needed information related to postsecondary goals (Izzo & Kochhar-Bryant, 2006, as cited in Richter & Mazzotti, 2011).

The SOP is relevant here because it starts with a summary of transition assessment results, then, with embellishment from the youth and the transition team, can become an opportunity to describe the student's experience, background, interests, and personal goals. As noted by Martin, Van Dycke, D'Ottavio, and Erickson (2007), "Identification of post–high school interests, skills, and limits, mediated by needs and cultural beliefs, produces a vision of post–high school life that will help students answer the question 'Where do I want to go to school, live, and work after leaving school?' " (p. 13).

Since IDEA (2004), different SOP templates have been developed. First, the National Transition Documentation Summit (NTDS; Richter & Mazzotti, 2011) recommended that the SOP contain (1) youth background information, (2) postsecondary goals, (3) results of transition assessments, (4) recommendations to assist in meeting postsecondary goals, and (5) youth input. The NTDS encouraged state and local education agencies to adopt the SOP template as a way of standardizing information to inform ASPs. Second, the self-directed SOP (Martin et al., 2007) called for the youth to develop the SOP to include postsecondary goals and the youth's perceptions of his or her disability, academic performance, and assessment information. These researchers recommended that this template be couched in first-person language and developed by (or with assistance of) the youth. That is, they envisioned the SOP to involve maximum self-direction, thus making the student responsible for organizing the contents.

The SOP relates to our earlier discussion about portfolio assessment. We believe that youth and their transition teams can fulfill the SOP requirement and, at the same time, create an individualized and highly informative portfolio. Although research is needed in this area, we find that youth who develop their own SOP promote their skill and assert a vision for their future. A portfolio-based SOP may be one way for youth to learn self-advocacy because they are better informed of their accomplishments and more attuned to their future plans. Audiences that peruse such a document, whether they are VR counselors, employers, or ASPs, may be positively impressed by the forward-thinking, constructive attitude of the youth.

We now present two case scenarios involving youth, selection of transition assessments, and the results. The cases illustrate how assessment can help guide the transition process.

CASE EXAMPLES: YOUTH IN TRANSITION AND THEIR ASSESSMENTS

Trang

A son of Vietnamese immigrants, Trang is a 16-year-old youth diagnosed with a specific learning disability. Although English is his native language, Trang struggles with reading comprehension, spending all of his energy decoding words. Trang aspires to work in a construction trade and possesses well-developed math and computer skills. Yet, his low reading levels, limited expressive language, and shyness in social situations are concerns for his teacher, Ms. Petrovic. "He has great potential," says Ms. Petrovic, "but I know he will need intensive work in reading, communication, and social skills."

Ms. Petrovic searched through Trang's files to find a recent psychological evaluation. According to the *Woodcock–Johnson III Tests of Achievement* (Woodcock, McGrew, & Mather, 2001), Trang had low scores on subtests measuring Reading Fluency, Passage Comprehension, and Letter-Word Identification. Scores on Math Fluency and Calculation were very high, whereas scores on Applied Problems (math problems requiring reading) were low. Because test results were consistent with her impressions, Ms. Petrovic decided to perform a CBA of Trang's vocabulary and reading comprehension so that she could pinpoint where to focus her instruction. Next, she arranged for Trang and his parents to fill out the *Ansell–Casey Life Skills Assessment–III* (Nollan et al., 2002) because this assessment measures independent living skills and is culturally sensitive. Results showed that Trang and his parents held high expectations for his career. Trang rated himself high in skills of communication, daily living, home life, housing and money management, self-care, and social relationships; however, his parents rated him much lower.

"I need to meet with Trang and his parents to see if we can all get on the same page," Ms. Petrovic thought. "Maybe I can get them to work at home on daily living and self-care skills."

Finally, Ms. Petrovic had Trang fill out the *Arc Self-Determination Scale* (Wehmeyer & Kelchner, 1995) to assess his level of independence and self-determination. Results indicated that Trang scored himself high on Autonomy, Self-Regulation, and Psychological Empowerment, but low on Self-Realization. That is, he wanted to be independent, in charge, and self-sufficient, but he needed to become more realistic in understanding his skill set. "The good news," Ms. Petrovic stated, "is that Trang really believes in himself and his potential. I need to maintain his self-esteem while I focus on his low areas. Time to start planning his transition."

Regina

Scheduled to exit from special education services in less than a year, Regina and her teacher, Mr. Kealoha, are in the final stages of transition planning. Regina is an 18-year-old with significant disabilities. She uses an electric wheelchair for mobility and a speech-generating device for communicating.

Regina had been on Mr. Kealoha's caseload since she entered Blackstone High School in ninth grade. At that time, Mr. Kealoha reviewed the existing formal and informal transition assessments but found nothing that seemed to pinpoint Regina's needs. He quizzed Regina on career interests by having her respond "yes" or "no" to a series of questions, and determined that she was interested in working in personal beautification. Mr. Kealoha then showed Regina a series of photos from beauty magazines to see if he could spark her interest. She seemed most animated in her responses to photos from beauty salons. Mr. Kealoha shared findings from this informal assessment with Regina's parents and IEP team. The team encouraged the teacher to look into getting Regina involved in a beauty salon, if possible.

With the help of his paraeducator, Maria, Mr. Kealoha contacted a local school of cosmetology and set up an appointment. As he explained Regina's interest, the owner indicated she would be receptive in having Regina visit and become familiar with the school's operation. During Regina's visit, Mr. Kealoha conducted an informal ecological assessment by examining the height of various work areas (sinks, tables, etc.), position of electrical outlets, and so forth. Some of the students in the beauty school struck up conversations with Regina and were surprised she could readily respond with her communication device. Next, Mr. Kealoha met with the owner to arrange a month-long situational assessment during the last hour of her school day. The paraeducator provided transportation for Regina to the school of cosmetology, then helped her catch the city bus to go home. For the first week, Regina observed others to become familiar with operations. After a week, the paraeducator asked Regina if she would like to wash combs and brushes, which was a much-needed task for the cosmetology students. The paraeducator set up Regina's wheelchair next to the sink, then conducted a direct observation to assess Regina's performance. Some parts of the task required adjustments, but soon Regina was performing the cleaning work. The paraeducator conducted a task analysis of the comb/brush cleaning procedure and collected data on the degree of prompting needed to complete each task. For each step, she scored no prompt, verbal, gesture, touch/tap, or hand-guided prompt. Mr. Kealoha taught the paraeducator to provide the least prompts necessary to encourage independent performance by Regina. Soon, Regina was performing the cleaning task on her own. The owner offered Regina a paid job cleaning materials at the school of cosmetology, if only for a few hours per week. In a final IEP meeting, the team agreed that planning over several years had resulted in a step toward successful transition to community employment for Regina.

SUMMARY

In this chapter, we examined transition assessment, the purpose of which is to gather and analyze relevant information on a student's skills, needs, preferences, and interests so that the student and his or her team can plan, implement, and evaluate transition activities. The goals of transition assessment are to help students (1) make informed choices that will enhance their postschool lives, (2) take charge of the transition process, and (3) understand and acquire the skills needed for postschool environments (Sitlington et al., 1997). Seven characteristics of transition assessment were discussed. We reviewed formal, or norm-referenced, standardized assessments as well as informal assessments. Specific examples of both formal and informal assessments were provided. Other assessment procedures included CBA, direct observation, ecological assessment, situational assessment, task analysis, and portfolio assessment.

REVISITING KENLEY

Mr. White started the transition planning meeting by introducing Kenley, Mr. and Mrs. Schneider (Kenley's parents), Ashton (Kenley's brother), Teresa Schmidt (VR counselor), and Alisha Jones (transition class paraeducator). Mr. White explained that the purpose of the IEP meeting was to plan Kenley's transition. He had invited Ms. Schmidt, a VR counselor from the Garden City Office.

"Kenley, please tell the team what you want to do after you leave school."

Kenley looked around the table. "That's my brother, Ashton." He said, pointing across the table. "And that's my mom and dad."

"Yes, Kenley, we're pleased to have your family here. What do you want to do after you leave school?"

"I don't want to leave school. I like school," he said, looking at his teacher. "But someday I have to leave school, right? So when I leave school, I want to work at the store with my mom and dad."

"And why do you want to work there?"

"Money," Kenley smiled.

"Tell us what you are really good at? What could you do at the store?"

"Groceries. I can put groceries in bags. Carts. I can get carts."

As the conversation continued, Kenley reported that he wanted to learn to bag groceries, retrieve carts from the parking lot, and stock groceries at Southridge Grocery. His mother was the cashier and his father worked in the deli. Ashton had talked to his parents about how Kenley could learn to perform tasks at the store through on-site, community-based instruction, with Mr. White's and Alisha's help. Conceivably, the community-based instruction experience might eventually lead to a job at the store. Kenley still had 2 years remaining at the high school, and his community training would have to involve rotating through other job sites as well as the grocery store.

"Teresa, from the VR perspective, is this a workable plan?" Mr. White asked.

"Yes, I think so. Mr. and Mrs. Schneider, I will need to meet with you and then I'll need to meet with Kenley, but I think we can get a VR case started. The only hesitation I have is Kenley's goal for employment. We may need to think a little more broadly than just focusing on a job at the store. We'll want to consider as many options as possible."

"But Ms. Schmidt," Ashton started, "there are very few options in Southridge. This is a small community and we don't have a lot of employment possibilities. There's the store, the mill, and the farm implement company."

"I understand." Ms. Schmidt responded. "But maybe we can think creatively. There are also jobs here at the school. I will need to look at Kenley's preference assessment, but maybe he has an interest in school cafeteria work, the library, or school office assistance. Another creative option might be to look at jobs Kenley could do online. We have some clients who go into business for themselves selling products over the Internet."

"But we have a family support system at Southridge Grocery," Ashton replied.

"I know," Teresa started. "And we can be creative about jobs at the grocery store. Some rural communities need people who can deliver groceries because their older citizens can't get out to go to the store anymore. Maybe Kenley could deliver groceries on his bike."

"I like my bike," Kenley said.

"I think the key thing, Kenley," Teresa began, "is to take the next 2 years and provide you with lots of experience learning about your community. You can learn about different kinds of jobs. Mr. White, Alisha, Ashton, and your folks can all help you learn in the community."

EXERCISE 5.4

- Review a transition assessment instrument. What are the administration procedures? What does the examiner do? What does the youth do? What data are generated? How are the data used? How do the data inform the support team?

- Look back to Chapter 1 at the case examples involving Josefina and Kenley: How would you select a transition assessment for each of them? What data do you need to assist with transition planning for each case?

- Consider your own transition from high school to college. Which of your skills needed to be assessed in order to identify teaching, accommodation, or support? What ecological or situational assessments would have been useful to determine the extent to which your skills met the demands of college environments? How might you have used the assessment data?

- What additional assessments would you recommend for Trang or Regina? What aspects related to SPIN or environments may still need to be assessed for either of them?

WEBSITES WITH ADDITIONAL INFORMATION

Career Occupational Preference System

www.edits.net

Transition Coalition

http://transitioncoalition.org/transition/assessment_review/all.php

NSTTAC

http://nsttac.org/content/age-appropriate-transition-assessment-toolkit-3rd-edition

http://nsttac.org/content/age-appropriate-transition-assessment-toolkit-3rd-edition#section1C

The Rhode Island Regional Transition Center Coordinators

www.ritap.org/ritap/content/mytransition/RI%20Transition%20Matrix%202012.pdf

CHAPTER 6

Transition Planning

This chapter addresses . . .

- The definition of transition planning.
- Participants in the planning process.
- Planning approaches.
- Five steps required in the development of an individualized transition plan.
- Measurable postsecondary goals, present levels of performance, and annual goals.
- Indicator 13 and the evaluation of transition plans.
- The planning process as it leads to employment, PSE, and independent living.
- Transition planning for students (1) at risk of dropping out of school, (2) with mental health care needs, (3) with significant health care needs, and (4) with profound multiple disabilities.

WHAT IS TRANSITION PLANNING?

Abraham Lincoln once said, "Give me 6 hours to chop down a tree and I will spend the first four sharpening the axe" (*www.brainyquote.com/quotes/quotes/a/abraham-lin109275.html*). Careful planning and preparation are of paramount importance in transition activities. The transition process requires that youth, parents, educators, and adult service professionals come together to create a match between youths' abilities, needs, preferences, and the demands of their adult environment (Hardman & Dawson, 2010).

Test and colleagues (2006) stated that planning should involve both depth and breadth. A cursory list of activities and services does not constitute an adequate transition plan. In addition to commonly identified areas of transition planning such as employment and PSE, planning for a particular youth may require consideration of numerous dimensions, such as health and medical needs, mental health services, transportation, mobility, occupational and physical therapy, social skills, sex education, speech and language therapy, socialization opportunities, recreation, leisure, residential living (e.g., apartment, dormitory, group home), and benefits and estate planning. Clearly, transition planning is complex and requires an individualized approach.

HOW DOES PLANNING "START WITH THE END IN MIND"?

In Chapter 2, we established that planning should start early. But now we want to reinforce a point made by Flexer and colleagues (2013): When planning transition for youth with disabilities, start with the end in mind. That is, from the outset, transition planning should conceptualize a successful outcome for a youth. Although most of us change our goals many times during adolescence, we have some idea of what we want to achieve. Broad questions can be considered by students and their parents as early as sixth grade, such as:

"Do I want to go to college? If so, what do I want to study?"
"Do I want to work so that I can make money? If so, what kind of job would I like to do?"
"Most people have several jobs before they get the job they really like. What would be my ideal career job? What jobs would I accept before I get my ideal job?"
"Where would I like to live? With whom do I want to live [self, family, friends, relatives]?"

Answers to these questions create a pathway to adulthood. Specific questions should be tailored to the needs of the youth, as well as the form of expressive communication used by the youth (e.g., verbal English, sign language, Picture Exchange Communication System).

WHAT ARE THE PLANNING APPROACHES?

We now describe two approaches: person-centered planning and courses of study. Although there are numerous transition planning approaches, we find that these two represent the options relatively well.

Person-Centered Planning

According to O'Brien (2002), person-centered planning was designed to be a systematic way to generate an actionable understanding of a person as a contributing community citizen. The process became one way to envision a person's goals and how to achieve them (Crockett & Hardman, 2010). The goal was to create an environment that "encourages the student to dream, supports the student, creates possibilities, solves problems, and enhances the student's overall present and future quality of life" (Test et al., 2006, p. 117). The planning process occurred *with* the individual, not *about* the individual (Butterworth, Steere, & Whitney-Thomas, 1997).

The person-centered approach is sometimes associated with individuals who have more significant disabilities. However, the processes are germane to individuals of all levels and ages. In addition to adults with significant disabilities, person-centered planning has been used in school systems for transition purposes (Forest & Pearpoint, 1992). There are numerous iterations of the original person-centered planning concept, including *personal futures planning* (Mount & Zwernick, 1988), *McGill Action Plan System* (MAPS; Forest & Pearpoint, 1992), and *outcomes-based planning* (Steere, Wood, Pancsofar, & Butterworth, 1990). As a planning strategy, person-centered planning is less formal than the IEP and clearly focuses on strengths, supports, and individual needs. Steere and colleagues (2007) described key features of person-centered planning:

1. A support team consists of the focal person, family, friends, and concerned community members. For youth in transition, this team should include educators, related-services staff, and representatives from adult services as well.
2. The team gets together in an environment that is comfortable and familiar to the youth with disabilities, such as his or her home or a favorite place in the community. The setting should be informal and comfortable for all participants.
3. The focal person and team develop a comprehensive personal profile emphasizing strengths, abilities, capacities, and gifts.
4. The team uses graphics to illustrate ideas (using easels, butcher block paper, PowerPoint projection, etc.).
5. The focal person is the "central member in the planning process" (p. 48). The team should ensure that the focal person can actively participate in the planning process.
6. A facilitator guides the process. This person should be "trusted by the members of the circle of support" (p. 48). Although the facilitator could be a teacher, the team may want to have someone guide the process who has less official authority. The teacher, youth, parent, and other transition team members can later take the content and complete the IEP.
7. Once the profile is developed, the youth and team develop a vision for the future. The facilitator and youth may want to get together beforehand so that a personal vision of the future is created and then shared during the planning meeting.
8. The team then identifies challenges and barriers to reaching the vision for the future, and actions the team can take to overcome impediments. These actions

are prioritized and individual members take responsibility for implementing them.

9. The team reconvenes as necessary to update progress.

Steere and colleagues (2007) noted that understanding the person-centered approach required one to abandon "preconceived ideas of programs and systems and, instead, [attempt] to look at the person's gifts, talents, and abilities rather than limitations" (p. 87). The approach values personal strengths and the efforts of family and advocates. Key ingredients are:

- Management and supervision to ensure that procedures are implemented with fidelity.
- Training team members in person-centered values.
- Communication and coordination of services across all support team members.
- Well-defined roles and responsibilities (Everson & Reid, 1999; Reid & Green, 2002).

Compared to standard client service provision, researchers found person-centered planning effective (e.g., Taylor & Averitt Taylor, 2013).

Relationship between Person-Centered Planning and the IEP

Person-centered planning is consistent with IDEA (2004) language focusing on a student's strengths, preferences, and interests as well as emphasis on active student involvement. IDEA language may be a bit more forceful in asserting "a results-oriented process," although all forms of person-centered planning acknowledge goal-directedness. To establish a person-centered transition plan, the LEA representative should first meet with the special education teacher, parent, and youth. School personnel usually welcome having a youth support team that can take responsibility for implementing parts of the action plan in home and community settings. The key to successful planning is making sure everyone is on the same page, working on the same goals, and meeting periodically to share progress or make corrections. Second, the LEA, teacher, youth, and parents decide which elements of the person-centered plan should be incorporated into the youth's IEP.

Courses of Study

Whereas person-centered planning is a goal-directed approach for envisioning the future for youth with disabilities, a course of study is the common planning mechanism for typical students and those who have IEPs. A *course of study* is a multiyear description of courses needed for high school graduation (Flexer et al., 2013). Although an IEP identifies goals and objectives, the course of study represents the pathway to a diploma. School counselors can assist the IEP team in determining academic courses and electives that best match a youth's strengths, preferences, and interests, as well as showing students how to apply for college or job training programs (Kochhar-Bryant et al., 2009).

*Balancing Courses of Study with Functional Skills
in Transition Planning*

One of the challenges in transition planning is deciding the most appropriate combination of a rigorous academic program leading to a diploma and the functional skills necessary for living as an adult in community environments. For many, the answer requires a careful eye on the youth's postschool goals and life aspirations. The first step is a comprehensive transition assessment involving a youth's academic skills and career preferences (see Chapter 5). The next steps involve either person-centered planning or a school-based transition meeting to consider the youth's vision of the future and the parents'/family's suggestions, at which point the team can create the pathway (Wehmeyer, 2002). The team should consider that academic skills play a critical role throughout adulthood, and that functional skills are vitally important because they allow the youth to access new environments.

WHAT ARE THE STEPS OF THE TRANSITION PLANNING PROCESS?

We describe specific steps transition educators follow in writing the individualized transition plan (ITP), which becomes a part of a youth's IEP. These steps are critical to (1) meet the requirements of IDEA (2004), (2) develop the ITP tailored to meet the needs of individual youth, and (3) increase the likelihood of successful postschool outcomes. As noted in Chapter 3, the ITP must be developed in the first IEP following a youth's 16th birthday and updated at least once per year. Some states require ITPs prior to age 16. Mazzotti and colleagues (2009) described five steps in the process, as shown in Figure 6.1.

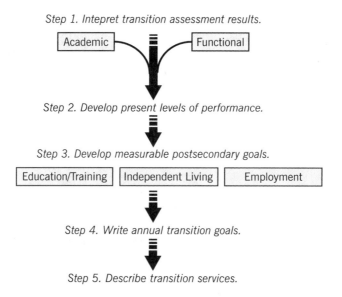

FIGURE 6.1. Steps of the transition planning process.

Step 1: Interpret Transition Assessment Results

Transition assessment results should inform planning efforts with respect to employment, PSE, and independent living (see Chapter 5). The data generated from assessment should help answer some of the initial questions about what the youth prefers and needs after special education services cease. The transition educator or student should list the assessments and data (e.g., standard scores, percentiles, grade or age-equivalence scores, preferences for adulthood, interest areas). By inspecting data, team members can begin to form judgments about these planning questions:

- To what extent do academic and skill assessment results support the youth's preferences for adulthood? That is, how close or far is the youth's present academic achievement in relation to levels that will be required in his or her preferred employment, PSE, and/or independent living?
- Based on assessments, what strengths does the youth possess to support his or her preferences?
- What family or community supports can facilitate the youth's preferences for adulthood?
- What barriers or limitations might impede the youth's preferences for adulthood?
- How fixated are the youth's preferences for adulthood? Is the youth focused on a certain path, strong but flexible, open to different options, undecided, or unaware of options?

Based on answers to the questions above, should additional assessment be conducted? Also, how often should transition assessment be updated?

Step 2: Develop the Present Level of Performance Statement

The *present level of performance* is a statement that objectively summarizes assessment results and describes the extent to which present levels relate to standards of performance. Using data from assessments, the transition educator, student, or other team member should compose this statement by providing an objective, neutral, and unbiased description of facts. For example:

"Based on results from the achievement tests, Laquita's vocabulary and reading comprehension are similar to a student at mid–fourth grade. Given that she is in eighth grade, these results are about three to four grade levels below current placement. Her reading percentile score was 11, which means that her performance equaled or exceeded 11% of all students her age who took the same test. She wants to be a pharmaceutical technician, which requires relatively high reading levels with specialized vocabulary . . . [present-level statement continues]."

The transition educator should not hesitate to describe scores that are substantially lower than expected levels. But on the other hand, the educator should be careful not to judge low performance, critique disparities, or deny a youth's aspirations. The youth and the entire transition support team should evaluate all data. We make the following recommendations for present-level statements:

1. Identify the assessment(s) used and include data in the written statement. Data accomplish two important "upshots." First, data show that the transition educator is describing performance from current assessments and not personal opinion, views of others, or hearsay. Second, data communicate a measured and objective evaluation of a youth's performance.

2. Provide statements of test results or observations measuring (a) skills the student has demonstrated (e.g., "Skylor can . . ."), (b) the skill deficit (e.g., "Skylor has not yet learned . . .), and (c) the area of need (e.g., "Skylor needs to . . ."). The statement should cover all relevant assessments and all likely areas to be addressed in a student's goals.

3. Make clear the relationship between assessment results and preferred employment, PSE, and independent living. Some statements identify test results and how they impact current performance in the classroom, but fail to relate results to long-term outcomes.

4. Avoid a specific target for improvement; this comes later in the form of transition goals, which should involve input from the student and the transition team.

The purpose of a present-level statement is to objectively summarize results in order to allow the student and team to make relevant judgments and set goals. The statement allows the transition planning team to create measurable goals and objectives that are "logically linked to the student's current abilities and postschool goals" (Polychronis & McDonnell, 2010, p. 93). An example of a present-level statement appears follows:

"Samantha is a 17-year-old junior who completed four job sample rotations (bussing tables, copy center help, preschool assistant, hospital aide) over a 16-week period. Observations indicate she is engaged in the required job tasks 80–90% of the time. Productivity in most job tasks is near the production level required by employees, according to supervisors at each job site. Teachers report that Samantha responds well to children/adults and displays good social skills. Teachers describe her as polite and attentive in response to correction. In math, writing, and language classes, she turned in 60% of her assignments and earned a 2.5 GPA overall (A = 4.0). Samantha participated in the XYZ Career Exploration Assessment and reported she would like to be a licensed professional nurse or child development professional. In order to gain entry into courses leading to one of these chosen fields, Samantha needs to increase her assignment completion rate and raise her GPA."

EXERCISE 6.1

Read the following hypothetical statements. Let's say they are excerpts from present-level performance statements for various students. Which statements meet the recommendations described above? If the statement needs improvement, identify what needs to be changed and edit it to meet the requirements.

Excerpts from present level of performance statements	Improved version
Andre told me he wanted to be a surgeon. Dream on.	
The preference assessment results indicate that Selicia is interested in being a physical therapist, but this is not possible because she lacks both fine- and gross-motor skill coordination required in the profession.	
Given results from the General Achievement Test, Orlando's math performance is similar to a student at mid–seventh grade. Given that he is finishing ninth grade, according to these results, his performance is about two grade levels below expected placement.	
Direct observations of Sophia's behavior indicate off-task behavior 60–70% of the time, which is excessive for a junior in high school. This behavior prevents her from finishing assignments in most classes.	

Step 3: Develop Measurable Postsecondary Goals

Measurable postsecondary goals are statements of the student's aspirations looking ahead at least 1 year after the end of special education services. According to IDEA (2004), "The IEP must include appropriate measurable post-secondary goals based on age-appropriate transition assessments related to training, education, employment and, where appropriate, independent living skills. . . ." (34 C.F.R. § 300.320[b]). The measurable postsecondary goal must be linked with transition assessment results and the present level of performance statement (Test et al., 2006).

Measurable postsecondary goals are probably the most visible and important part of an ITP, because they represent the vision for the youth's future. The student and transition team should spend time and effort to carefully plan measurable postsecondary goals. Some transition educators use first-person language in goals (i.e., "I will . . ." as opposed to "[the youth's first name] will . . .") in order to personalize the statements and emphasize that goals are developed *by the student*. Identifying measurable postsecondary goals allow us to plan a student's transition with the end in mind, then work backward toward shorter-term and more specific benchmarks, called *annual goals*.

Postsecondary goals should be:

1. *Measurable.* That is, one must be able to determine whether the goal has been successfully met or not. Typically, postsecondary goals are simply scored "+" (yes, successfully met) or "–" (no, not successfully met).

2. *Time-limited.* That is, the period within which the goal must be reached should be specified. Measurable postsecondary goals typically set the time limit at 1 year following the end of special education services.

3. *Specific and well defined.* The goal should identify specifically what the student and the transition team envision, not name a generic outcome. For example, "Ben will get a job" is not appropriate because the goal is generic. "Ben will apply for employment as a retail salesperson at a department store" is more appropriate.

4. *Identified typically for both employment and PSE.* Goals for independent living are optional, but recommended. A transition plan usually has two or more measurable postsecondary goals. Each goal statement should target only one area. So, "Hao will apply to take classes from a community college and get a job on the college campus" is inappropriate because it targets two goals. Instead, separate the goal into two statements.

5. *Stated so the goal is reached after a student exits special education services.* "Sean will graduate from high school" is inappropriate, for example, because the goal is reached at the point of completing school. However, "After graduating from high school, Sean will apply to the community college" is appropriate.

6. *Based on age-appropriate transition assessments.* The transition educator must make it clear that measurable postsecondary goals are based on assessment results from an age-appropriate assessment and the results are reported in the present level of performance statement.

7. *Aligned with (and the focus of) the course of study.* The student's course of study should logically lead to the measurable postsecondary goals.

Components of Measurable Postsecondary Goals

Measurable postsecondary goals consist of three components: (1) a time frame, (2) the behavior to be performed, and (3) a measurable criterion of success (i.e., the required level of performance). The behavior to be performed should be specific and stated in future tense. The required level of performance should be specified. Measurable postsecondary goals should be designed using the format shown in Figure 6.2 (*www.nsttac. org*).

EXERCISE 6.2

Read the following hypothetical list of measurable postsecondary goals. Which goals are consistent with the recommendations described in the preceding material? If the goal is not consistent with recommendations, identify what needs to be changed and edit it accordingly.

Measurable postsecondary goals	Improved version
One year after high school, Asad will get a job in the community.	
One year after high school, Asad will give strong consideration to his future and think seriously about the importance of a career.	
One year after high school, Asad will accurately and independently complete an application for his preferred job.	
One year after graduating from high school, Asad will independently complete an interview with the manager/human resources department for his preferred job.	

Time frame **III▶** The student or "I" **III▶** will **III▶**

describe the behavior to be performed **III▶** state the measurable criteria

Example

One year after finishing high school (**the time frame**), Alejandro will accurately and independently complete all work tasks as required by his immediate supervisor in his current job as office assistant (**the behavior to be performed**), as determined by a positive supervisor report (**measurable criterion**).

Postsecondary Measurable Goals

Employment-related

One year after graduating from high school, Rosa will apply for employment in her preferred field of graphics arts, as measured by a complete and submitted application.

Postsecondary education-related

One year after graduating from high school, Brynly will apply to enter occupational therapist training, as measured by a submitted application to a community college.

Independent living-related

One year after Sabrina completes the post-high school program, she will move into an apartment with a roommate, as determined by a paid deposit and street address.

FIGURE 6.2. Format and example of a measurable postsecondary goal (*www.nsttac.org*).

Step 4: Write Annual IEP Goals

Annual goals are designed to assist the student in making progress toward measurable postsecondary goals. Goals should represent a coordinated set of activities focused on improving academic achievement or functional performance. Like measurable postsecondary goals, annual goals must relate to assessment results in the present level of performance statement. They may be written in first-person language.

One or more annual goals should be composed to address each measurable postsecondary goal. For example, the measurable postsecondary goal "One year after finishing high school, Stewart will accurately and independently complete all work tasks as required by his immediate supervisor in his current job as office assistant, as measured by a positive supervisor report" should be divided into a sequence of three annual goals:

- *Goal 1*: Given a school-based situational assessment in the main office of the high school and instruction from the clerical assistant, Stewart will independently complete all work tasks as required by his immediate supervisor in his current job as office assistant, as measured by a positive supervisor report.
- *Goal 2*: Given a situational assessment as an office assistant trainee in a community business, Stewart will independently complete all work tasks as required by his immediate supervisor in his current job as office assistant, as measured by a positive supervisor report.
- *Goal 3*: Given a job application form, Stewart will apply for an office assistant position, as measured by an accurately completed application form.

Goals 1, 2, and 3 should logically lead to successfully addressing the measurable postsecondary goal.

Components of Annual Goals

Annual goals usually contain three components: (1) a condition statement, (2) a behavior to be performed, and (3) a measurable criterion of success. These components are similar to those of measurable postsecondary goals, except that the condition statement of an annual goal describes the specific circumstances under which the goal is met. Conditions can encompass teaching strategies, community or school locations, job tasks, college preparation courses, or other events that set the context for the goal. Annual goals should also specify the desired behavior and the criterion for measuring the behavior. See the format for annual goals and an example in Figure 6.3.

Ambiguous language should be avoided because it (1) raises questions about which specific behavior is performed and how it is measured; (2) invites misinterpretation of goals by parents, transition team members, and others reviewing transition plans; and (3) prevents determination, at a later time, of whether the goal was successfully met (see Table 6.1).

The criterion statement should be measurable and require a high standard of performance. Many times, the transition educator will identify both a level of performance

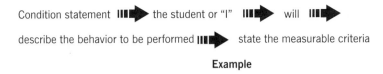

Condition statement ▮▮▶ the student or "I" ▮▮▶ will ▮▮▶

describe the behavior to be performed ▮▮▶ state the measurable criteria

Example

Given math worksheets with 50 problems involving pre-algebra questions to "solve for *x*" and direct instruction teaching strategies, Trevor will complete all problems with at least 90% accuracy for three consecutive math sessions.

FIGURE 6.3. Format and example of an annual goal (*www.nsttac.org*).

and a time criterion. For example, "at least 90% accuracy" is a level of performance criterion and "for three consecutive sessions" is a time criterion. Examples of annual goals are shown in the following list:

- Given a list of signs used on the public bus route, Savanna will verbally name the correct bus route for at least 90% of flash cards for three consecutive sessions.
- Given my list of survival vocabulary terms in employment settings, I will verbally name the correct term for at least 40 of 50 words for five consecutive sessions.
- Given a task analysis for scanning different kinds of documents and a scanning machine or photocopier, Jamaal will independently perform all steps (100%) of the task analysis across five different kinds of documents, each for three consecutive sessions.

TABLE 6.1. Ambiguous versus Observable, Measurable Language in Annual Goals

Ambiguous terms	Observable, measurable terms (examples may vary depending on condition statement and context)
To identify	To point to (or verbally name)
To match	To place matching objects side by side
To arrange	To place objects in sequence
To choose	To orally name a choice between two alternatives
To use	To make movements with the tool to solve the problem
To measure	To place a yardstick on the fabric and orally name the correct length
To demonstrate	To engage in a sequence of physical and verbal actions related to forwarding a telephone call

Dividing Annual Goals into Short-Term Objectives

Transition educators or team members sometimes break annual goals into short-term objectives that are even more specific. Objectives should lead to successful completion of the annual goal. For example, the annual goal "Given a job application form, Eric will apply for an office assistant position as measured by an accurately completed application form" could be divided into a series of short-term objectives:

1. Given a job application form, Eric will complete the section requiring personal information as measured by accurate completion of all requirements.
2. Given a job application form, Eric will complete the section requiring work history as measured by accurate completion of all requirements.
3. Given a job application form, Eric will complete the section requiring description of educational background as measured by accurate completion of all requirements.

EXERCISE 6.3

Read the following hypothetical list of annual goals. Which goals are consistent with the examples above? If the goal needs improvement, identify changes and edit it to meet the requirements.

Annual goals	Improved version
Given a checking account, Jed will accurately balance the account with at least 90% accuracy across 50 checking account entries.	
Ned will work at a restaurant to earn money so he can go to college.	
Fred will successfully pass his algebra class.	
When taken to the rail stop closest to the high school by a teacher or paraeducator, Ted will independently and accurately take the train to destinations for five consecutive trips.	

Step 5: Describe Transition Services

The ITP must describe transition services to be implemented to improve the academic, functional, and independent living skills that will enable the student to meet annual and measurable postsecondary goals. Transition services usually relate to strengths or needs identified in the present level of performance statement, and are designed to help the student make progress toward annual goals. Services depend on individual circumstances and vary widely. Examples include mnemonic strategies to improve study skills, teaching procedures to increase social skills, physical therapy to bolster stamina, speech therapy to improve communication, community-based training to enhance employability skills, menu planning to improve independent living potential, and so forth. In Table 6.2, we categorize transition services into six areas.

If assessment results reveal that gaps exist between a student's current skill levels and the skills needed for employment, PSE, or independent living, transition services must address these gaps. Close alignment must exist between assessment data, summary of assessment results in the present level of performance, and services. (See *www.nsttac.org* for descriptions of evidence-based transition services.) Beyond the categories of transition services described in the preceding material, most IEP forms allow the transition educator to check or describe optional or required services, which may include the following:

Involvement of Other Service Representatives

Examples of other services include VR, centers for independent living, workforce services, or disability service offices at colleges or universities. For example, if a student needs assistance obtaining employment, VR services may be described. If a student needs assistance with community transportation or independent living, the independent living center services may be described.

Transfer of Rights Discussed 1 Year Prior to Age 18

At least 1 year prior to the student's 18th birthday, IDEA (2004) requires parents/guardians and the student to be informed of rights under IDEA transferring to the student at age 18. Once students reach 18 years of age, they assume legal rights for certain decisions

TABLE 6.2. Types and Examples of Transition Services

Type of Service	Example
Academic instructional services	Core curriculum, concurrent enrollment in a college course, peer tutor assistance to learn a skill, online instruction, etc.
Career-related services	Career awareness and exploration, career counseling, etc.
Community-based employment or other instructional services	Employment-related training, job coaching, apprenticeship, internship, job site training, community-based job samples, situational assessment, public transportation training, etc.
Independent living instructional services	Services leading to independent performance of daily living activities (self-care and domestic) such as hygiene, laundry, clothing care, diet and nutrition, meal preparation, budgeting, paying bills, task analysis of a functional skill, etc.
Functional vocational services.	Career technical service courses, task analysis of a functional skill, etc.

unless guardianship has been awarded by a court. Transition educators must discuss transfer of rights with parents/guardians before the student's 17th birthday. Discussion of transfer of rights must be noted in the ITP.

Invitation of the Youth to the IEP Meeting

IDEA (2004) requires that a student be invited to the IEP meeting if the purpose is to consider postsecondary goals and transition services. The student must sign the IEP to document attendance. If the student does not attend the meeting, the transition teacher must describe how the student was involved in developing the ITP. If a student is unable to sign the IEP due to functional limitations of his or her disability, the teacher can make a note on the IEP form describing the circumstances.

Graduation, Certificate of Completion, or Alternative Forms of Exit

The ITP should identify how the student will exit special education services. The transition educator must describe this form of exit to the student, parents, and transition team, including its implications and consequences. For example, if a student will leave special education services with a certificate of completion (not a graduation diploma), the student and parents should be fully informed what this means. The type of exit must be stated on the ITP. Test and colleagues (2006) noted that approximately 80% of states provide an alternative exit document (not a diploma) upon completion of high school, usually a certificate or alternative diploma that verifies attendance. Youth, their parents, and families need to be clear about what exit document is being received and what implications it carries for future plans. Test and colleagues recommended that, during the planning process, "students and their families must receive honest and clear advisement regarding curriculum options and exit documents so that they can make informed decisions" (p. 50).

There are numerous components to an ITP. An example of a complete ITP for a hypothetical student appears at the end of this chapter.

HOW DOES INDICATOR 13 EVALUATE A TRANSITION PLAN?

As we described in Chapter 3, there are 21 Part B Indicators in IDEA (2004). One of them, Indicator 13, evaluates the ITP. To assist states in collecting data to meet Indicator 13, NSTTAC (*www.nsttac.org*) developed the following checklist:

1. Is there an appropriate measurable postsecondary goal or goals that covers education or training, employment, and, as needed, independent living?
2. Is (are) the postsecondary goal(s) updated annually?
3. Is there evidence that the measurable postsecondary goal(s) were based on age-appropriate transition assessment?

4. Are there transition services in the IEP that will reasonably enable the student to meet his or her postsecondary goal(s)?

5. Do the transition services include courses of study that will reasonably enable the student to meet his or her postsecondary goal(s)?

6. Is (are) there annual IEP goal(s) related to the student's transition services needs?

7. Is there evidence that the student was invited to the IEP Team meeting where transition services were discussed?

8. If appropriate, is there evidence that a representative of any participating agency was invited to the IEP Team meeting with the prior consent of the parent or student who has reached the age of majority?

As you can see, when these questions are answered affirmatively, they indicate that the ITP has been developed adequately. Transition educators can use the Indicator 13 checklist to score their performance in developing transition plans. NSTTAC developed sample transition plans to illustrate how they are evaluated using the Indicator 13 checklist. See *www. nsttac.org.*

IN WHAT AREAS SHOULD THE TEAM PLAN TRANSITION SERVICES?

In this chapter, we have addressed planning participants, approaches, and steps in developing the ITP. But *in what areas* should the student and transition team plan focus? We recommend planning transition in areas of employment, PSE, and (if applicable) independent living. The following sections provide brief overviews of transition planning in these areas.

Planning Transition to Employment

Transition research supports providing services in community-based job samples and paid employment because they often lead to successful postschool outcomes (Benz, Lindstrom, & Yovanoff, 2000). The closer the transition team can come to placing a youth in paid community employment during high school, the more likely the youth will remain employed after high school. For youth with moderate to significant disabilities, McDonnell (2010) suggested that transition teams focus on planning (1) in-school employment training (e.g., office, library), and (2) community-based job sampling (i.e., students placed in actual work experiences). Providing transition services in the community is challenging, given that participation in credit-bearing courses and high standards in educational achievement are likewise crucially important, thus producing "congestion" in scheduling a course of study. Yet, many researchers (e.g., Benz et al., 2000; Test, Richter, & Walker, 2012) stressed the importance of providing instructional services in the community in order to enhance postschool employment outcomes. See Chapter 8 for more information.

Planning Transition to PSE

Planning for transition should start early, particularly if the student is interested in PSE such as vocational, technical, 2-year, or 4-year college admittance. Steere and colleagues (2007) suggested starting PSE planning by ninth grade, if not sooner. They stated:

> The IEP/Transition Planning Team must be aware of the courses colleges look for when considering applicants. For example, most four-year colleges look for success in course sequences of English, mathematics, the sciences, social studies, and foreign languages. . . . Starting in the freshman year of high school, an academic schedule should be developed for all the years of high school. (p. 193)

By ninth grade, the student and family should (1) design a class schedule for all 4 years and (2) begin exploring career options (Kochhar-Bryant et al., 2009). Each subsequent year, planning should continue and culminate with the high school senior's skills in time management, self-advocacy, understanding the time and place to disclose disability, independent living, and preparation for college. See Chapter 9 for details.

For students requiring extra supports, such as those with significant intellectual disabilities or low-functioning autism, college options may seem remote and unlikely. Yet, as we describe in Chapter 9, increasing numbers of students who require significant supports are participating in inclusive college programs by taking credit-bearing or audited courses (Grigal & Hart, 2010; Kochhar-Bryant et al., 2009; McDonald, MacPherson-Court, Frank, Uditsky, & Symons, 1997). But in rare cases where college is not considered possible, community education courses or vocational training may be options (Morgan, Kupferman, & Sheen, 2012). Stakeholders involved in transition planning should not rule out PSE and instead explore the wide spectrum of options available.

Planning Transition to Independent Living

Planning transition to independent living depends on the characteristics, needs, and preferences of the individual. Pierangelo and Giuliani (2004, pp. 65–66) suggested a wide-ranging continuum of living options to consider in transition planning:

- Independent living, such as an apartment.
- Semi-independent living with separated units or apartments.
- Foster homes with families providing some care and support.
- Group homes.
- Boarding or supervised facilities with extensive support.
- Intermediate care facilities.
- If comprehensive medical care is necessary, nursing homes.

The continuum of living options can encompass the needs of a wide variety of students of varying functioning levels and characteristics. See Chapter 10 for more information.

WHAT IS TRANSITION PLANNING FOR STUDENTS AT RISK OF SCHOOL DROPOUT, WITH MENTAL HEALTH NEEDS, WITH SIGNIFICANT HEALTH NEEDS, OR WITH PROFOUND DISABILITIES?

As we mentioned in the Prologue, the focus of this text is mainly on low-incidence developmental disabilities (e.g., intellectual disability; autism) and high-incidence disabilities (e.g., specific learning disabilities, emotional disturbance). Many times, these same students exhibit additional characteristics that magnify their challenges in transition planning and service delivery. Or, other children who do not have low- or high-incidence disabilities but exhibit one or more of these characteristics encounter challenges in their own transition. We briefly address transition planning for individuals with these characteristics. For students in transition with low-functioning autism, we refer the reader to another source (Hendricks & Wehman, 2009) where extensive information is provided. Also, see the list of websites at the end of the chapter for transition planning for students with other characteristics.

Transition Planning for Youth at Risk of School Dropout

According to the U.S. Department of Education, Office of Special Education Programs (2010), 28.3% of students with disabilities drop out of high school. Rates vary widely across types of disabilities. For example, dropout rates were nearly twice as high for students with emotional disturbance/behavior disorders (48.2%) as for students with any other type of disability. However, about one-fourth of students with other types of disability drop out of school. Factors associated with dropping out include suspension/expulsion, grade retention, and low grades. Zablocki and Krezmien (2012) examined data from NLTS-2 to analyze variables affecting dropouts and found higher than average dropout rates among (1) students with emotional disturbance, (2) African American and Native American students, (3) females, and (4) students from households with lower than average income.

Considerable research exists on dropout indicators and prevention (e.g., Dockery, 2012). Pyle and Wexler (2012) examined dropout prevention for students with disabilities by reviewing recent research on dropout prevention and implications for practice. These authors made several recommendations for educators involved in transition planning for potential dropouts:

Academic Support

1. Actively engage students in instructional tasks by matching curriculum to their level, culture, and interest. Provide effective instruction that is individualized and explicit, with multiple opportunities for success in order to encourage students' potential.
2. Offer small-group or individual support in study skills, test-taking strategies, and content-area classes to increase student success in courses.

3. Advise students who are at risk of failing a promotion or graduation test well in advance. Provide them with appropriate instruction to increase chances of passing.
4. Provide extra study time and opportunities for credit recovery.

Behavioral Support

1. Teach students how to positively and effectively communicate with peers and adults.
2. Promote constructive problem solving.
3. Include cognitive components in behavioral interventions.
4. Establish behavioral goals and recognize students when they accomplish them.

Personalized Instruction

1. Vary instructional methods to engage students by structuring different formats for grouping or participating in learning.
2. Provide student choice in curricula, time schedules, and assessments to increase motivation and self-efficacy.

Rigorous and Relevant Instruction

1. Design instruction to engage students in active participation in activities, enhance the rigor of assignments, and align curricula with standards.
2. Incorporate career-related curricula and opportunities for students to apply essential concepts and skills for a functional purpose.
3. Provide accessible information to students about their disability, their rights, and their responsibilities. Bring awareness to students regarding how their disability affects their daily activities (pp. 285–287).

Transition Planning for Youth with Mental Health Needs

According to Merikangas and colleagues (2011), a relatively large segment of youth in the United States meet the criteria for mental health problems, including 11.2% with mood disorders, 8.3% with anxiety disorders, and 9.6% with behavior disorders. These findings were generated from a nationally representative sample of 6,483 adolescents ages 13–18 who participated in a survey. Only 36.2% of adolescents who reported mental health problems had received treatment.

Over 4,000 individuals between the ages of 10 and 24 die by suicide each year (Centers for Disease Control and Prevention, 2012). Many others injure themselves or contemplate suicide. These findings speak to the high prevalence of youth with mental health needs and the importance of support during transition years. In some cases, school professionals are not well trained in providing mental health or suicide prevention programs (Walsh, Hooven, & Kronick, 2013). Yet, as Walsh and colleagues (2013) noted, behaviors associated with suicide were those that school personnel regularly encounter, including depression, anxiety, and substance abuse. Consistent with Pyle and Wexler (2012), we recommend that supports be established in school settings—not outsourced to community programs that depend on the referred youth or a parent to make an appointment. In many studies, efforts by school professionals trained in basic mental health problem detection, counseling, and preventive measures correlated with improved outcomes (e.g., Gould, Greenberg, Velting, & Shaffer, 2003).

Transition Planning for Youth with Significant Health Care Needs

According to the Maternal and Child Health Bureau (MCHB), children with significant health care needs are those at increased risk for a chronic physical, developmental, behavioral, or emotional condition (McPherson et al., 1998). In Table 6.3, we list chronic health conditions experienced by these children. Twenty-one percent of today's youth have a chronic condition producing significant health care need. Given the huge population of youth with needs, educators must understand the importance of encouraging parents and youth to contact health care providers early to plan for adulthood, and to assist youth in becoming self-sufficient in medical management.

Transition Planning for Youth with Profound Multiple Disabilities

Educators use the term *profound intellectual disability* to refer to individuals who are untestable or those with estimated intelligence quotients of less than 25 (mean = 100; standard deviation = 15) (Grossman, 1983). Other terms include *multiple disabilities* or *profound multiple disabilities*. Whereas children with profound intellectual disabilities typically have some degree of expressive and receptive language, children with profound *multiple* disabilities rely on assistive technology to communicate, assuming they can be taught to activate technological devices (e.g., Mechling, 2006). Children with profound multiple disabilities have some definable characteristics. First, they perform few, if any, of the tasks included on intelligence tests (Bailey, 1981). Second, they may exhibit signs of neuromuscular dysfunction, such as muscle rigidity or skeletal differences (Landesman-Dwyer & Sackett, 1978). They may be nonambulatory and have little or no control over motor movements (Guess et al., 1988). Third, they often have medical complications relating to seizure disorders or difficulties with food ingestion (Korabek,

TABLE 6.3. Chronic Conditions That Produce Significant Health Care Needs for Some Children

• Asthma	• Eczema/other skin disease	• Other respiratory problems
• Anemia	• Epilepsy	• Persistent bowel problems
• Arthritis	• Fetal alcohol syndrome	• Physical differences
• Autoimmune disorders (e.g., AIDS)	• Hernia	• Repeated ear infections
• Brain tumor	• High blood pressure	• Severe allergies
• Cerebral palsy	• Other birth defect (e.g., cleft palate)	• Sickle cell anemia
• Chronic heart condition	• Other blood disorder	• Spina bifida
• Diabetes		

Note. From *www.acf.hhs.gov/sites/default/files/opre/special_health.pdf.*

Reid, & Ivancic, 1981). Because of these issues, they are often considered children with significant health care needs (described above).

A person-centered planning approach is often employed because it relies on stakeholder support and focuses on strengths of the youth. Assistive technology, particularly as it relates to expressive communication, should be considered (Cook & Hussey, 2002). The degree of match between the youth's strengths/preferences, health status, communication, and the demands of an environment are critical in planning. Youth may not be able to perform entire jobs because of health, skill, or stamina issues, but they may be able to perform a particular task. In this case, perhaps a team of youth can be assembled to perform one job. Similarly, youth may not be able to take college courses, but they may participate in a course by performing certain functions, such as answering specific questions. If health issues result in frequent absence, arrangements should be made to involve the youth via distance technology. Transition planning should be carried out with the intention of maximizing the individual's participation, involvement, and ultimately, quality of life.

SUMMARY

In this chapter, we examined various aspects of transition planning. Each transition team member plays a role in the planning process, but the student's role should be pivotal. To the extent possible, the student should play a key role in determining goals and creating the direction for the planning process. Once goals have been established, planning should start "with the end in mind" and work backward to the current circumstances. Two approaches discussed in detail were person-centered planning and courses of study. Five steps were described in transition planning. Indicator 13 provides a method for evaluating the adequacy of ITPs. We described transition planning in areas of employment, PSE, and independent living. Finally, we considered transition planning for students at risk of dropping out, with mental health needs, with significant health care needs, or with profound multiple disabilities.

REVISITING JOSEFINA

"I would love to have a job. But I will be happy at home taking care of the kids. Thank you." Josefina opened her person-centered planning meeting with a statement of her plans. She had already discussed them with Ms. Martin, her teacher, and her parents, Raul and Mariana Hernandez. She turned to Vanessa, her cousin whom she had asked to "facilitate" her meeting.

"Thanks, Josefina," started Vanessa, "We appreciate you and we want you to have a happy future. Now we're going to develop what we call a personal profile, which means your strengths, abilities, and gifts. Who wants to tell me about Josefina's strengths?"

Over the next few minutes, Josefina's parents, family, close friends, and teacher described her talents. Josefina was well liked by family and classmates from Ignacio High School.

"What I hear everyone say," started Vanessa, "is that Josefina, you are a great helper. You love helping others to do good things. It sounds like you will be good taking care of the kids at home." Several in the support team nodded their heads.

"Excuse me," Mateo said as he raised his hand. Mateo was Josefina's older brother. "Sorry, I was just wondering. Josefina, you are a good helper, but you also have many skills. Why don't you want to get a job? Imagine what you could do if you were helping others on a job? She can work, right? I mean she's in a wheelchair and all, but she can work, right?"

Mateo and others turned toward the teacher, Ms. Martin. Josefina's teacher joined the person-centered planning meeting but wanted to maintain a low profile, preferring instead to hear what the support team planned.

"What do the rest of you think?"

Some team members agreed with Mateo that Josefina should explore a career in a helping profession. But Josefina's parents, Raul and Mariana, insisted the family needed her at home. They had been counting on Josefina returning home after finishing high school to tend her two sisters. The group again turned to Ms. Martin.

"At Ignacio, we had a plan for Josefina to become a teacher's assistant and work in a school. She could definitely do the work. But I want to respect the family's wishes."

"Ms. Martin, why can't she do both?" asked Mateo.

"What do you mean?" asked Ms. Martin.

"Why can't she sit the kids at home and teach them too? Like a day care assistant. She could make some money sitting for other kids along with her sisters."

"She would have to take some classes to become a child development specialist. It will take some time and will cost money. But she could work at home to supervise children."

Eyes turned toward Josefina and her parents. Josefina appeared excited. Her mom asked about the expense of taking classes. Ms. Martin knew of some scholarships for which Josefina would be eligible and offered to investigate. One of Josefina's friends said that her mother was a child development specialist and could offer assistance. The group continued to discuss Josefina's career path to become a specialist, while at the same time, helping at home.

"Thank you, everyone, for your help," Josefina smiled.

After the person-centered planning meeting, Ms. Martin scheduled Josefina's final IEP transition planning meeting. Also, Ms. Martin told Josefina and her parents that she would build the person-centered plan into the transition plan. Ms. Martin invited the parents and met with Josefina to prepare for the IEP transition planning meeting.

At the meeting, Josefina introduced herself and her parents to members of her IEP transition planning team. She described her postsecondary goal and her annual goal for her senior year. Ms. Martin provided some results from transition assessments. Team members offered suggestions and asked Josefina questions about her future plans. In a short time, the meeting concluded and team members signed the document. Josefina breathed a sign of relief.

See Josefina's hypothetical ITP in Figure 6.4.

INDIVIDUALIZED TRANSITION PLAN

Student: Josefina Hernandez   **Grade**: 12   **Date**: September 12, 2015

Age-Appropriate Transition Assessments (Dates of Assessment):

Education: Woodcock–Johnson Tests of Achievement (9/1/15), Vineland Adaptive Behavior Scale (9/2/15)

Employment: Transition Planning Inventory (9/5/15), Career Ability Placement Survey (CAPS) (9/5/15)

Independent Living: The Arc Self-Determination Scale (9/8/15)

Present Level of Academic and Functional Performance:

Based on results from the achievement tests, Josefina's vocabulary and reading comprehension are similar to a student at sixth grade. Given that she is in 12th grade, these results are six grade levels below current placement. Her reading percentile score was 9, which means that her performance equaled or exceeded 9% of students her age who took the same test. She wants to be a child development specialist, which requires high reading levels with specialized vocabulary. (Achievement present levels continue.) The Vineland Adaptive Behavior Scale measures student's functioning level in areas of communication, daily living, socialization, and motor skills. Josefina's standard scores were between 85 and 101, with percentile ranks ranging from 34th percentile to 54th percentile. The low score was in communication. These adaptive scores are relatively high. The TPI-2 requests information from the student/parents/guardians, and school personnel in order to identify areas of need that allow the transition team to develop services. Like previous years, the TPI-2 showed that Josefina has strengths related to helping professions and socialization. These results are consistent with the CAPS. Dimension scores on the CAPS indicate strengths in spatial relations. On the Arc Self-Determination Scale, Josefina rated herself high in self-realization and psychological empowerment. She wants to be independent but maintains a close relationship with her family. All assessments were administered by Ms. Rebecca Martin.

Measurable Postsecondary Goals Based on the Student's Needs, Strengths, Preferences, and Interests:

Employment-related: One year after graduating from high school, Josefina will apply to work as a child development intern.

Postsecondary education-related: In the year after graduating from high school, Josefina will apply to take classes leading to a child development specialist degree at Ignacio Community College.

Independent living-related (as needed): Not developed, as Josefina plans to live at home.

(continued)

FIGURE 6.4. Josefina's hypothetical ITP.

Annual Goals:

(1) *Given blank application forms from preschools and day care centers, Josefina will independently and accurately complete 100% of form sections, as measured by teacher review. (2) Given an application form for Ignacio Community College, Josefina will independently and accurately complete 100% of form sections, as measured by teacher review. (3) Before the end of the senior year, Josefina will independently call and make an appointment with the child development department advisor at Ignacio Community College, as measured by teacher verification.*

Transition Services: What transition services, experiences, and/or specialized instruction are needed during the period of this IEP for the student to develop the skills and knowledge to facilitate movement toward the postsecondary goals?
Employment: *Academic, functional vocational, and career-related services*

Person responsible: *Ms. Martin, Special Education; Mr. Piazza, Career Technical Education*

Postsecondary education: *Academic instructional services*

Person responsible: *Ms. Martin*

[Other services are described.]

Course of Study Addressing Postschool Transition Needs for Postsecondary Adult Activities:
Language arts (4 units), mathematics (3 units), science (3 units), social studies (3 units), arts (1.5 units), physical/health education (2 units), career technical education (0.5 units), electives (6.0 units). Students with disabilities served by special education programs may have changes made to graduation requirements through IEPs to meet educational needs. A student's IEP shall document the nature and extent of modifications and substitutions or exemptions made to accommodate a student with disabilities.

  X Course of study and current transcript attached   X SEOP attached

Transfer of Rights: Not later than 1 year before the student's 18th birthday, the student and parent must be informed of any rights under IDEA that will transfer, or have transferred, to the student. Adult students must be informed of their procedural safeguards at least annually.

Date student reaches the age of majority: *11/21/15*

The student and parents(s) were informed of the transfer of rights notice on: *8/25/14*

Graduation: Anticipated graduation/school completion date: *6/3/16*

  Anticipated exit document: X diploma   ___ certificate of completion

Student participation: If the student did not attend the IEP meeting, describe how the student participated in the transition planning process: *Student participated in meeting.*

FIGURE 6.4. *(continued)*

EXERCISE 6.4

Review the assessment data for Raenia, provided later in this exercise. How would you use Raenia's data to plan her transition? Write a present level of performance statement based on the assessment data. Write one or more measurable postsecondary goals and one or more annual goals. Describe transition services consistent with the annual goal. Finally, apply the Indicator 13 checklist to your present level of performance and goals. How did you evaluate your work?

Raenia is a 16-year-old girl living in a large U.S. city who wants a career working in the theater. She has two additional years at South City High School before she plans to graduate with a diploma. Her parents are supportive of her career. Raenia receives special education services for specific learning disabilities in her general education classes. She attends a resource room for intensive academic assistance in math and reading. Her resource teacher, Ms. Gutierrez, describes Raenia as needing to improve her social skills. Her other high school teachers report that Raenia is motivated to learn but tends to stay silent when she needs help on assignments or when she does not understand instructions.

Achievement test results:
- Math grade-equivalence score: fourth grade
- Science grade-equivalence score: seventh grade
- Reading grade-equivalence score: fifth grade
- Language arts grade-equivalence score: eighth grade

Current grade level: 10

Summary of results of social skills rating scale (completed by Ms. Gutierrez): Raenia's performance was rated high in peer interaction. She scored low on social greetings, asking questions for clarification, and self-expression to adults.

Preference assessment results: Raenia's highest preference was in theatrical arts working as a costume designer. She enjoys painting, designing clothing, creating costumes, and dancing.

Career Ability Placement Survey (CAPS) summary: Highest scores were obtained in Spatial Relations (how well a person visualizes in three dimensions and can form mental pictures of objectives from a diagram or picture) and Perceptual Speed and Accuracy (how well a person perceives small details rapidly and accurately). Lowest scores were in Mechanical Reasoning, Verbal Reasoning, and Numeric Ability.

Requirements for theatrical careers: Artistic talent (spatial relations, musical understanding, choreography), social skills, and reading.

EXERCISE 6.5

Review the cases involving Demarius and Kenley in Chapter 1: How would you plan their transition? What information would you need to write a present level of performance statement?

WEBSITES WITH ADDITIONAL INFORMATION

NSTTAC Indicator 13 (Select the links for descriptions of students.)

www.nsttac.org/content/nsttac-indicator-13-checklist-form-b-enhanced-professional-development

Student-Directed Transition Planning

www.ou.edu/education/centers-and-partnerships/zarrow/trasition-education-materials/student-directed-transition-planning.html

IEP and Transition Planning

www.ncset.org/topics/ieptransition/default.asp?topic=28

National Parent Center on Transition and Employment

www.pacer.org/tatra/planning/transitionemp.asp

Transition Planning for Students with Hearing Loss

www.asha.org/aud/Articles/Teens-and-Young-Adults—Achievement-With-Hearing-Loss/

Transition Planning for Students with Visual Impairments

www.afb.org/info/programs-and-services/professional-development/teachers/career-education/1235

Transition Planning for Students with Deaf-Blindness

https://nationaldb.org/library/page/2282

CHAPTER 7

Student Involvement and Self-Determination to Guide Transition

This chapter addresses . . .

- Student expectations for postschool outcomes.
- Research on student involvement and self-determination in transition.
- Strategies to promote student involvement during transition planning.
- Educational programs to teach self-determination and self-management.

WHAT POSTSCHOOL OUTCOMES DO STUDENTS EXPECT?

As described in Chapter 2, researchers conducted interviews with students with disabilities in the NLTS-2 to determine, in part, their expectations for the future (Wagner, Newman, Cameto, Levine, & Marder, 2007). The students, who at the time were 13–15 years old, were asked whether they expected to get a paid job or attend a PSE program. Students responded to indicate whether they definitely would, probably would, or definitely/probably would not reach the targeted goal. In cases where the student was unable to respond to questions due to expressive or functional limitations, parents responded for their child. About 5,000 students or parents responded to the survey. In Table 7.1, we provide information on their expectations. Relatively high percentages of students expected to get a paid job (ranging from 77.7% [autism] to 97.1% [specific learning disabilities]). Also, relatively high percentages of students indicated they definitely planned to get involved in a PSE program. Generally, the findings show that students had high expectations for the future.

TABLE 7.1. Expectations of Youth with Disabilities, by Disability Categories, Regarding Postschool Outcomes

Percentage expecting to . . .	LD	SLI	ID	ED	HI	VI	OI	OHI	AUT	TBI	MD	DB
Get a paid job												
Definitely will	97.1	95.7	86.3	92.9	96.1	92.6	83.8	95.8	77.7	92.5	86.1	92.2
Probably will	2.6	4.3	9.7	5.8	3.1	7.2	11.3	4.2	9.8	6.7	11.2	17.8
Definitely or probably won't	0.2	[a]	4.0	1.3	0.8	0.2	4.9	[a]	2.6	.08	2.7	[a]
Get PSE												
Definitely will	53.3	58.8	37.7	56.2	79.9	69.9	62.2	49.6	47.2	66.9	47.1	55.4
Probably will	34.5	30.6	41.6	30.1	15.4	24.1	24.0	35.8	37.2	24.3	37.8	[b]
Definitely or probably won't	12.7	10.6	20.7	13.7	4.7	6.0	13.7	14.6	15.6	8.8	15.1	19.1

Note. LD, learning disability; SLI, speech/language impairment; ID, intellectual disability; ED, emotional disturbance; HI, hearing impairment; VI, visual impairment; OI, orthopedic impairment; OHI, other health impairment; AUT, autism; TBI, traumatic brain injury; MD, multiple disability; DB, deaf-blindness. From Wagner et al. (2007b). Reprinted with permission from SRI International.
[a] Rounds to zero.
[b] Fewer than 30 respondents.

In Table 7.2, we present reported outcomes of the same youth with disabilities from the NLTS-2 sample up to 8 years after high school. That is, data in Table 7.2 are from the same individuals who reported their expectations in Table 7.1 (minus some attrition), but now well out of high school and in their 20s. The data are from Wave 5 of NLTS-2 (Newman et al., 2011). The numbers in parentheses show the differences, by disability category, between expected and actual outcomes. A close examination reveals differences between expectations and outcomes for both employment and 4-year college involvement. For all categories of disability, outcomes fell short of expectations. For example, whereas 97.1% of 13- to 15-year-olds with specific learning disabilities expected to get paid employment, only 67.3% were actually employed at the time of the interview up to 8 years after high school, for a difference of 29.8%. Some difference scores were near 50%, such as intellectual disability (employment), orthopedic impairment (employment), other health impairment (employment), multiple disability (employment), hearing impairment (4-year college), and traumatic brain injury (4-year college).

One might argue that these data merely show that high expectations of 13- to 15-year-olds with disabilities are not realized, a finding that probably mirrors data of typical youth. In other words, we all have high expectations and, upon reaching post–high school age, we settle for something less (or different). Comparison data from typical youth are not available. Nonetheless, we are concerned that these findings do indicate that youth with disabilities generally want to achieve valued adult outcomes, but those outcomes do not usually match their expectations.

EXERCISE 7.1

Respond to the following questions:

- What were your expectations for the future at age 13?
- Did you expect to get a paid job after high school?
- Did you expect to go to college?
- To what extent were your expectations realized?
- To what extent did your expectations change?
- How do you account for the changes?
- What role did career awareness and education play?
- How do you think your experience might compare to that of a student with a disability?

HOW CAN STUDENTS GET INVOLVED IN PLANNING THEIR TRANSITION?

Starting early in their educational careers, students with disabilities should be given opportunities to explore their interests, define their values, identify their desires and dreams, and analyze their strengths, preferences, and interests related to postschool adult living. Without student input, transition from school to adulthood may be misguided or without substance. But beyond input, as much as possible, students should become the driving force in shaping their futures. That is, they should have input in determining the pathway to their independence. Although it is true that their pathway

TABLE 7.2. Reported Outcomes of Youth or Their Parents/Guardians, by Disability Categories

Percentages who . . .	LD	SLI	ID	ED	HI	VI	OI	OHI	AUT	TBI	MD	DB
Got a paid job												
At the time of the interview	67.3 (−29.8)	63.7 (−32.0)	38.8 (−47.5)	49.6 (−43.3)	57.2 (−38.9)	43.8 (−48.8)	35.0 (−48.8)	35.0 (−60.8)	37.2 (−40.5)	51.6 (−40.9)	39.2 (−46.9)	30.1 (−62.1)
Were involved in PSE: 4-year college												
At the time of the interview	21.2 (−32.1)	32.5 (−26.3)	6.7 (−31.0)	10.8 (−45.4)	33.8 (−46.1)	40.1 (−29.8)	26.1 (−36.1)	26.1 (−23.5)	17.4 (−29.8)	18.5 (−48.4)	7.4 (−39.7)	23.7 (−31.7)

Note. Percentages in parentheses show differences between expected and actual outcomes. Abbreviations as in Table 7.1. From Newman et al. (2011). Reprinted with permission from SRI International.

may change course several times, it is important to respect students as decision makers and as the ones who must live with the results. In this chapter, we describe a two-part process we view as critical for transition to successful postschool outcomes: (1) student self-involvement in the IEP process and (2) student self-determination of his or her future.

WHAT IS SELF-INVOLVEMENT?

Test and colleagues (2004) conducted a literature review of student involvement in transition practices. They defined *self-involvement* as

> (a) describing one's disability, strengths, legal rights, and present level of performance; (b) evaluating one's progress, weighing alternative goals, and engaging in goal-setting and goal-attainment activities; (c) preparing for a formal presentation and advocating for oneself in a formal setting [such as an IEP meeting]; (d) communicating one's preferences and interests; (e) accepting responsibility for areas where improvement is needed; (f) participating in discussions regarding one's post-school plans and needs; and (g) determining one's accommodation needs and securing appropriate accommodations. (p. 393)

Self-involvement, then, is a broad term referring to actions that serve as a foundation for developing self-determination. From an early age, educators can teach students skills in a variety of activities and contexts leading to self-determination.

WHAT IS SELF-DETERMINATION?

In Chapter 1, *self-determination* was defined as volitional actions enabling one to act as the primary causal agent in one's life (Wehmeyer, 2005). According to Wehmeyer (2005), *volition* refers to the power to make conscious choices about one's actions. *Causal agency* implies that actions are purposeful or performed to achieve an end. An individual who is self-determined makes conscious choices enabling purposeful actions to achieve an end result.

Misinterpretations of Self-Determination

The construct of self-determination may be prone to misinterpretation. As it relates to individuals with significant disabilities, Wehmeyer (2005) described several potential misinterpretations. These are important to understand because they may apply to all youth and their stakeholders. First, self-determination is not a program or a curriculum, nor is it a process (e.g., teaching a skill) or an outcome (e.g., graduating from high school). Instead, it is a *characteristic* of the person. Actively participating in an IEP meeting is an example of self-involvement, but not of self-determination. Second, self-determination is not a set of skills. If it were, we might erroneously conclude that youth requiring significant supports have limited or no self-determination. However, if it is a characteristic of a person, we may be able to teach skills to enhance one's self-determination. Third, self-determination is not the same as independent performance. Again, it should be viewed as a personal characteristic, not a repertoire of behaviors. Finally, and perhaps most importantly, self-determination is not a matter of making a simple choice. Although transition educators, parents, and other stakeholders should encourage choice making out of respect for a youth, making a choice (e.g., choosing a blue or red binder or choosing pizza or soup for lunch) does not constitute self-determination.

The Role of the Educator in Self-Determination

Wehmeyer, Agran, and Hughes (2000) surveyed 1,219 special education teachers from 50 states to find out if they promoted self-determination and self-directed learning. Sixty percent of respondents were familiar with the term *self-determination*, but only 22% reported that students had goals in this area. The survey is now several years old; hopefully, today's educators promote self-determination at higher levels. So what should an educator do to recognize, value, and promote self-determination? Wehmeyer (2005) stated:

> The role of teachers is not to teach students to control their lives. It is to enable students with severe disabilities to become more self-determined, even if it is just a little bit more. We can achieve this by enabling students to express preferences, by implementing instruction that promotes involvement in problem solving and decision-making, and by promoting self-advocacy and student-directed learning. We can do this through student involvement in educational planning meetings; through the provision of supports, self- or other-directed, including technology, which augment capacity; through effective communication instruction; and through person-centered planning. (pp. 119–120)

Educators play important roles in facilitating self-determination. The opportunities that avail themselves in school and community environments to enable self-determination are abundant (e.g., selecting elective courses, considering career options, weighing one's values). The more educators take advantage of these opportunities for their students, the more they will understand how particular students make decisions on their own.

The Role of the Student in Self-Determination

When we were first afforded an opportunity to make important decisions as adolescents, our responses may have been tentative and lacking in confidence. From the student's standpoint, making decisions to shape his or her future may come with uncertainty, anxiety, and self-doubt. Although students are often excited to have the opportunity to take a lead role, their initial actions may lack polish and sophistication. We see this tentativeness frequently with students who have disabilities and consider it a normal learning process. Some may even be defensive or aggressive. Educators should support the student throughout the process of acquiring self-determination, expecting a wide range of behavior.

Case example: Bianca. One of the authors recalls "Bianca," a 19-year-old girl in transition to adulthood referred to a university employment clinic designed to assist transition-age youth obtain employment. Bianca had been labeled "unemployable" by an ASP agency. She described herself as a "ret—d" who was like "a third grader." Although the author countered her claim, saying that she was a young adult, Bianca retorted loudly:

"I said I'm a third grader! So get used to it!"

Bianca demonstrated little awareness of the world of work except to say it involved "people sweating" and "getting up early." She made repeated statements (with increasing volume) that she could not work, hold a job, or find employment. After a few initial sessions during which clinic staff administered job preference and other assessments, Bianca stopped coming to appointments. Phone calls were not answered. When clinic staff went to her house and knocked on her door, they received no response other than curtains being closed from within. On the second visit to the house, Bianca abruptly opened the door and yelled "Leave me alone!" However, a conversation ensued about how the clinic wanted only to have her visit some job sites corresponding with preferred activities she had identified in assessments. She agreed to resume sessions as long as clinic staff would not ask her to work.

"I told you I can't work. I'm a ret– –d."

Bianca accompanied staff to several job sites where others performed her preferred activities. At first, Bianca appeared disinterested, frequently looking at her watch and asking when she could leave. On the third visit, she visited a bakery. She seemed upset when asked to wear a hair net and wash her hands to enter the baking area, but she complied when one of the bakery staff engaged her directly a conversation. On repeated trips to the same bakery, Bianca developed a relationship with some of the employees and started performing tasks, such as bagging bread and moving trays. Clinic staff and employees focused on tasks that Bianca could perform and avoided new, unfamiliar ones. Bianca started volunteering to learn new tasks. Also, clinic staff discussed with employees various ways they could involve Bianca in work and break-time activities. Eventually, she filled out an application and obtained employment at the bakery—which, by the way, involved a lot of perspiration and getting up very early in the morning.

Initially, Bianca displayed numerous problem behaviors. When these behaviors were ignored and people engaged her in conversation, she began to respond. The focus turned from the problem behaviors to valuing Bianca as an individual. Although it was still necessary to implement a behavior intervention plan, Bianca became respected as a full-fledged, contributing member of the bakery. Her ability to self-determine was always a part of her character. What changed was how people respected and valued her.

EXERCISE 7.2

Respond to the following questions:

- Have you worked with a youth like Bianca?
- If so, what did you do to encourage his or her self-determination?

- If not, how would you proceed?
- What experiences might be pivotal for youth such as Bianca to recognize their strengths and potential? What actions should be avoided?

If you are taking a course on transition, discuss these questions as a group.

WHAT RESEARCH EXISTS ON STUDENT INVOLVEMENT AND SELF-DETERMINATION?

Research on IEP Meeting Involvement

Test and colleagues (2004) reviewed research designed to increase students' involvement in IEP processes. They found that students with various disabilities, including those requiring significant support, could be taught to become actively involved in the IEP meeting and associated activities. Yet, without partaking in programs designed to teach involvement, IEP meeting participation of students with disabilities was generally low. Martin and colleagues (2006) observed 109 middle and high school IEP meetings. Participants included students with disabilities, special and general education teachers, family members, administrators, and support staff. The majority of students had mild disabilities (78%). No student had been taught to actively participate in meeting discussions. Researchers found that, across all meetings, students talked 3% of the time; special education teachers talked 51% of the time; family members talked 15% of the time; and administrators, general education teachers, and support staff talked between 6 and 9% of the time. Researchers concluded that students needed to be taught effective meeting participation skills.

Martin, Marshall, Maxson, and Jerman (1997) developed a program to increase student involvement in meetings, called the *Self-Directed IEP*. This program is described later in this chapter. In a number of research studies (e.g., Martin et al., 2006), researchers found that the program increased student involvement. For example, students in the Self-Directed IEP intervention group participated more frequently in IEP meetings than students in a control group.

Thoma, Rogan, and Baker (2001) found that although many students were physically present at formal transition IEP meetings, those with more significant disabilities were not active participants. The authors reported that meetings often focused on deficits and that student voices were unheard.

Research on IEP meetings provide data indicating that students need specific instruction to develop skills to become actively involved in group discussion. Across various disability categories, instruction designed to increase involvement proved effective.

INVOLVING STUDENTS WITH SIGNIFICANT SUPPORT NEEDS IN THEIR IEP MEETINGS

Given training, support, and perhaps technology, students requiring significant supports may be taught to become involved in their IEP meetings. Stringham (2013) taught four 18- to 21-year-old post–high school students to participate in their IEP meetings using an iPad equipped with an application that allowed scripts to be narrated describing students' self-identified preferences. All students had profound intellectual disabilities and low-functioning autism. Generally, students verbalized only 10–20 words that were understood by persons familiar with their speech and could respond vocally to indicate "yes" or "no." All student verbalizations were made in response to questions or prompts from adults. Participants rarely initiated expressive communications. Other forms of expressive communication, such as American Sign Language or the Picture Exchange Communication System (PECS; Bondy & Frost, 2001), were used by some participants but not fluently.

The procedure first involved teaching the participants to lead and participate in an IEP meeting using modified Self-Directed IEP curriculum lessons (Martin et al., 1997). Procedures also included developing a script in which a familiar person served as a narrator who read statements to introduce team members or express the participant's desires/needs. The participant touched buttons on an iPad2® with a Stories-2Learn application (*https://itunes.apple.com/us/app/stories2learn/id348576875?mt=8*) to activate narrated scripts. During a mock IEP meeting (a pretest), the four participants averaged 42% of modified Self-Directed IEP program steps performed independently. After training and the use of the electronic script, participants averaged 83%. In the mock IEP pretest, participants verbalized or used signs/gestures an average of 8.5% of sampled 10-second intervals. In the actual IEP meeting, participants activated the scripted voice between 17.4 and 23.9% of intervals. The researcher reviewed audiotapes of IEP meetings and found that participants attempted to embellish the narrator's script with their own verbalizations, signs, or gestures. After IEP meetings, parents noted the increased participation of their sons or daughters, particularly their embellishments.

Research on Skills Related to Self-Determination

Considerable research indicates that youth who engage in behaviors related to self-determination have better postschool outcomes (e.g., Test et al., 2009; Wehmeyer & Palmer, 2003). For example, Wehmeyer and Palmer (2003) conducted a follow-up study with young adults with intellectual disability or specific learning disabilities 1 and 3 years after they exited school. Forty-seven young adults with high scores and 47 with low scores on a self-determination measure were interviewed after exiting high school. Self-determination was measured using the Arc Self-Determination Scale (Wehmeyer & Kelchner, 1995). The authors reported that young adults who had high self-determination scores were more successful in employment, health, financial independence, and independent living. Similarly, Williams-Diehm, Wehmeyer, Palmer, Soukup, and Garner (2008) examined 276 students' self-determination measures who had shown different levels of involvement in IEP meetings. The authors used three different self-report measures on self-determination: (1) the Arc Self-Determination Scale, (2) the AIR Self-Determination Scale (Wolman et al., 1994), and (3) a questionnaire designed to measure involvement in IEP meetings. The results suggested that students who were more actively involved in transition planning meetings scored higher on measures of self-determination.

WHAT ARE EDUCATIONAL PROGRAMS THAT FACILITATE STUDENT INVOLVEMENT AND SELF-DETERMINATION?

In previous chapters, we described the importance of starting early in transition instruction. For example, in Chapter 2, we described Nielsen's (2013) research on transition skills in a sixth- to 12th-grade timeline. In Chapter 6, we described transition planning by "starting with the end in mind" and asking questions of students about their future plans as early as sixth grade. However, the process of conceptualizing "what should be taught" and identifying actual programs to teach self-determination can be a daunting task. Peterson, Sedaghat, Burden, Van Dycke, and Pomeroy (2013) developed a continuum of self-determination instruction from sixth through 12th grade. In Figure 7.1, we present the continuum for broad categories of instruction. According to Peterson and colleagues, instruction in self-determination can provide students with:

1. Knowledge of the impact of their disability in relationship to potential postsecondary education and employment involvement
2. Skills necessary to participate in transition assessments
3. Skills to lead IEP meetings
4. Skills to participate in writing of one's Summary of Performance
5. Knowledge of when/how to use a transition portfolio
6. Knowledge to identify adults who will support them as well as supports needed after leaving the high school setting
7. Skills to use self-evaluation tools to determine college and career readiness
8. Skills and knowledge to assist in developing connections with postsecondary settings

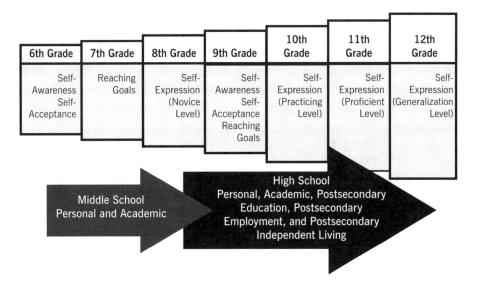

FIGURE 7.1. A sixth- to 12th-grade continuum of broad categories of self-determination instruction. From Peterson, Sedaghat, et al. (2013). Reprinted with permission from the authors.

9. Skills to use disability disclosure as needed in potential PSE and employment involvement

10. Skills to discuss needs with PSE, employment, and independent living personnel

11. Skills to request accommodations as needed in instructional, vocational, and independent living settings

The continuum developed by Peterson and colleagues (2013) was established for students with mild to moderate disabilities. For students with more significant disabilities, instruction should start sooner or accommodations should be established for teaching self-expression. Some, but not all, of instructional programs in this sequence have strong evidence from empirical research supporting practice. More research is needed.

Peterson and colleagues (2013) described self-awareness, self-acceptance, reaching goals, and self-expression in a developmental sequence. For example, self-awareness involves (1) discussing preferences, interests, dreams; (2) identifying strengths and needs; (3) making informed decisions; (4) discussing learning differences and disability awareness; (5) participating in assessments of transition-related skills; (6) describing the impact of one's disability; and (7) discussing accommodations. These skills should be addressed beginning about sixth grade.

In Figure 7.2, we present specific educational programs designed to teach self-determination from sixth to 12th grade (Peterson et al., 2013). These programs, many of which are described later in this chapter, correspond with the broad categories of skills described in Figure 7.1. Transition educators may need to adjust the grade level of instruction, depending on the skills of the student and opportunities to practice skills. However, the continuum across grade levels provides a scope and sequence for instruction that may foster self-determination.

We describe programs and guidebooks to facilitate self-determination. These include (1) *Possible Selves*, (2) *Self-Determination Strategies*, (3) *Student-Led IEPs*, (4) the *Self-Directed Learning Model of Instruction*, (5) *STEPS to Self-Determination*, (6) *ChoiceMaker*, and (7) *411 on Disability Disclosure*. See websites for these programs at the end of this chapter.

Possible Selves

This program was designed to increase motivation by having students examine their futures and think about goals that are important to them. Starting in about sixth grade, the program allows students to describe their characteristics and expectations for the future. Students set goals, create plans, and begin working toward their goals.

Self-Determination Strategies

The book *Self-Determination Strategies* (Parker, Field, & Hoffman, 2012) is designed to guide educators, counselors, disability service providers, and college instructors who work with youth in transition. Specific to youth considering PSE, the 56-page book assists instructors by providing case studies and advice.

6th Grade	7th Grade	8th Grade	9th Grade	10th Grade	11th Grade	12th Grade
Possible Selves (Initial Instruction) *Self-Determination* (Initial Strategies Instruction)	*Student-Led IEPS* (Initial Instruction) *Self-Determined Learning Model of Instruction* (Initial Instruction)	*Student-Led IEPS* (Review) *Advocacy Presentations* (Initial Instruction)	*Steps to Self-Determination* (Initial Instruction) *Take Action* (Initial Instruction) *Self-Advocacy Strategy* (Initial Instruction)	*411 on Disability Disclosure* (Initial Instruction) *Choosing Educational Goals* (Initial Instruction) *Choosing Employment Goals* (Initial Instruction) *Self-Directed IEP* (Initial Instruction)	*Self-Directed IEP* (Review) *411 on Disability Disclosure* (Review) *Choosing Educational Goals* (Review) *Choosing Employment Goals* (Review)	*Student-Directed Summary of Performance* (Initial Instruction) *Transition to Postsecondary Education: Strategies for Students with Disabilities* (Initial Instruction) *Adult Agencies: Linkages for Adolescents in Transition* (Initial Instruction)

FIGURE 7.2. A sixth- to 12th-grade continuum of educational programs designed to foster self-determination. From Peterson, Sedaghat, et al. (2013). Reprinted with permission from the authors.

Student-Led IEPs

This book for transition professionals, by McGahee, Mason, Wallace, and Jones (2001), describes the advantages of student-led IEPs, obstacles to implementation, and teaching activities that foster student-led meetings. The book can be used by educators as they design instruction for student-led IEPs.

The Self-Directed Learning Model of Instruction (SDLMI)

Designed to assist students in becoming self-regulated problem solvers and causal agents in their lives, the *Self-Directed Learning Model of Instruction* (SDLMI; Wehmeyer, Palmer, Agran, Mithaug, & Martin, 2000) is a framework consisting of three instructional phases, including goal setting, taking action, and adjusting the goal or plan. Each of these phases presents a problem to be solved by the student through a series of four questions. For example, in Phase 1, *goal setting*, students are presented with questions and corresponding instructional objectives. Question 1 asks students what they would like to learn. Corresponding instructional objectives are designed to enable students to identify strengths and needs; communicate preferences, interests, beliefs, and values; and to teach them how to prioritize needs. In addition, there are specific objectives for all phases, leading to instruction in (1) self-scheduling, (2) self-instruction, (3) antecedent cue regulation, (4) choice making, (5) goal attainment strategies, (6) problem-solving instruction, (7) decision-making instruction, (8) self-advocacy instruction, (9) assertiveness training, (10) communication skills training, and (11) self-monitoring.

STEPS to Self-Determination

Starting at about ninth grade, *STEPS to Self-Determination* (Field & Hoffman, 1996) is designed to assist students in defining goals important to self-determination. Materials include an instructor's guide, CD-ROM, DVD, student activity book, and self-determination knowledge scale. Areas include (1) assessing self-determination by using a knowledge scale; (2) identifying strengths, weaknesses, needs, and preferences; (3) developing decision-making skills; (4) identifying rights and responsibilities; (5) setting goals; (6) anticipating consequences of one's actions; (7) enhancing creativity; (8) developing communication skills; (9) accessing resources and supports; (10) developing negotiating skills, and (11) experiencing and learning from outcomes.

ChoiceMaker

The *ChoiceMaker* series (Martin & Marshall, 1996) includes *Take Action, Choose and Take Action, Choosing Employment Goals, Choosing Personal Goals, Choosing Education Goals,* and *The Self-Directed IEP*. Starting at about 10th grade, *The Self-Directed IEP* teaches students to lead their IEP meetings by describing their strengths, preferences, interests, goals, and needs. The *Self-Directed IEP* shows a video of students with different disabilities using skills in their classes as they talk about their experiences. The video is used to introduce the concept of a self-directed IEP to students, parents, educators, and administrators. Another video shows a student named "Zeke" who describes how he leads his IEP meeting to a friend. Lessons include mnemonic learning strategies, vocabulary-building exercises, role-playing activities, and reading and writing tasks. See the website at the end of this chapter for information on the series.

411 on Disability Disclosure

This eight-unit workbook (National Collaborative on Workforce and Disability for Youth, 2005) was developed to teach students how and when to disclose their disability. The program assists youth in making informed decisions about whether or not to disclose disability, understand the impact of such a decision, and practice the disclosure process. Workbook sections include self-determination ("The BIG Picture"), disclosure ("What Is It and Why Is It So Important?"), advantages and disadvantages of disclosure, rights and responsibilities under the law, accommodations, postsecondary disclosure ("Why? When? What? To Whom? How?"), disclosure on the job, and disclosure in social and community settings. In addition to the workbook, there are two additional documents, including a workbook for families and a workbook on cyber disclosure (i.e., disability disclosure in the context of social networks).

Additional Programs Related to Self-Determination

Beyond the programs described above, we review four additional ones: (1) *Take Charge of the Future*, (2) *Whose Future Is It Anyway?*, (3) *Beyond High School* model, and (4) *Student-Directed Transition Planning*.

Take Charge for the Future

Developed by Powers, Turner, Westwood, Matuszewski, and Phillips (2001), *Take Charge for the Future (TAKE CHARGE)* was designed to facilitate student-directed participation during the transition process. Using this program, students learn that they have a responsibility in achieving success and are exposed to different strategies to "take charge." The program coaches youth to apply student-directed planning skills to achieve transition goals, peer-based mentorship and parent support, and in-service education for school transition staff. Activities include (1) biweekly coaching sessions; (2) monthly community-based workshops for youth, parents, and adult mentors; (3) community activities preformed by mentors and students; (4) telephone and home visit supports for parents; and (5) in-service education for transition staff.

Whose Future Is It Anyway?

Wehmeyer and Lawrence (1995) designed this curriculum to assist students in exploring the self-awareness and skills related to problem solving, decision making, goal setting, and small-group communication. According to Wehmeyer, Lawrence, Garner, Soukup, and Palmer (2004), the curriculum assumes that (1) students who are educated in planning their future will be more likely get and stay involved, (2) students of all abilities can learn planning skills, and (3) students who believe that their voice will be heard will more likely participate in planning and education decisions. The curriculum is designed for students ages 14 through 21 and is comprised of six sections and 36 sessions. Transition educators or students read scripted lessons and complete activities.

Beyond High School Model

Developed by Wehmeyer and colleagues (2006), the *Beyond High School* model encourages student involvement and self-determination for transitioning 18- to 21-year-old students with disabilities. The model consists of three distinct stages. Stage 1 is comprised of three phases. During the first phase, students participate in targeted instruction designed to develop short- and long-term goals similar to *Whose Future Is It Anyway?* Next, students learn to self-regulate problems using the SDLMI. Finally, students learn how to advocate for themselves. During each of the stages, students answer specific questions (e.g., "What Is My Learning Goal?," "What Is My Plan?," and "What Have I Learned?"), which are used to support student-directed learning. With this information, students apply self-regulated problem solving to identify goals in transition areas, such as employment, recreation, and leisure. Stage 2 requires that a student-directed, person-centered planning meeting be convened during which the team works with individual students to refine goals and supports. At the end of this stage, the student goals are finalized and an action plan developed to achieve goals, including identification of supports. Finally, in Stage 3, students implement the plan, monitor progress in achieving goals, evaluate the plan, and make necessary revisions.

Student-Directed Transition Planning

This program consists of lessons that provide students with the knowledge and skills needed to develop and use their summary of performance (Woods, Sylvester, & Martin, 2010). Transition educators use eight lessons to teach students to actively engage in transition-focused IEPs. Woods and colleagues (2010) conducted a study to determine whether student-directed transition planning increased student knowledge of transition terms, concepts, and self-efficacy in the planning process. The authors reported that students who participated in the program had significantly increased knowledge and self-efficacy scores.

HOW DOES AN EDUCATOR SELECT THE MOST APPROPRIATE SELF-DETERMINATION PROGRAM?

Clearly, there are numerous options for fostering self-determination. The good news is that with self-determination being a point of considerable emphasis in curriculum development for youth with different types of disabilities in transition to adulthood, numerous options exist. We appreciate the continuum proposed by Peterson, Sedaghat, and colleagues (2013) for sixth through 12th graders (see Figure 7.2) for providing a logical sequence of programs. Furthermore, we anticipate researchers will soon create additional taxonomies and continua of instructional programs to accommodate diverse learners. In the meantime, we direct readers to the websites at the end of this chapter to gather information on individual programs and match them to characteristics of learners. Finally, for open source materials on self-determination, go to the Zarrow Center for Learning Enrichment at the University of Oklahoma (*www.ou.edu/education/centers-and-partnerships/zarrow.html?rd=1*).

HOW IS SELF-DETERMINATION MAINTAINED OVER TIME?

Because self-determination is a lifelong endeavor, skills must be maintained over time and across environments. For example, many of us have found that skills we learned in high school or college (solving problems, making decisions, setting a daily schedule and sticking to it) turned out to be valuable for years to come. Rather than run the risk of involving students in curricula for short periods only to discover lack of maintenance over time, transition educators must teach students to monitor their skills related to self-determination.

Self-Monitoring

Teaching a student to define certain behaviors (e.g., staying on-task during a lesson, solving a problem using a series of steps), self-checking the behaviors using a checklist or tracking form, collecting data on behavioral performance, and evaluating progress has been called *self-monitoring*. Monitoring one's own behaviors has been conceptualized as leading to self-determination (Hughes et al., 2002). For youth in transition, learning to self-monitor behavior and daily routines should occur before, during, or after instruction in self-determination. The combination of skills related to self-determination and behaviors related to self-monitoring produce strong habits leading to self-support and independence in adulthood.

Research on Self-Monitoring

Researchers (e.g., Wehmeyer, Agran, & Hughes, 1998) examined teaching self-monitoring and found positive outcomes. In Table 7.3, we list some of the transition-related skills taught through self-monitoring research. For example, Hughes and colleagues (2002) taught high school students with intellectual disabilities to use self-monitoring systems in general education classrooms by increasing behaviors such as saying "Thank you" and initiating an activity or responding to an initiation from a peer. Self-monitoring was individualized for each of four students and included such prompts as picture cards or checking a form. After baseline levels showing low levels of performance of these behaviors, students were taught to monitor their behaviors in general education settings. Behaviors then increased to near 100% correct in most sessions and maintained without additional training up to 20 data collection sessions.

TABLE 7.3. A Sample of Studies on the Effects of Self-Monitoring with Transition-Related Skills

Transition-related skills	Studies
Active classroom participation (general education classroom)	Agran, Wehmeyer, Cavin, & Palmer (2008); Agran, Sinclair, Alper, et al. (2005); Hughes et al. (2002)
Organizational skills (e.g., recording assignments, using a day planner)	Agran, Blanchard, Wehmeyer, & Hughes (2001)
Work performance, sequencing of job tasks, and social skills	Lagomarcino & Rusch (1988)

Teaching Self-Monitoring

Hughes and Carter (2012) described a series of teaching steps for promoting self-monitoring. Although the teaching process was initiated by an educator, the outcome consisted of students monitoring their own performance. These procedures and recording forms can be adapted to the characteristics of students.

1. Identify the problem or skill to be taught. Define the behavior operationally. For example, using a day planner means (a) typing tasks and appointments into an electronic planner, (b) checking the planner before leaving the house in the morning, (c) checking the planner at hourly intervals throughout the day, (d) completing all tasks and attending all appointments according to the daily schedule, and (e) evaluating before leaving for home that all tasks and appointments have been fulfilled.

2. Determine acceptability of the behavior/skill to be taught. Ensure that the student understands the expectation and that it is reasonable.

3. Identify natural supports in the environment. As Hughes and Carter (2012) pointed out, there are often natural supports that prompt students to begin, continue, or end an activity on their own. For example, if a student is to check the planner at hourly intervals throughout the day to monitor tasks/appointments, setting a timer on the electronic device may cue the occasion.

4. Select a strategy for teaching: self-instruction, permanent prompts, self-monitoring, or self-reinforcement. *Self-instruction* means vocally stating the instructions to oneself. *Permanent prompts* can be pictures, task lists (e.g., those used in defining the behavior in #1), or natural cues in an environment (e.g., a note to oneself on the door when leaving the house). *Self-reinforcement* refers to recognizing one's success in performing a task or reaching a goal. Select the strategy or combination of strategies most likely to be successful.

5. Teach the skill. First, identify the steps that comprise the task. Second, teach each step and the self-monitoring strategy. Third, start withdrawing assistance when the student begins performing the task independently. For example, the educator may introduce the task of using a day planner. The educator demonstrates the first task (typing

tasks and appointments into an electronic planner). The student then practices that task. Once completed, the student fills out a self-monitoring checklist (see Figure 7.3). Subsequent steps are then taught. For checking the planner before leaving the house in the morning, the student may need to send a text to the educator when the step is complete (as well as fill in the self-monitoring checklist).

6. Evaluate performance. This can be done jointly, with both the educator and the student using a checklist to see if all tasks are completed accurately. For example, a student may be using a day planner but occasionally missing tasks or not attending appointments according to the daily schedule. In this case, the step would be targeted for more intensive teaching. The student and educator would co-check whether the student completed tasks or attended appointments. Once the student is independently responding and using the self-monitoring checklist, the educator should gradually and systematically reduce prompts.

SUMMARY

In this chapter, we first considered student expectations of postschool outcomes. Next, we defined self-involvement and self-determination. Misinterpretations of self-determination were reviewed to enable the reader to establish a specific, targeted understanding of the concept. We reviewed research on student involvement in IEP meetings. Generally, researchers have found that, with specific instruction, students became actively involved as participants in IEP meetings. Also, we reviewed research on postschool outcomes of students with different levels of self-determination. We described Peterson, Sedaghat, and colleagues' (2013) continuum of educational programs for fostering self-determination, which provides a scope and sequence across grade levels for delivery of instruction leading to self-determination. Beyond the continuum of programs proposed by Peterson and colleagues, additional programs were reviewed. Finally, self-monitoring was addressed as a way of solidifying self-support and independence in adulthood.

Step	M	T	W	Th	F
Type tasks and appointments into an electronic planner	✓	✓	✓	✓	✓
Check the planner before leaving the house in the morning	✓	✓	✓	✓	✓
Check the planner at hourly intervals throughout the day	✓	✓	✓	✓	✓
Complete tasks and attend all appointments according to the daily schedule	✓	—	—	✓	—
Evaluate before leaving for home that all tasks and appointments have been fulfilled	✓	✓	✓	✓	✓

FIGURE 7.3. Sample self-monitoring checklist for using a day planner.

REVISITING DEMARIUS

"Say what?" Demarius seemed surprised.

"I said, I want you to come with me to the sports academy," Gabriel said.

"I don't go nowhere with strangers," Demarius responded.

"I'm Gabriel. Your grandmother asked that I—"

"My gramma talked to you?" Gabriel interrupted. "Leave me alone!"

"Just come with me, Demarius. Your gramma will meet us at the sports academy."

"You say she's at the sports academy?"

"She's there waiting for us."

"I'm not going nowhere with you. Besides, I know who you are. You're a drug addict."

"I was a drug addict. But I cleaned up. I got my life together. I'm a personal trainer at East Bay Sports Academy. Come on, I'll show you."

"I don't trust a drug addict. I'm not going with you nowhere!"

"This is not about me. It's about you. I need you at the sports academy. I need your help. I got a job for you. You can work after school. People come to work out in the evenings. I can't keep up. I need your help."

Demarius paused. "You're tellin' me that my gramma sent you here to talk to me and you have a job for me? And I'm supposed to believe some drug addict?"

"I got my life together. Your gramma wants you to get yours together."

"My life is fine."

"Really? What you doin' with your time? Hanging out? You don't make no money."

"Don't have to make nothin.' Least I ain't makin' some rich guy richer."

"Your gramma wants what's best for you. She wants you to be your own man and pay your own way. That's what my gramma wanted for me. It turned my life around. Now it's your turn. Let's go." Gabriel started walking.

"Wait a minute. You lived with your gramma? What did she say to you?"

"She said 'Get a job and stay in school because you can't live on the street.' "

"You believe that?"

"What?" Gabriel looked at Demarius, speaking in a high-pitched voice, "Now you're asking what a drug addict believes?"

"Well," Demarius started, "I'll walk to the sports academy. But only to tell my gramma she shouldn't trust you."

EXERCISE 7.3

Consider the following scenario. Abdul is a 21-year-old male with Prader–Willi syndrome and mild intellectual disabilities who exhibits problem behaviors (e.g., darting, physical aggression, and noncompliance). His transition teacher has been working with him on ways to express what he wants without engaging in these behaviors and has been using a self-determination curriculum to help him plan for his future. During this process, Abdul made considerable progress in reducing his problematic behaviors and indicated that he would like to work in a library after his transition from school. He has a waiver for adult services with a service provider agency and is assigned a case service coordinator. The last time the service coordinator saw

Abdul was during an episode of physical aggression and noncompliance. The special education teacher invited the case service coordinator to Abdul's transition planning meeting. During the meeting, Abdul expressed his desire to work in a library. After the meeting, the case service coordinator pulled the special educator aside and expressed concerns about Abdul's behavior. She stated some hesitations in placing him in community employment and, specifically, the library option. Consider these questions: What strategies can transition professionals use to educate other professionals, such as the case coordinator, about self-determination and student involvement? About Abdul's desire to work in a library?

WEBSITES WITH ADDITIONAL INFORMATION

Possible Selves

www.ku.crl.org

Self-Determination Strategies

www.proedinc.com/customer/productView.aspx?ID=5150

Student-Led IEPs

http://journals.cec.sped.org/tecplus/vol3/iss5/art4

STEPS to Self-Determination

www.proedinc.com/customer/productView.aspx?ID=3601

ChoiceMaker Series

http://store.cambiumlearning.com/choicemaker-self-determination-series

411 on Disability Disclosure

www.transcen.org

Self-Directed IEP

http://store.cambiumlearning.com/ProgramPage.aspx?parentId=19005526&functionID=009000008& site=sw

Take Charge for the Future (TAKE CHARGE)

http://nsttac.org

Whose Future Is It Anyway?

www.ou.edu/education/centers-and-partnerships/zarrow/trasition-education-materials/whos-future-is- it-anyway.htm

CHAPTER 8

Transition to Employment

with TASHINA MEAKER

This chapter addresses . . .

- Types of employment options.
- Research on transition to employment.
- Tools available to assist students in career awareness and exploration.
- Community-based instruction.
- Risk management issues in community-based instruction.
- How transition professionals assist in obtaining employment for youth.

WHAT ARE EMPLOYMENT OPTIONS FOR YOUTH IN TRANSITION?

Employment is a key ingredient defining one's quality of life (National Organization on Disability, 2004). Several avenues lead to obtaining and maintaining employment for individuals with disabilities, including competitive integrated, supported, and customized employment. We describe each below.

Competitive Integrated Employment

As mentioned in Chapter 3, the Workforce Innovation and Opportunity Act (WIOA, 2014) amended the Rehabilitation Act of 1973 and provided a number of key definitions related to the employment of people with disabilities. WIOA defines competitive

---

Tashina Meaker, MS, is a special education teacher at Logan High School, Logan, Utah.

integrated employment as work performed on a full- or part-time basis, including self-employment, that (1) is compensated at least at minimum wage, (2) is in a location where the employee interacts with people who do not have disabilities, and (3) presents opportunities for advancement similar to those available to employees without disabilities (Public Law 113-128 § 404, 2014).

Supported Employment

WIOA defines supported employment as competitive integrated employment or employment in an integrated work setting in which individuals are working on a short-term basis toward competitive integrated employment. Supported employment involves an integrated community job where an individual is paid at minimum wage or better and is supported by a job coach. Although the goal is for the supported employee to work independently, the assumption is that long-term support may be necessary. Job coaches may work for school districts or ASP agencies. Students can begin supported employment in high school and continue after high school.

Customized Employment

Although WIOA (2014) includes customized employment within supported employment, important distinctions are made between the two models. *Customized employment* refers to developing an individualized relationship between an employee and employer to meet the needs of both parties. WIOA states that "customized employment means competitive integrated employment, for an individual with significant disability that is based on an individualized determination of the strengths, needs, and interest of the individual with a significant disability, is designed to meet the specific abilities of the individual with a significant disability and the business needs of the employer and is carried out through flexible strategies" (WIOA, Public Law 113-128 § 404 [7], 2014). Flexible strategies include job carving (i.e., performing selected job tasks), customized job descriptions, and using services of a professional to facilitate placement.

According to Griffin, Hammis, Geary, and Sullivan (2008), the hallmarks of customized employment are (1) identifying specific job duties or employer expectations to be negotiated; (2) targeting individualized job goals based on needs, strengths, and interests of the employment seeker; (3) meeting the needs of both the employment seeker and the employer; (4) starting with the individual as the source of potential employment options; and (5) finding employment in integrated environments of the community at prevailing wages (p. 135).

IS EMPLOYMENT AN OUTCOME FOR ALL STUDENTS WITH DISABILITIES?

Many states have adopted Employment First policies requiring that integrated employment placements be the first option for individuals with disabilities, including those requiring significant supports (Hoff, 2013). This policy means that there is an expectation for stakeholders who assist students with disabilities to first attempt their transition to integrated employment. As of 2015, there were 32 states with formal policy actions and 46 states with some type of policy action related to Employment First (Association of People Supporting Employment First [APSE], 2015). Because of policies like Employment First, it becomes increasingly important to provide instruction and support strategies that promote integrated employment for all students with disabilities. In addition, given strategies such as supported employment, customized employment, and self-employment, more students requiring significant supports can be employed in integrated community businesses (McDonnell, 2010; Wehman, 2011). Realistically, employment may not be an outcome for some students because of profound/multiple disabilities or health impairments. However, with high expectations and consistent support from stakeholders, one of the employment options may be viable for students who were considered unemployable in previous generations.

WHAT ARE RESEARCH FINDINGS ON TRANSITION TO EMPLOYMENT?

Researchers have consistently demonstrated that participation in variety of work experiences during high school is one of the most consistent and reliable predictors of postschool employment for youth with disabilities (e.g., Benz et al., 2000; Carter et al., 2010). Moreover, Luecking (2009) reported that students with disabilities who participated in community-based employment preparation showed improved self-esteem and an understanding of the workplace culture and expectations. Employment experiences can consist of various options, including job shadowing (touring and observing jobs), community-based job sampling (rotations through different jobs while receiving instruction), and participating in paid employment during high school, vocational education, or work–study experiences. Researchers have recommended community-based employment experiences, especially for students requiring significant supports (Mank, Cioffi, Yovanoff, & Taylor, 2003).

WHAT ARE CAREER AWARENESS AND DEVELOPMENT?

Career theorists explain how and why people choose careers. Frank Parsons (1909), one of the most notable early theorists, surmised that career awareness and exploration involved considering the person, examining work settings, and making a match. Parsons wrote:

> In the wise choice of a vocation there are three broad factors: (1) a clear understanding of yourself, your aptitudes, interests, ambitions, resources, limitations, and their causes; (2) a knowledge of the requirements and conditions of success, advantages and disadvantages, compensation, opportunities, and prospects in different lines of work; (3) true reasoning on the relations of these two groups of facts. (p. 5)

Parsons's theory was the catalyst for a number of theorists who examined the reasons why individuals choose work. Contemporary theorists have suggested that career development (1) occurs over the lifespan (Super, 1980), (2) is based on congruence between personality types and work environments (Holland, 1996), and (3) is based on the mutual interaction between the individual and the work environment (Dawis & Lofquist, 1984). Most contemporary career theorists did not explicitly include individuals with disabilities in their theory. We believe that future research should explore the process of career development for youth and young adults with disabilities. Research in this area is important because one common thread in contemporary career theories is that the type of employment one chooses is based on life experiences, exposure to different work opportunities, and a strong match between employment interests and skills. Many theories reinforce the notion that career development is not a static, one-time event, but rather an ongoing process. This assumption underscores the importance of exposing students with disabilities to a wide range of meaningful work and employment-related experiences throughout the transition years. High school students with disabilities may need substantial coursework and meaningful experience in community-based employment environments to be prepared for careers.

WHAT IS THE PREFERRED TIMELINE FOR CAREER AWARENESS AND EXPLORATION?

During transition years, students with disabilities should engage in various career exploration experiences, develop skills to adapt to the social and environmental demands of a job, and learn the essential functions of each job. Each of these experiences should accumulate to help students develop a career pathway. The earlier a student with a disability starts the career development process, the better the prospects for successful employment (Cimera, Burgess, & Bedesem, 2014; Test et al., 2009).

In Figure 8.1, we provide a timeline showing when specific work-related activities should ideally occur. As illustrated, career awareness should start as early as middle school, followed by career exploration activities and job shadowing in 10th grade.

Each career awareness and exploration experience can be documented using a student portfolio. Students can collate documents, photos, and videos into their portfolio

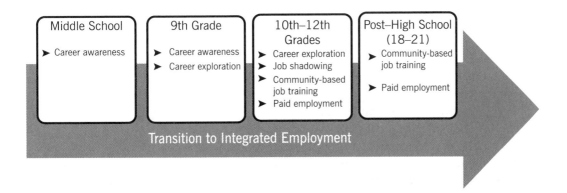

FIGURE 8.1. Timeline for work experiences for transition-age students.

and place them in their summary of performance file. (The summary of performance is described in Chapter 5.) Early career awareness experiences allow students with opportunities to identify different types of careers and specific roles, responsibilities, and tasks of individuals working in those environments. During the middle school years, educators can help students explore different career options by visiting employment sites, overseeing job-shadowing activities (i.e., tours of job sites with youth observing tasks and their functions), inviting employers to class so that they can describe their occupations, and teaching work-related behaviors. In late middle or early high school years, students can begin researching and compiling information on specific occupations, enrolling in career classes, and engaging in community-based instruction. The ultimate goal of a coordinated career development plan is to equip students with the information and skills necessary to obtain meaningful paid employment prior to exiting school.

WHAT TOOLS ARE AVAILABLE FOR STUDENT CAREER EXPLORATION?

The Occupation Information Network (O*NET; *www.onetonline.org*), a database sponsored by the U.S. Department of Labor, can be used to compile occupation-specific information. The O*NET database contains hundreds of occupation descriptors usable as a career exploration tool. O*NET defines key features of an occupation, such as the day-to-day aspects of the job, qualifications and interests, and national and state wage data. An interesting feature is a web-based interactive tool called *My Next Move* (*www. mynextmove.org*), which allows individuals to explore over 900 careers and review information on skills, tasks, salaries, and employment outlook. My Next Move asks students what they would like to do and allows them to search careers by key words, browse occupations by industry, or complete an interest profiler to help focus on specific occupations. The profiler contains 60 questions about the type of work the student enjoys. Once the questions are answered, the profiler generates results. My Next Move provides information on the student's work and RIASEC personality code (Holland et al., 1997). RIASEC stands for *realistic, investigative, artistic, social, enterprising,* and *conventional.* Holland and colleagues (1997) developed this code to identify six different personality types. In Table 8.1, we provide information on the RIASEC code.

My Next Move provides information on five job zones that are groups of careers requiring the same level of experience, education, and training. Job zones range from 1 (little or no work-related skill, high school status or GED required) to 5 (extensive preparation, graduate education required). Finally, My Next Move provides a list of careers that align with the RIASEC code and job zone, providing detailed information about the knowledge, skills, abilities, personality, technology, education, salary, and job outlook. This information can be used to help the student and the IEP team to identify potential job-shadowing and training opportunities.

The My Next Move profiler is appropriate for students who can read with or without an accommodation and can generalize written material to applied settings. The tool can also be used to help teachers think about how to carve (i.e., modify) or negotiate jobs for students with profound disabilities. That is, some students requiring significant supports may not be able to utilize the report as presented by O*NET and instead need

TABLE 8.1. RIASEC Code Definitions

Personality type	Definition	Types of occupations
Realistic	People like work that includes practical, hands-on problems and answers.	Skilled trades (plumber, electrician, machine operator); technician skills (mechanic, photographer, drafting, park ranger).
Investigative	People like work that has to do with ideas and thinking rather than physical activities or leading people.	Chemist, physicist, mathematician, laboratory technician, computer programmer.
Artistic	People like work such as acting, music, art, and design.	Sculptor, painter, designer; teacher or musician; writer, editor, critic.
Social	People like working with others to help them learn and grow.	Teacher, educational administrator, college professor, social worker, sociologist, rehabilitation counselor.
Enterprising	People like starting and carrying out business projects.	Managerial positions, sales, lawyer, travel agent.
Conventional	People like work that follows a set pattern of procedures and details rather than ideas.	Clerical worker, librarian, bank teller.

Note. From *www.mynextmove.org/explore/ip.*

applied experiences to gain information about employment. Teachers of such students can use My Next Move to identify basic job requirements. Once initial information is obtained, the teacher and the student can engage in community-based job exploration by conducting informational interviews with members of community businesses. The purpose of these interviews is to learn more about jobs and determine if there are job carving or job creation possibilities within a specific business.

CASE EXAMPLE

Jerry is a 16-year-old student with IDD. Jerry obtained an IQ score of 65 on the Wechsler Adult Intelligence Scale—Fourth Edition (WAIS-IV; Wechsler, 2008), a standard score of 45 on the Comprehensive Assessment of Spoken Language (CASL; Carrow-Woolfolk, 1999), and a standard score of 47 on the Expressive Vocabulary Test, Second Edition (EVT-2; Williams, 2007). Jerry has good receptive language skills but has some expressive language delays. His teacher has been helping him explore a variety of career options. Because of his love for animals, Jerry expressed interest in working in a veterinary office. The transition teacher assisted Jerry with My Next Move by researching the requirements for jobs working with animals and found information on *Veterinary Technologists and Technicians*. The following information was provided:

VETERINARY TECHNOLOGISTS AND TECHNICIANS

What they do:
Perform medical tests in a laboratory for use in the treatment and diagnosis of diseases in animals; prepare vaccines and serums for prevention of diseases; prepare tissue samples, take blood samples, and execute laboratory tests, such as urinalysis and blood counts; clean and sterilize instruments and materials; and maintain equipment and machines. May assist a veterinarian during surgery.

On the job, they:
- Care for and monitor the condition of animals recovering from surgery.
- Maintain controlled drug inventory and related logbooks.
- Administer anesthesia to animals under the direction of a veterinarian, and monitor animals' responses to anesthetics so that dosages can be adjusted.

Knowledge

Business
- Customer service
- Administrative service

Arts and Humanities
- English language

Math and Science
- Biology
- Arithmetic, algebra, geometry, calculus, or statistics

Health
- Medicine and dentistry

Skills

Basic Skills
- Listening to others, not interrupting, and asking good questions.
- Thinking about the pros and cons of different ways to solve problems.

Problem Solving
- Noticing problems and figuring out the best way to solve it.

Abilities

Verbal
- Communicate by speaking.
- Listen and understand what people say.

Ideas and Logic
- Notice when problems happen.
- Use rules to solve problems.

Hand and Finger Use
- Put together small parts with your fingers.
- Hold or move items with your hands.

Attention
- Do two or more things at the same time.

Personality

People interested in this work like activities that include practical hands-on problems and solutions. They do well at jobs that need cooperation, attention to detail, dependability, integrity, self-control, and initiative.

Technology

You might use software like this:

Medical Software
- Animal intelligence software
- McAllister Software systems®

Data Base User Interface and Query Software
- Filemaker Pro®
- Microsoft Access®

Spreadsheet software
- Microsoft Excel®

Education	Job Outlook
Associates degree or high school diploma or GED.	Bright: New job opportunities are very likely in the future. Salary: about $30,500 per year.

Jerry may have difficultly performing many of the essential functions outlined in the My Next Move description. However, he is passionate about working with animals and has numerous strengths and skills that would benefit a veterinarian. For example, Jerry stated that he occasionally gets paid to independently care for dogs and cats (walking dogs, cleaning animal waste, feeding and watering, and administering oral pet medication) while neighbors are out of town. He is meticulous and maintains clean living environments.

Customized employment is one option for Jerry. In this case, the customized employment process requires conducting informational interviews of members of animal-themed businesses to determine if there is a potential to carve or create a position for Jerry.

EXERCISE 8.1

Based on this information, how would you advise Jerry about his desire to work with animals? What might he need to learn? What courses should he take? Are there ways you might expose Jerry to different roles and responsibilities of working with animals? Can you think of ways to carve or create a position in a veterinarian office or other animal businesses? Are there other types of jobs working with animals that he might pursue? Is self-employment an option?

HOW CAN TRANSITION PROFESSIONALS USE JOB SHADOWING AS AN EXPLORATION TOOL?

Job shadowing is an important career development tool because it allows students to see first hand what tasks a professional performs (Test et al., 2006). Job shadowing can involve individual or small-group activities and can last a few hours, all day, or multiple days. Site selection should be based on information obtained from job preference assessment/interest inventories of students and should be structured to provide them with the opportunity to explore all aspects of occupations. Transition professionals (either teachers or transition specialists) should oversee job-shadowing activities, including scheduling, keeping records of student job- shadowing sites and contacts, and obtaining feedback from employers (see Figure 8.2).

Students should be actively engaged in selecting employers to job-shadow and developing questions to ask employers. Specific questions for employers may include:

"On a typical day in this position, what does the worker do?"
"What training or education is required for this type of work?"
"What personal qualities or abilities are important to being successful in this job?"
"What part of this job do you find most satisfying? Most challenging?"

JOB SHADOW FEEDBACK FORM		
Student: _____ Date of Job Shadow: _____		
Job Shadow Site: _____ Phone: _____ Email: _____		
Job Shadow Contact: _____		
1. Did you have any concerns or comments about the student's behavior?	Yes	No
2. Would you be willing to have another student job-shadow?	Yes	No
3. Would you like to be a job training or internship site for students?	Yes	No

FIGURE 8.2. Job Shadow Workplace Supervisor Feedback Form.

From *Promoting Successful Transition to Adulthood for Students with Disabilities* by Robert L. Morgan and Tim Riesen. Copyright 2016 by The Guilford Press. Permission to photocopy this figure is granted to purchasers of this book for personal use only (see copyright page for details). Purchasers can download a larger version of this figure (see the box at the end of the table of contents).

"How did you get your job?"

"What opportunities for advancement are there in this field?"

"What is the salary range for this position?"

"How do you see jobs in this field changing in the future?"

"Is there a demand for people in this occupation?"

"What types of training do companies offer persons entering this field?"

Students should also complete a Job Shadow Worksheet (see example in Figure 8.3) to be reviewed and discussed with the transition educator. Students can use the information to identify tasks and features of employment they like and dislike.

An important component of a comprehensive job-shadowing program is soliciting employer feedback. The feedback should be shared with the student, used to target skills needing instruction, and maintain positive relationships with each employer.

HOW DO TRANSITION PROFESSIONALS DEVELOP COMMUNITY EMPLOYMENT SITES?

Developing community-based sites requires transition professionals to spend time visiting places of employment. The purpose of these visits is to build partnerships with businesspersons. While meeting with employers, transition professionals should clearly articulate the purpose and benefit of community-based vocational activities; that is, to teach work-related skills by allowing students to receive on-site training. The benefit to the employer is advertisement to the community that the business promotes job instruction for youth with disabilities.

Transition professionals should answer employer questions related to liability. Generally, as long as there is a clear and explicit training goal in the student's IEP, unpaid job training is considered an extension of school and the school district is liable. However, it is a good idea to check with school administration to get an accurate description of the policy on liability. Further information regarding liability is provided later in this chapter.

When employers allow students to participate in unpaid job training, transition professionals should outline roles, responsibilities, and general supervision. The National Center on Secondary Education and Transition (NCSET; 2005) developed an agreement form that highlights roles, responsibilities, and expectations (see *www.ncset.org/publications/essentialtools/flsa/NCSET_EssentialTools_FLSA.pdf*). The form should be reviewed and signed by the student, employer, and parents prior to engaging in unpaid job training. An agreement should be developed for each student participating in nonpaid job training. At a minimum, the agreement should ensure that employers, students, and parents understand and agree to the following:

- The employer derives no financial benefit from the activities of the student.
- The student does not displace a regular employee and is closely supervised.
- All parties understand that the student is not entitled to receive any wages during the agreement time.
- All parties understand that the student is not entitled to a job at the end of the experience (NCSET, 2005).

JOB SHADOW WORKSHEET

Student: _____   Date of Job Shadow: _____

Job Shadow Site: _____

Job Shadow Contact: _____   Number of Hours on the Job Shadow: _____

Experience Summary

1. What type of job did you observe? _____

_____

2. What types of job tasks did the employee complete? _____

_____

3. Where tasks do you think you would enjoy completing? _____

_____

4. What tasks do you think you would not enjoy completing? _____

_____

5. What type of training or education is required for the job you observed? _____

_____

FIGURE 8.3. Job Shadow Worksheet.

WHAT RISK MANAGEMENT ISSUES SHOULD BE CONSIDERED?

Risk management refers to identifying, assessing, and prioritizing risks to minimize problems (Hubbard, 2009). With ever-tightening school budgets and increased rates of litigation, school administrators are understandably concerned about minimizing risks. For some administrators, conducting instruction in a community may signal increased risk. There are numerous uncontrolled variables that make it potentially risky. The prospect of injuring oneself, getting lost, or encountering other hazards makes it necessary for educators to be diligent and well prepared. Transition educators should carefully prepare proposals to administrators by showing that they will minimize risks in community activities. Educators need to communicate to administrators that they will account for all predictable problems and that remaining ones are no more likely than if students had stayed in the school building. Transition educators should consider the following:

- Parents/guardians should provide written, informed consent regarding all community settings to be visited along with activities at each site, transportation to be used, and at least general information about the types of employees their youth will likely encounter. Copies of written consent should remain in the student's file and be sent to parents/guardians.

- What the student is learning, what ITP goal it is related to, and where it will be learned should be specified in a written ITP and signed off by the parent/guardian. All community activities must be related to clearly linked ITP goals. Students should not be taught in community settings unless there is a written rationale and signed consent (Test et al., 2006).

- Transition professionals should closely examine school liability insurance policies for coverage. Educators and students are usually covered by school liability policies even when they go to community sites. However, work-based learning activities sponsored by community businesses or campus-based activities compel transition professionals to check liability policies. Ensure coverage before initiating community activities.

- Transition educators should bring to community settings information on student health conditions, medications, and treatment procedures. Parents should provide written consent so that staff members accompanying students to community settings have access to relevant health records. All records must remain secure and in the possession of supervising staff. Educators should also hold the names and communications for emergency contact individuals.

- All staff accompanying students to community settings should receive training in emergency procedures (e.g., administration of cardiopulmonary resuscitation [CPR], evacuation, and any other pertinent procedures).

- Community activities must comply with limitations placed by the FLSA described in Chapter 3. In a nutshell, students can participate in community employment training if it is beneficial to them and is associated with their ITPs. However, if the work of students is benefiting a company or organization, the student must be compensated. Also, there are time limits placed on training activities.

- Staff working with students in the community must be trained to a level of competency in supervising students. Competencies should include delivering instruction, accounting for student whereabouts, and responding to emergencies. Intermittently, supervisors should directly observe staff in community settings. Also, staff should know emergency policies and procedures adopted by the organization serving as the site for community activities.

- Students with disabilities should be taught to recognize safety hazards and respond by reporting the hazard to a supervisor (Morgan & Salzberg, 1992). This training lesson should occur immediately upon entering the community setting, and training should continue until each student demonstrates mastery. Researchers found that students requiring significant supports can learn hazard recognition and work safety skills (Martella & Marchand-Martella, 1995).

- Students with disabilities and their supervising staff should wear safety equipment at all times as required in particular work environments. Transition professionals should ask employers about the wearing of required safety equipment.

WHAT IS COMMUNITY-BASED INSTRUCTION?

To adequately prepare students with disabilities for the postschool employment world, especially students requiring significant supports, community-based instruction (CBI) is necessary. As McDonnell (2010) stated, "Researchers have recognized for years that instruction for students with disabilities should be anchored to real-life situations and the applied problems that they will face as employees and citizens" (p. 173). Researchers have demonstrated the importance of using CBI to teach functional employment skills to students with disabilities (Bates, Cuvo, Miner, & Korabek, 1999; Cihak, Alberto, Kessler, & Taber, 2004). McDonnell cited two reasons for CBI. First, it makes the school curriculum relevant. That is, it demonstrates to students the real-world applications of lessons learned in school. Second, it assists in generalizing skills that students learn in school to the demands of the community (p. 173). Those students who know how to get around town, ask for help when needed, request services, fill out job and college applications, socialize with others, and perform tasks independently are better equipped to work and learn in their communities than those who do not have experience. Similar community skills, such as crossing streets, finding items in a supermarket, and navigating a college campus, are best taught in the environments in which skills are displayed.

We believe that CBI may have additional benefits. It teaches students about the complexity and dynamics of a community environment. Students realize the importance of adaptability and learning skills to a mastery level. For example, after students use a few ATM machines, they soon learn that there are subtle but important differences in how to operate them. Card entry points, keyboards, and display boards vary across machines. Students must be alert and adapt to differences. Also, CBI sends an important message to the business community that schools are committed to on-site training of relevant employment skills to students. Finally, CBI demonstrates to employers the skills that students with disabilities possess and how they can learn.

One of the authors recently observed a 21-year-old student requiring significant supports get hired for a job because the employer was impressed with his skills and motivation to learn. The student was receiving CBI at the employer's place of work. The hire would not have occurred if the transition professional had merely presented the student's resumé and described the student's interest to the employer. Being involved in CBI at the site sealed the deal.

Westling, Fox, and Carter (2015) stressed that CBI offers a promising approach for sampling different aspects of community life and helping students develop preferences about what they want to do. CBI allows students with disabilities to sample environments associated with adult activities such as jobs and college courses, as well as recreational, civic, service, and leisure opportunities. Because typical high school students and adults without disabilities are actively engaged in these environments for substantial periods of time, CBI allows students with disabilities an equal opportunity. The challenge, of course, is to infuse CBI into courses of study for students. We address this issue later in the chapter.

Five Principles of CBI

McDonnell (2010) described five principles of CBI for students with disabilities in transition to adulthood. Although future research is needed to establish an evidence base, we think each of these principles deserves emphasis here.

1. Expected outcomes of CBI should reflect the values, preferences, and expectations of individual youth and their families.
2. CBI is most effective when it is done in the neighborhoods and communities where students live rather than where their schools are located, because it allows students to practice their skills in familiar environments.
3. The effectiveness of CBI may be increased if students are supported by peer tutors.
4. The complexity and demands of CBI require that instructional time and staff resources be focused on establishing reliable performance in community settings.
5. CBI must be designed to build on the natural supports offered by peers, family members, coworkers, or community members. (pp. 174–175)

WHAT IS COMMUNITY PRESENCE?

The concept of community presence is basic: It means sharing community locations with others who do not have disabilities in order to produce reciprocal interaction (O'Brien & Lyle, 1987). Similar to the concept of school inclusion, community presence supports opportunities for individuals with disabilities to live, work, recreate, and be educated in community environments (Test et al., 2006). Simulated activities in schools and on computers can teach skills to students, but they do not facilitate interaction with people, places, and things in the community. Actively participating in community environments makes students in transition an integral part of the community as active participants who assume rights and responsibilities. Learning in the community brings with it risks, uncertainties, and trepidations, so learners must be alert at all times. We view learning in the community as a natural and vital opportunity for students with disabilities.

Transition professionals can establish a community presence. In some cases, they should establish themselves in the community in advance of youth with disabilities by assessing environments and advocating for community settings as learning environments. To establish community presence, professionals must be strategic. When working with community organizations and businesses, they must answer the question "What's in it for the organization/business?" And in many cases, the answer is that having students present in the organization/business fulfills a need or solves a problem. Not only can students learn valuable skills, but they may also fulfill a need or solve a problem that otherwise might have persisted for the employer. Consider an example:

CASE EXAMPLE

Mr. Gouviea was shopping one evening with his wife at the local mall. His wife stopped at City Dress Shoppe to look for clothes on sale. While his wife sampled items from the sales racks, Mr. Gouviea struck up a conversation with the manager. Although a sale at the boutique had been successful, the manager explained that customers often returned clothes items to the wrong locations, did not replace items on hangers, and generally left the sales rack areas in disarray. The manager had insufficient sales staff to keep up with the customer activity. Mr. Gouviea, a transition teacher at the high school, had a couple of ideas. First, he had four students in his class who could return items to the correct rack locations and replace them on hangers. They could work individually on different sales racks of City Dress Shoppe so they would not stand out as a "special education class." Second, these four students were working on three-digit subtraction, decimal placement, and computation of percentages, so they could fulfill their math lesson requirements (computing dollars saved on sales items, percent of total price, etc.) while assisting at the boutique. Mr. Gouviea worked out the details with the manager to place students for CBI.

Establishing a community presence may require that transition professionals set the stage by communicating the importance of CBI to a variety of community groups. For example:

- High school alumni and boosters are often willing to help students attending their alma mater. Alumni who become business owners may be willing to assist students with disabilities in CBI because a connection already exists (i.e., allegiance to the school).
- Chambers of commerce often have projects to assist the community. Educators can contact chamber members and ask about opportunities for students with disabilities to fulfill community functions while learning skills.
- Communities often have volunteer projects whose organizers may be interested in providing opportunities for students with disabilities. Although volunteer

projects do not represent employment, they may be good starting points for CBI. Educators should contact organizers.

EXERCISE 8.2

Answer the following questions:

- How could transition professionals in your area establish a community presence?
- In your community, what activities could be developed for student involvement?

HOW DO TRANSITION EDUCATORS SCHEDULE CBI?

One of the most frequently asked questions is how to schedule CBI, given that transition educators are often faced with course demands and limited scheduling flexibility. Scheduling CBI requires that transition educators first assess their school priorities. To help plan for CBI, we offer the following recommendations to educators.

1. Create master schedules for each student with consideration to IEP/ITP goals and programs of study (see the example in Figure 8.4). Start with students who exhibit problem behavior and/or students who are medically fragile because they demand the most staff resources.
2. Write school events (lunch, assemblies, therapy services, etc.) into the master schedule.
3. Identify staff who work with individual students each period. At this stage, the schedules should reveal periods of the day when CBI could be arranged.
4. Color-code the master schedule according to physical location (setting). Include all community locations and consider time in transit to/from school.
5. Require teachers and staff to keep the master schedule with them at all times because it identifies locations and activities of both students and their supervisors. Make sure the master schedule includes staff cell phones, business phones, etc.
6. Teach the students to describe details in their daily schedule. Quiz them on details. Use pictures if necessary to facilitate student comprehension.
7. Code student ITP goals into the schedule to emphasize the importance of CBI.

Transportation to the Community

A significant barrier to community participation for youth with disabilities is often transportation (Test et al., 2006). The ideal community location for CBI is one that is on a bus or train route. Even when an ideal location exists, catching a bus, transferring at the bus station, conducting CBI at a site, then reversing the process to get back to school can take considerable time. Despite these issues, whenever possible, transition professionals should rely on transportation systems that will remain available when students exit from school services so that they can get around as adults (McDonnell, 2010). School

Student	1st hour	2nd hour	3rd hour	4th hour	Lunch	5th hour	6th hour	7th hour
Andy	News-2-You *Heather*	Language Arts *Alyssa*	Math *Tammy*	Reading *Javier*	Lunch	Vocational *Mikayla*	Ceramics *Erasto*	CBI *Breanna*
Isadora	News-2-You *Heather*	Language Arts *Lochan*	Math *Sierra*	Reading *Javier*	Lunch	CBI *Raul*	CBI *Raul*	CBI *Breanna*
Matthew	CBI *Raul*	Language Arts *Lochan*	Physical Education *PE Staff*	Reading *Javier*	Lunch	Ceramics *Pulotu*	Social Skills *Tawni*	Math *Tammy*
Michelle	CBI *Raul*	CBI *Raul*	Math *Tammy*	Reading *Javier*	Lunch	Vocational *Mikayla*	Ceramics *Erasto*	Social Skills *Tawni*
Megan	News-2-You *Heather*	Language Arts *Lochan*	Math *Tammy*	Reading *Javier*	Lunch	Employment	Employment	Employment

FIGURE 8.4. Example of a master schedule. Color-code according to location.

buses or school-owned vehicles are probably more efficient, but their availability may be limited and they will no longer exist when students leave the school system. Local transportation or taxi companies may be interested in providing free transportation directly to CBI sites in exchange for media about their efforts to assist youth. Parents and family members may be valuable resources in transporting youth to or from community sites. They can transport students efficiently and economically, although appropriate permissions must be signed and insurance liability established upfront (Test et al., 2006).

WHAT SKILLS ARE TARGETED AND HOW ARE THEY TAUGHT IN COMMUNITY SETTINGS?

The skills targeted for instruction depend on the job tasks and the skills needed by the student. In addition to job tasks, community employment settings require that employees (and youth) adhere to rules set by the employer. These rules may not be explicit; they are often implied and relate to "soft skills" in the workplace, such as following instructions and accepting correction. In Table 8.2, we list and describe research on soft skills.

Transition professionals should first observe students performing job tasks to determine how proficient they are and, if necessary, develop instructional programs. Many employment activities can be divided into a task analysis. Such an analysis involves breaking a job task down into smaller, teachable steps. (See Chapter 5 for information on task analyses.) In Figure 8.5, we provide an example of a task analysis for making a deep-dish pizza.

WHAT INFORMATION SHOULD BE INCLUDED IN AN INSTRUCTIONAL PROGRAM?

After a transition professional has collected data in one or more observations using a task analysis, he or she can develop an instructional program. An instructional program should include an objective, stimuli, response prompting and fading procedures, and data collection procedures. One common problem in CBI is the lack of clear instructional objectives. Without clear objectives, students may simply rotate through job training sites and not acquire new skills leading to potential employment outcomes. Clear objectives allow the transition team to monitor progress and move to other tasks when the student achieves the objective criterion. Each objective should be written in terms that are both observable and measurable. The objective should include the conditions under which the skill will be performed and criteria to evaluate performance. Consider an objective written for a student training at a take-out pizza store: *Given a deep-dish pizza pan, a 4-ounce ladle, and a 6-ounce cheese cup, Jerry will independently make a pepperoni deep-dish pizza with 100% accuracy for five consecutive pizzas according to the steps outlined in the task analysis.*

TABLE 8.2. Examples of "Soft Skills" in the Workplace

Name and definition of skill	Research citation
Following directions: making eye contact, acknowledging the direction, performing all tasks within 10 seconds of a supervisor's instruction, then returning to announce completion of direction.	Chadsey-Rusch & Gonzalez (1996)
Accepting criticism: Turning one's body toward the supervisor, keeping eye contact, talking with a normal voice, responding with head nods, and expressing willingness to correct the problem.	Eckert (2000)
Asking questions (for clarification on tasks): Approaching a supervisor, saying "Excuse me," and using a question and specific language to seek clarification about how to perform a task.	Chadsey-Rusch, Karlan, & Riva (1984)

Student Alias: _Jerry_   Date: _2/21_

Measurable Objective: _Given a deep-dish pizza pan, a 4-ounce ladle, and a 6-ounce cheese cup, Jerry will independently make a pepperoni deep-dish pizza with 100% accuracy for five consecutive pizzas, according to the steps outlined in the task analysis._

Settings: _restaurant kitchen_

Materials: _deep-dish pan, pizza dough, 6-ounce cup, sauce, ladle, cheese, pepperoni_

Step #	Stimulus	Task/Response	Speed
1	Prep station and deep pan.	Place square deep-dish pan on prep station.	5 seconds
2	Pizza dough.	Punch dough down into pan with two fingers.	20 seconds
3	Ladle, pizza sauce, deep-dish pan with dough.	Ladle pizza sauce on each deep-dish section (4-ounce ladle) (four "quadrants" of deep dish).	20 seconds
4	Sauce & dough in pan.	Spread sauce evenly on each section with bottom of ladle.	20 seconds
5	Cheese cup, cheese.	Fill 6-ounce cheese cup with cheese.	5 seconds
6	Deep-dish pan.	Evenly spread cheese on each deep-dish section.	20 seconds
7	Quadrants of deep dish.	Place four pepperonis on section 1.	5 seconds
8–10	Quadrants of deep dish.	Place four pepperonis on sections 2–4.	5 seconds each

Teaching procedures: Fade prompts using least-to-most prompt strategy. Begin fading as soon as a student responds independently on a step.

FIGURE 8.5. Example of a task analysis for making a deep-dish pizza.

WHAT ARE RESPONSE PROMPTS?

For some students, especially those with more significant support needs, it may be necessary to provide specific response prompts during instruction. Response prompts are teaching strategies that are presented to increase the probability of a correct response (Wolery, Bailey, & Sugai, 1988). Response prompts are designed to make learning more positive and increase the efficiency of instruction by eliminating student errors. Typically, an array of prompts, called the *prompt hierarchy*, is used to help the student respond correctly. In Table 8.3, we provide an example of the types of response prompts in the hierarchy.

According to Wolery and colleagues (1988), there are four guidelines for using response prompts:

1. *Select the least intrusive but effective prompt.* The educator should allow the student to perform the target response as independently as possible and prompt only if necessary. Use the least intrusive prompt that produces the correct target response.
2. *Select natural prompts and those related to the behavior.* Educators should use prompts that reflect natural events in the work environment. That is, prompts should resemble behaviors that occur naturally in environments.
3. *Prompt only when the student is attending.* Response prompts are designed to assist the student in performing a specific target response; therefore, it is important the student is attending to the task when the educator is delivering the prompt. If the student is not attending, then he or she will not perform the target response.
4. *Provide prompts in a supportive manner.* The purpose of response prompting is not to punish or adversely affect student behavior. Instead, prompts should facilitate learning.

Least-to-Most Prompts Strategy

One common strategy used to teach students with disabilities is called least-to-most (LTM) prompts, which allows students with disabilities to respond at the level of prompt they need to complete the task (Wolery, Ault, & Doyle, 1992). There are two important points when using LTM. First, the student must have the opportunity to respond without a prompt. Second, the educator must use the least prompt necessary to produce the correct response. According to Wolery and colleagues (1992), specific steps should be followed when using the LTM prompting strategy:

1. *Identify the stimulus that cues the individual to respond.* The stimulus should be an environmental cue, such as dirty dishes in a sink or a customer requesting help.
2. *Select the number of levels in the hierarchy.* Include at least three levels of prompts, beginning with independent level and progressing to most assistance.
3. *Select the types of prompts to be used in the hierarchy* (see Table 8.3).
4. *Sequence the LTM prompts.* Begin with independent performance and conclude

TABLE 8.3. Prompt Hierarchy

Prompt	Example
Indirect verbal	Indirect verbal prompts are hints about expected behavior. For example, if a student is learning to mop, the instructor asks, "What do you do now?"
Verbal	Verbal prompts are direct statements that help the student perform the correct response. For example, the instructor says, "You need to mop the floor."
Gesture	Gestures are cues for the student to complete a task. For example, the instructor points to the floor.
Model	A model is a demonstration of the correct behavior. For example, the instructor mops the floor and then asks the student to mop.
Partial physical	A partial physical prompt, if/when appropriate, involves touching the student's hands or arms. For example, the instructor taps the student on the elbow to prompt mopping.
Full physical	A full physical prompt, if/when appropriate, is hand-over-hand assistance so the student performs the behavior. For example, the instructor, with hand over hand, guides the mop.

with the controlling prompt (the prompt with the most assistance that results in the student performing the task).

5. *Determine the length of the response interval.* Allow a sufficient amount of time for the student to respond (e.g., 10 seconds) before providing the next level of prompt.

6. *Provide appropriate feedback for correct (independent) and incorrect (prompted) responses.*

7. *Implement and adjust prompts based on data patterns.* Collect data on performance.

Students should repeat a task until it is performed independently. As students begin to perform tasks on their own, prompts should be systematically faded. Completing a task with prompts from the educator is not a "finished product." Student should learn to recognize natural cues serving as the occasion to perform the task, not perform just because of an educator request. Employers expect employees to complete assigned tasks quickly and independently. Therefore, educators must fade prompts as students learn to independently respond to natural cues.

HOW DOES ONE IMPLEMENT INSTRUCTION AND DATA COLLECTION?

Transition educators should consistently collect data on student performance of community employment tasks. Without systematic data collection, the instructional team is unable to make informed decisions about student progress toward meeting the objective. In Figure 8.6, we provide an example of a data collection system for making a deep-dish pizza. In this example, the instructor documents the prompts needed to complete each step.

After each instructional session, the educator summarizes the student's performance by calculating the percentage of independent (I) student responses. The information can be displayed graphically to track student performance (see Figure 8.7). In this example, the percentage of independent responses is graphically displayed for each teaching session. Graphing data is a useful tool for helping educators make adjustments to an instructional program and determine when the student meets a criterion set for independent performance.

HOW DO TRANSITION PROFESSIONALS ASSIST IN SECURING EMPLOYMENT?

Many of the strategies for securing paid employment for individuals with disabilities come from the field of VR, particularly in the area of supported and customized employment (Brooke, Inge, Amstrong, & Wehman, 1997; Griffin, Hammis, & Geary, 2007). In supported and customized employment, professionals use the term *job development* to describe how to engage employers and place individuals on the job. To develop jobs, transition professionals establish partnerships and create a network of employers. There is a variety of connections that can be used as a starting point for networking, including families, friends, neighbors, past employers, former coworkers, churches, chambers of commerce, clubs, and local businesses.

If a student has identified a preferred job and CBI has resulted in a relatively sound match between the student's skill set and the requirements of that preferred job, the transition professional is ready to assist in securing employment. The student may be able to work part-time after school, on weekends, or during summer. In post–high school programs (for students fulfilling high school requirements during ages 18–21), school schedules can usually be reduced to accommodate work. Transition professionals can assist in securing employment as follows.

- Encourage the student or family to contact employers using the student's network.
- If one's school district or region has a transition specialist or other professional who assists in job placement, contact that professional.
- Contact the local VR office to request an "open case" for the student seeking employment.
- Contact the state agency overseeing developmental disabilities for an application and a referral to an adult service organization (i.e., a community rehabilitation provider) that specializes in job placements.

In any case, understand that supports (in the form of a job coach, coworker, family member, or other) will be necessary for a student to successfully learn the tasks, master the skills, ask questions when necessary, and develop the stamina and endurance

Key: I = Independent   IV = Indirect Verbal   V = Verbal   M = Model   P = Physical

DATA COLLECTION SHEET								
Student: Jerry	Instructional Objective: Given a deep-dish pizza pan, a 4-ounce ladle, and a 6-ounce cheese cup, Jerry will make a pepperoni pizza with 100% accuracy according to the steps outlined in the task analysis for three consecutive probes.							
Steps		**Sessions**						
		1	**2**	**3**	**4**	**5**	**6**	**7**
1. Place square deep-dish pan on prep station.		V	V	IV	I	I	I	I
2. Punch dough down with two fingers.		V	IV	I	IV	I	I	I
3. Ladle pizza sauce on each deep-dish section (4-ounce ladle).		V	V	I	IV	I	I	I
4. Spread sauce evenly on each section with bottom of ladle.		M	V	IV	I	I	I	I
5. Fill 6-ounce cheese cup with cheese.		IV	I	I	I	I	I	I
6. Evenly spread cheese on each deep-dish section.		IV	I	I	I	I	I	I
7. Place four pepperonis on section 1.		V	V	IV	IV	IV	I	I
8. Place four pepperonis on section 2.		V	IV	I	I	I	I	I
9. Place four pepperonis on section 3.		V	I	I	I	I	I	I
10. Place four pepperonis on section 4.		I	I	I	I	I	I	I
% unprompted independent responses		10%	40%	70%	70%	90%	100%	100%

FIGURE 8.6. Example of a data collection sheet.

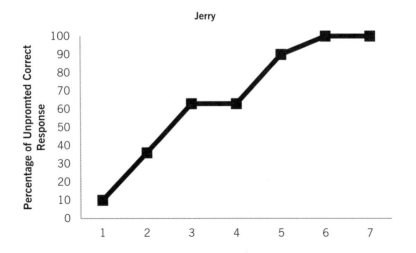

FIGURE 8.7. Example of a graph tracking student performance across seven sessions.

necessary to work for a period of time. Transition educators can assist in ensuring that these supports are in place.

SUMMARY

In this chapter, we examined types of employment options, including competitive integrated, supported, and customized employment. Research on employment of individuals with disabilities was briefly reviewed. We described four stages of career development and timelines for each. Tools for career exploration were described, including O*Net, job shadowing, and CBI. Five reasons for CBI were provided. McDonnell's (2010) principles of CBI were also described. Regarding CBI, we described community presence, scheduling, and transportation. We then described what skills can be targeted and how they can be taught in CBI. Response prompting and data collection were described and illustrated. We stressed the point of fading response prompts so students can perform tasks independently. The role of transition professionals in assisting with employment placement was examined. Finally, risk management issues were considered, along with ways that transition professionals can prepare for them.

REVISITING KENLEY

Kenley's transition planning meeting concluded with the plan to provide him with experience learning about his community through job rotations. In the next year, Kenley tried various jobs, including grocery bagger at Southridge Grocery. He and his family had hoped the experience at the grocery would work out, but Kenley had issues adjusting to bagging and other tasks. He struggled to keep up. Rules for bagging groceries were hard for him to follow, especially when lines formed at the checkout counter, requiring that he bag at a fast pace. Also, when Kenley focused on the bagging rules, he neglected to greet the customers. The manager was reluctant to consider employment after high school. Kenley's brother Ashton had tried to rally support for him, but to no avail.

At the same time, Ashton was going through a transition himself. Having graduated from high school, he had taken some college courses online. The college experience had been quite successful for Ashton. He became interested in a bachelor's degree at a distant college. After he talked to his parents, it was time to break the news to Kenley. As dinner was finishing up, Ashton started nervously.

"Kenley. I need to tell you something."

"OK, brother," Kenley responded.

"Kenley, I'm going away to college. I'm going to move away. I won't be here except when I come home for holidays."

"What?"

"I've been accepted into college. I'm moving away."

"What you say? Move? No. No, no, *no*! You *can't* move!"

Kenley was clearly upset with what he was hearing. It was the last thing he expected from his brother who had always been there for him. When others refused to accept Kenley, Ashton was always at his side.

"Kenley, I'll come visit you. We can talk on the phone. It won't be that different."

"No, no, *no*! You're my *brother*!"

Kenley abruptly stood up and ran out of the house. The words reverberated through Ashton's head. He sat with his elbows on the kitchen table and ran his hands through his hair.

"Look, Ashton, you had to tell him," said Kenley's father, Mr. Schneider. "There's no easy way to do this. He had to hear it. Now he has to get over it."

"But he's right. *I'm* his brother. I've always been here for him. Maybe this is a mistake."

"No! It is not a mistake!" Mr. Schneider retorted loudly. "You need to do this. It is an opportunity for you. My folks didn't go to college and neither did your mom or dad. You're going to college."

"Look, Son," Mrs. Schneider started. "Don't worry about Kenley. We'll be OK. You need to get on with your life. And so does Kenley."

"But, Mom, what will Kenley do?"

EXERCISE 8.3

Research two local businesses in your community. Contact each business and schedule an informational interview. Ask the following questions:

- What is the greatest employment need of [name of the business] at this time?
- Does [name of the business] have any positions open at this time?
- Are there tasks at [name of the business] that are currently not being accomplished?
- Is [name of the business] familiar with transition programs?
- Would [name of the business] being willing to serve as a situational assessment site?
- Has [name of the business] considered allowing students with disabilities to participate in an assessment on the work site (assuming school supervision)?
- What needs does [name of the business] have that might be filled by youth?

What did you learn about each business? About each employer's needs? About how youth with disabilities may fulfill those needs?

WEBSITES WITH ADDITIONAL INFORMATION

National Center on Secondary Education and Transition Agreement Form

www.ncset.org/publications/essentialtools/flsa/NCSET_EssentialTools_FLSA.pdf

Job Accommodation Network

http://askjan.org

O*NET

www.onetonline.org

National Association of Councils on Developmental Disabilities

www.dphhs.mt.gov/dsd/ddp/selndocuments/NationalCouncilonDevelopmentalDisabilities.pdf

The Arc

www.thearc.org/what-we-do/public-policy/policy-issues/employment

National Dissemination Center for People with Disabilities

http://nichcy.org/employment-and-people-with-developmental-disabilities

Real People, Real Jobs

www.realworkstories.org

Federal Jobs Network

www.federaljobs.net/disabled.htm

Disability Job Exchange

www.disabilityjobexchange.com

Ability Jobs

http://abilityjobs.com

Careers for People with Disabilities

http://careersforpeoplewithdisabilities.org/employer-info/types-of-jobs

Center for Reintegration

www.reintegration.com/reint/employment/workplace.asp

National Alliance for Mental Illness

www.nami.org/Content/NavigationMenu/Inform_Yourself/About_Mental_Illness/About_Treatments_and_Supports/Supported_Employment1.htm

CHAPTER 9

Transition to Postsecondary Education

with Scott Kupferman

This chapter addresses . . .

- The rationale for PSE for students with disabilities.
- Characteristics of PSE options.
- Types of PSE programs and how to select compatible ones.
- Differences in expectations in PSE compared to secondary education.
- Preparations needed by students with disabilities to enter or to adapt to PSE.
- Challenges that can be anticipated in PSE.
- Accommodations and Universal Design for Learning.

WHY CONSIDER PSE?

This chapter examines PSE, or "all learning options available to students following high school, including credit and noncredit or continuing education courses in community colleges, four-year colleges, vocational–technical colleges, and other forms of adult education" (Grigal & Hart, 2010, p. 4). In the United States, there has long existed a shared belief that education continues after high school and brings with it rewards of career pathways, self-fulfillment, and quality of life. For many, PSE has been the educational fulcrum where a learner goes from having established foundational knowledge and

Scott Kupferman, PhD, CRC, is an Assistant Professor in the College of Education at the University of Colorado, Colorado Springs.

skills in the K–12 system to exploring new fields and pursuing a career. PSE is a time to test and define oneself. Many of us think of college as a time when we pushed ourselves to the limits and discovered that those outer boundaries were illusory and self-made. We discovered that we could go further. Clearly, those opportunities, trials, and tribulations should be afforded to everyone, including those who are most challenged in learning environments.

Students with sensory disabilities (such as those with deafness, hearing loss, blindness, or low vision) and physical disabilities have been accessing PSE for decades (Kochhar-Bryant et al., 2009). More recently, students with specific learning disabilities, attention-deficit disorder, traumatic brain injury, emotional disturbance, and mental illness have made their way to PSE in increasing numbers (Uditsky & Hughson 2008). But now, students with intellectual disabilities, autism, and other developmental disabilities are also following suit (Grigal & Hart, 2010). Today, individuals of diverse characteristics seek lifelong learning opportunities. However, access to PSE for all students with disabilities can present challenges. This chapter addresses those challenges, particularly for students with developmental disabilities.

As much as any young adult, students with disabilities deserve ongoing, post–high school opportunities to participate in educational experiences with high expectations, rigorous standards, and intense performance requirements. To become contributing citizens of communities, students with disabilities may need additional time and support to maximize their knowledge and hone their skills. PSE for young adults with developmental disabilities was rarely considered until the first generation of children growing up with free and appropriate public education in the least restrictive environment reached college age. Even then, many students found closed doors, closed minds, and plenty of reasons why they were not welcome in college (i.e., failure to meet minimum academic requirements for entrance, low probability of meeting high academic standards in college coursework; Kochhar-Bryant et al., 2009). Some were told to be satisfied with the privileges and rights they had been afforded in previous educational opportunities. Essentially, some were told not to assert themselves or use their creativity and intelligence, even though these traits worked relatively well for their peers without disabilities who received an open door to PSE. As Will (2010) stated:

> Another factor contributing to unemployment and lack of independence for persons with intellectual disabilities lies in the flawed social contract that exists between our society and people with disabilities. The common understanding of this contract is that a person with a disability who needs support should receive public assistance. But in exchange for public assistance, the person with a disability must be contented with a life of enforced poverty and an absence of freedom. . . . For many reasons, postsecondary education is a most important key to shaping a new reality for people with disabilities. It has the exciting potential to create a future based not on low expectations, the can'ts and shouldn'ts, but on the high expectations of productivity and personal and economic freedom. (pp. xi–xii)

For students with disabilities and their families who choose to embrace high expectations, why not consider PSE? There is dignity in taking a risk and exposing oneself to the consequences (Perske, 1972). Despite risk of failure, focusing one's efforts on succeeding in PSE can be a valuable learning experience. For most of us, it is better to have tried than to have made no attempt. Failed attempts, in some situations, generate motivation and exploration of new alternatives. Some youth with disabilities demonstrate incredible persistence and tenacity. Perhaps the real question is whether PSE is ready for students with disabilities.

WHAT EVIDENCE SUPPORTS INVOLVEMENT OF STUDENTS WITH DISABILITIES IN PSE?

Researchers have found that involvement in PSE, even if not associated with attainment of degrees or certification, results in increased employment rates and higher wages for students with disabilities (e.g., Migliore, Timmons, Butterworth, & Lugas, 2012; Moore & Schelling, 2015). Think College (*www.thinkcollege.net*), which serves as a national organization dedicated to inclusive higher education options for people with intellectual disability, reports increased levels of independent living, social connections, and linkages to adult support systems. More research is needed to identify additional benefits to PSE for students with developmental disabilities, how employment was obtained, what types of jobs were acquired (on-campus vs. other), and supports that were needed on jobs.

Research should also address whether strong, well-supported PSE programs result in a "ripple effect" that affects systems. For example, students with developmental disabilities who otherwise would not have considered a PSE program may become energized and motivated to get involved. In turn, their parents may start asking questions and looking into programs. Importantly, schools may be affected as teachers and administrators begin to examine their curricula, policies, and student goals. They may become cognizant of the successes of former students in PSE programs, and say, for example, "If he [she] can do it, maybe. . . ." Finally, communities may begin to question their assumptions of limited expectations of individuals with developmental disabilities. Perhaps entire systems can be positively influenced when PSE programs become accessible.

ARE MORE STUDENTS WITH DISABILITIES ENTERING PSE?

Students with disabilities are entering PSE in increasing numbers. Between 1990 and 2005, students with disabilities increased their involvement 18.8% in 2-year community colleges, 9.1% in 4-year colleges, and 12.8% in vocational, business, and technical schools (Newman et al., 2011). These percentage data relate to all types of disabilities. Prentice (2002) attributed increased involvement to various factors, including enhanced assistive and instructional technology, expanded support services, emphasis on self-determination, and greater public awareness of the capabilities of individuals with disabilities.

Grigal and Neubert (2004) found that parent expectations might be an additional factor. They conducted a survey of 234 parents of secondary-level students with various disabilities in two urban school systems bordering a large metropolitan city. Researchers asked about postschool expectations of parents regarding their students with disabilities. Almost half of the parent respondents identified either 2- or 4-year college as the postgraduation plan for their children with high-incidence disabilities (e.g., specific learning disability, mild intellectual disability, emotional disturbance). For parents of children with low-incidence disabilities (e.g., moderate/severe intellectual disability, multiple disabilities), 21.7% named 2-year college and 36.2% named 4-year college as the postgraduation plan. We should note that growth in PSE involvement occurred during the same general period as legislation supporting college for individuals with disabilities, such as the Americans with Disabilities Act Amendments (ADAA; 2008) and the Higher Education Opportunity Act (HEOA, 2008).

WHAT ARE COLLEGE-BASED PROGRAMS FOR STUDENTS WITH DISABILITIES?

There are circumstances in which students with disabilities, particularly those who are highly motivated and resourceful, can succeed in college courses with minimal supports. However, many students with disabilities need specialized and intensive support in at least some aspects of the college experience. Obviously, the type of support varies depending on what the learner needs to be effective in the educational setting of choice. Recognizing this need and in response to Section 504 requirements, institutions of higher education have developed support programs. Two types of supports are described: (1) disability service offices (DSOs), and (2) PSE programs for students with intellectual disability (ID).

Disability Service Offices

Institutions of higher education receiving funding from the federal government must provide reasonable accommodations and physical/program access to students with disabilities. DSOs have many different names (e.g., Disability Resource Centers, Centers for Disability Services). DSOs are charged with the responsibility of conducting assessments and providing reasonable accommodations for students with disabilities. By law, the college student must initiate the request for an accommodation. To do so, the student must disclose a disability. The DSO may ask for an assessment of a developmental disability. The institution can require third-party documentation of the disability (Cory, 2011; Simon, 2011). After an assessment is completed, the DSO works with the student to consider whether accommodations are necessary in the classroom and/or living environments. Once accommodations are finalized, the DSO representative provides a letter to the student describing the needs. In turn, the student must deliver the letter to course instructors, teaching assistants, housing personnel, and others who need to know. At this point, accommodations must be initiated. DSO representatives remain available to consult with instructors or others should accommodation questions arise. Accommodations provided by DSOs are described later in this chapter.

PSE Programs for Students with ID

In recent years, school districts and institutions of higher education have collaborated to produce programs offering more intensive supports to college students with disabilities, particularly students with ID or other developmental disabilities. Think College (*www.thinkcollege.net*) reported there were 229 PSE programs located in 41 states. Grigal, Hart, and Weir (2012) conducted a national survey on PSE programs for students with ID. The surveyed programs provided a range of support services, such as advising, teaching of study skills, and assistance with independent living. They found:

- 40% of programs were located in 2-year colleges, 51% in 4-year colleges, and 10% in trade or technical schools.
- 53% of students accessed courses through the typical college registration process.
- Half the respondents reported that students with ID did not access academic advising or DSO services through the typical college channels, but instead received specialized services offered by program staff.
- 56% of programs were for young adults who had completed K–12 programs, and 22% were dual enrollment (i.e., secondary special education plus college enrollment). Another 22% offered both types of programs.
- 45% of programs indicated that instruction was provided only to students who had ID. The remaining 55% reported some degree of integration with typical college students.
- 81% of programs addressed employment training or career preparation.
- 33% of programs did not provide residential living services, but the remaining programs involved dorms (19%), on-campus apartments (10%), off-campus apartments (19%), fraternity/sorority houses (3%), and special sections of dorms or other housing (4%).
- The majority of programs reported that students with ID did not receive college credit in inclusive college courses (or only in some courses).

Grigal and colleagues (2012) called for increased inclusion of college students with ID and interagency collaboration to support such programs. They noted their survey data captured practices at "a moment in time for a field that is rapidly changing" (p. 232). For more information, go to *www.thinkcollege.net*.

Transition Programs for Students with ID

At about the same time as the Grigal and colleagues (2012) survey, Congress appropriated $10.6 million for model demonstration programs called *transition programs for students with intellectual disability*, or TPSIDs. Five-year grants were awarded to 27 institutions of higher education in the United States to assist students with ID. Each TPSID was required to assist students to transition to (and fully participate in) inclusive higher education leading to gainful employment (Grigal et al., 2013).

According to the 2011–2012 annual report (Grigal et al., 2013), TPSIDs provided services to 792 students, including 90% with ID, 23% with ASD, 13% with specific learning disabilities, 13% with developmental delay, and 12% with other health impairment (multiple diagnoses cause percentages to exceed 100%). These students included 318 who attended a TPSID from the outset and 474 newly enrolled students. The majority (74%) was white, 18% were black, and 9% were Hispanic.

After 2 years of operation, data from TPSIDs indicated relatively high levels of employment and earned wages (Grigal et al., 2013). For example, 30% of students were employed, and about half of the employed students were in their first paying job. At least 82% of jobs paid at or above minimum wage (8% of employed students did not report wages). Over half of employed students reported receiving supports from coworkers (i.e., natural supports) and about one-third reported working with a job coach. Types of jobs varied from a public relations intern at a medical university to a dietary aide at an assistive living facility. Additionally, data indicated that 47% of college courses taken by students were inclusive (Grigal et al., 2013). The remaining 53% of courses were *specialized*, that is, taken only by students in TPSIDs. The majority (58%) of students in inclusive courses earned standard college credit, whereas 86% of students in specialized courses earned credit only toward the TPSID credential. Students averaged just over seven courses per year.

College-Based PSE Programs for Students with Other Disabilities

Inclusive PSE and transition programs exist for students with specific learning disabilities, attention-deficit disorder, emotional disturbance, and mental health issues (Brinckerhoff, McGuire, & Shaw, 2002), although most are small and not highly organized like TPSIDs. College students with these disabilities typically get individual assistance from DSOs or develop their own study groups (Eckes & Ochoa, 2005).

WHAT ARE PSE OPTIONS FOR STUDENTS WITH DEVELOPMENTAL DISABILITIES?

We find that students, parents, and teachers often think of PSE as an undifferentiated category. When asked about PSE options, they might say, "College is not an option because of the significance of the disability." In reality, there are numerous programs and subprograms within the "college" category or any other PSE category that need to be understood before a decision is made. Even as we explored the PSE options in the preceding section, we found that in some institutions of higher education, college courses could be taken for credit, audit, or informally. Courses were sometimes inclusive and other times segregated. Even for an individual student with disabilities participating on a college campus, there are variations in credit options and degree of involvement (Eisenman & Mancini, 2010; Flexer et al., 2013; Grigal, Neubert, & Moon, 2002). Interested students, parents, and teachers must take a closer look. We consider the following PSE options: 4-year college or university, 2-year colleges, vocational–technical colleges, internships/apprenticeships, and community/adult education classes. Each option is summarized in Table 9.1.

TABLE 9.1. PSE Options: Descriptions of Characteristics, Advantages, and Disadvantages

Description	Advantages	Disadvantages
Four-year college or university		
The focus is on students planning to complete a bachelor's degree or graduate school. Admission requires successful completion of high school programs of study, grades, aptitude tests, etc. Some 4-year programs have "open admission" (i.e., open to any student over age 18 with a high school diploma or GED), but most do not. Despite admission requirements, there are usually several "remedial classes" available to develop academic preparation and study skills. Tuition is costly, although may be less for in-state students. Tuition at public institutions is less than private institutions.	Multiple opportunities for integration and inclusion in campus activities. Variety of course offerings. Numerous social groups and organizations. Most 4-year institutions have departments of education and/ or social science, and students majoring in these fields need practical experiences and may be available to assist students with disabilities.	Four-year institutions are less prevalent so accessibility may be limited; relocation may be necessary. Admission requirements may be prohibitive (although check with advisors for alternative routes). Some faculty may view admission of students with disabilities as a compromise to academic rigor and high scholastic standards. High cost of tuition may be prohibitive.
Two-year college		
The focus is on students planning to complete an associate degree or establish a vocational interest. Admission requirements are usually less rigorous than 4-year institutions. Most 2-year colleges are open admission. Students in need of academic preparation can take developmental coursework, although the options are not as plentiful as in 4-year institutions. Two-year colleges are usually nonresidential institutions. Students usually live at home or on their own in the community. There are usually several 2-year colleges available, often located closer to home.	Smaller classes and campus size. Credits usually transfer to 4-year institutions. Tuition is less than universities. Focus is on individual student career development.	Student population is transient (i.e., 2 years maximum). This may limit study partnerships, social interaction, etc.
Vocational–technical colleges		
Specific emphasis is placed on training in one or more technical fields (e.g., trades, business, nursing, data processing, information technology, cosmetology, automotive). Some colleges offer programs leading to an associate degree. Some courses may be offered concurrently with high school programs through CTE. Tuition costs vary widely. Some colleges are private or "for-profit."	Good for students who are certain of career preferences. Because on-the-job training is a focal point, this appeals to hands-on learners.	DSO and support services are often limited. Credits may not transfer to 2- or 4-year colleges. Check tuition costs, as rates vary.

(continued)

TABLE 9.1. *(continued)*

Description	Advantages	Disadvantages
Internships/apprenticeships		
Internships are time-limited, on-the-job training opportunities that permit the intern to sample work. Apprenticeships involve learning on the job under supervision of an expert. Sponsors are usually companies, a public agency, or a union (Pierangelo & Giuliani, 2004, p. 93).	Good for students who are certain of career preferences. On-the-job training is a focal point, so this appeals to hands-on learners.	DSO and support services are often limited or unavailable. Credits may not transfer to 2- or 4-year colleges. Costs vary.
Community/adult education		
Courses may be offered through school districts, community colleges, or volunteer organizations and are usually intended for individuals 16 years and older. Adult education courses are best suited for those with no high school diploma. Course offerings vary and include vocational, recreational, and academically focused ones.	Classes are small and personalized. Students participate based on interest. Good place to start for those who want to sample PSE prior to more involvement. Opportunity to learn specific skills. Inexpensive.	No DSO or support services other than those an instructor may choose to provide. No credential or certificate available. Courses do not offer credit leading to 2- or 4-year colleges.

Students, parents, and teachers should scrutinize various college and PSE options. One size certainly does not fit all. Once again, it comes down to matching student interests and skills with the appropriate setting. If we start with a given student's ITP—specifically, the present level of performance and measurable postsecondary goal—we can compare and contrast options.

HOW DOES ONE SELECT A COMPATIBLE PSE PROGRAM?

Students, parents, and teachers should inquire about various PSE programs. The ease with which answers are obtained from advisors, college instructors, or websites is a good indication of the receptivity of a program. A useful assignment for students interested in PSE is to write answers to questions about the characteristics of PSE programs. The student and the transition team can then examine answers to identify the most compatible program. There are several lists of questions about PSE programs (e.g., Barr, Hartman, & Spillane, 1995; Higher Education Consortium on Learning Disabilities, 1996; Test et al., 2006). We adapt questions from these lists and add our own in Table 9.2.

TABLE 9.2. Questions to Ask about PSE Programs

Question	How to interpret answer
1. Does the PSE program require a high school diploma? Are there any exceptions?	Determine the student's status on these questions.
2. Does admission require an SAT or ACT test? If so, has the student taken the test and scored above the PSE's minimum requirement? If not, are there exceptions for admission?	Determine the student's status.
3. Does admission require a minimum GPA?	Determine student's status.
4. Does admission require foreign language credits or math credits? If so, how many credits?	Determine student's status.
5. Can courses be taken for credit? Will credits count toward a major or degree? If not, do courses lead to a certificate?	Determine student's status.
6. Contact the DSO. Did the DSO representative describe accommodations? Was the DSO staff receptive to questions? Did the DSO provide thorough answers?	Evaluate responses to the questions.
7. Does the DSO work with other relevant agencies to provide services or accommodations (e.g., VR; CILs; services to students who have vision or hearing loss, mobility needs, or assistive technology)?	Evaluate response to the question.
8. Can the student be admitted to this PSE as a general status student? If not, will this prevent free application for federal student aid (FAFSA) or other benefits?	If the student can be admitted as a general status student, then move ahead. If not and if FAFSA is needed, make a note regarding this PSE.
9. If part- or full-time employment is sought in conjunction with the PSE program, do employment opportunities exist within the PSE?	Determine if the PSE program can assist in finding employment opportunities.
10. Are residential living arrangements planned? Did the housing representative respond favorably on accommodations and access requirements that may be necessary? Are living areas fully accessible?	If "yes" on the first question, contact housing at the PSE. Evaluate response to the latter questions.
11. Is there an orientation for incoming students? Did the orientation representative describe accommodations and access?	If "yes" on the first question, contact the PSE and ask to participate.
12. Talk to an academic advisor. Did the academic advisor respond favorably on accommodations and access requirements that may be necessary?	Evaluate response to the question.
13. In addition to the DSO and academic advisor, is individual tutoring available (if needed)? Are study skills classes available (if needed)?	Evaluate responses to the questions based on student's needs.

(continued)

TABLE 9.2. *(continued)*

Question	How to interpret answer
14. What modifications are faculty or administrators willing to make for students with disabilities at this PSE? What is the track record for appropriate modifications?	Direct your question to an independent person or organization with sufficient experience with the PSE.
15. Are there opportunities to become involved in extracurricular activities, organizations, or social activities?	Determine the student's status on these questions.
16. Are there opportunities for courses, recreational activities, workout facilities, athletics, or other events?	Determine the student's status on these questions.
17. Did representatives of the PSE answer the student's questions directly or did they respond to a parent or teacher as the student's representative?	Consider whether the representative was respectful of the student.
18. Did representatives of the PSE provide contact information, should questions arise?	Consider the representatives' openness.

EXERCISE 9.1

If possible, get to know a student with a disability who is attending a PSE program. If necessary, obtain written permission from a parent or guardian. Show the student the list of questions and obtain responses. Ask, "What additional questions would have been important in your experience? What else would you have asked about the PSE program?" Summarize your findings.

WHAT ARE THE DIFFERENCES IN EXPECTATIONS BETWEEN SECONDARY SCHOOLS AND PSE?

Clearly, there are major differences in expectations between secondary education and PSE. The differences exist in terms of both performance expectations of students with disabilities and the characteristics of educational programs. These differences are summarized in Table 9.3 and have been adapted from a variety of sources (e.g., Kochhar-Bryant et al., 2009; Townsend, 2007; Weir, Fialka, Timmons, Nord, & Gaylord, 2011; *www.thinkcollege.net/topics/highschool-college-differences)*.

EXERCISE 9.2

Respond to the following questions:

- Given your experience in transitioning from secondary education to higher education, what additional differences exist between secondary schools and college?
- What would you add to the list and how would you distinguish the differences?

TABLE 9.3. Differences in Expectations between Secondary Schools and PSE

Expectation	Secondary School	PSE
Motivation to learn	Advantageous for the student to be self-motivated.	Imperative that the student be self-motivated.
Self-determination	Advantageous for the student to be self-determined. If not, self-determination skills can be taught in coursework.	Student must demonstrate self-determination (e.g., self-advocacy, self-disclosure, self-assertion, decision making, and problem solving), although some courses may be available to learn these skills.
Identification, documentation, and disclosure of the student's disability	Special education services are responsible for identifying disability, given IDEA categories.	Student is responsible to disclose disability and accommodations needed, describe how disability affects performance, inform instructors, and provide documentation from the DSO. PSE requires a formal disability diagnosis. The special education evaluation may not suffice.
Financial responsibility for evaluation and documentation of disability	Special education services are responsible for evaluation and documentation of disability.	Student is financially responsible for an evaluation justifying/describing disability that meets requirements of the PSE. Some PSEs may provide evaluations or cover costs.
Identification of educational needs	Special education services are responsible for identifying educational needs and providing services to meet educational goals according to each student's IEP.	Student is responsible for identifying needs, goals, and monitoring of progress. PSE provides feedback on progress through quizzes, tests, and assignments. There is no IEP.
Knowledge of needs for reasonable accommodations, access, and modifications	Special education services are responsible for providing reasonable accommodations, access, and modifications	Student is responsible for knowing and communicating needs for reasonable accommodations, access, and modifications.
Monitoring performance in courses and educational activities	Special education services are responsible for monitoring, evaluating, and providing feedback on performance.	Student is primarily responsible for monitoring performance. PSE provides feedback, although less frequently than in secondary schools. College courses may involve only a midterm test and final. The student is responsible for more frequent self-monitoring and soliciting feedback from college instructors, when needed.

(continued)

TABLE 9.3. *(continued)*

Expectation	Secondary School	PSE
Attendance in classes	Student is responsible for attending classes, although excessive absences may result in consultation with parents/legal guardians.	Student is responsible for attending classes.
Independence: navigating site, finding services, attending study groups, etc.	Student is generally responsible for navigating the school, finding information, and attending meetings. However, student may get direct and immediate assistance from the school office, teacher, etc.	Student is responsible for demonstrating independence.
Advocacy from parents/ guardians	Parents/guardians are encouraged to advocate for their child through participation in IEP meetings and communications with teachers and other members of IEP team.	College instructors and DSO staff can communicate with parents only if parents have established legal guardianship so that educational records may be released, or if student provides written release of information to parents.
Self-management	Student is generally responsible for self-management (in terms of behavior, adherence to a daily schedule, hygiene, dressing, and other matters), although issues can be addressed in the student's IEP.	Student is entirely responsible for self-management. Consequences may exist (expulsion) for violation of academic integrity policies related to classroom civility, assault, or cheating.

HOW PREPARED ARE STUDENTS WITH DISABILITIES FOR PSE?

Preparation for PSE requires careful planning starting at an early age. In secondary education, PSE preparation should start in earnest by ninth grade (Flexer et al., 2013). Decisions about PSE programs should occur early so a course of study can be established. Although accommodations can be made in PSE, the importance of preparation in terms of academic, self-advocacy, social, and independent living skills cannot be overemphasized.

Authors have addressed college preparation skills (Grigal & Hart, 2010; Hamblet, 2011; Patrick Holschuh & Nist-Olejnik, 2011; Townsend, 2007), among others. In Table 9.4, we synthesize their information and add observations from our own experience.

HOW CAN STUDENTS WITH DISABILITIES PREPARE FOR PSE?

Based on her experience as a special educator, Hamblet (2011) described key skill areas for college-bound students with disabilities. She analyzed nine focus areas for students preparing for college, including (1) writing, (2) reading, (3) note taking, (4) study, (5) organization and time management, (6) compensatory strategies, (7) technology, and (8) independent living skills.

TABLE 9.4. What Students Should Anticipate as They Enter College Programs

What to anticipate

1. The workload will be heavier and more difficult than in high school. Studying will require more time and organization. Greater commitment will be required.
2. College instructors assume that students study effectively and consider fine details.
3. College instructors require more than memorization of facts. Students are required to exhibit *critical thinking*, that is, analysis and critiquing of information such as a scientific study, literary passage, or an essay.
4. College courses move at a faster pace. Many college instructors require that students read and comprehend three, four, or more chapters per week.
5. College instructors expect independent learning. Instructors often lecture about a small segment of a reading assignment and expect students to read and understand the rest.
6. A college course syllabus dictates everything that follows for the entire quarter or semester. Students must read the syllabus thoroughly and reread it during the term.
7. There may be fewer tests in a college course than in high school. With longer readings and fewer tests, it means that tests cover more material. Fewer tests also mean that students may not know how well they are doing until halfway (or more) into the term.
8. Students will find themselves making moral decisions. They must consider the consequences of actions in advance and act as a mature adult.

What to do

1. Attend all classes.
2. Sit near the front of class. This helps the student to hear the instructor and not be distracted. (Exception: For students with hearing loss, sitting in the front row may prevent them from understanding the questions raised by students sitting behind them.) Sitting in front also helps because the best-performing students may sit in the first few rows. The student can develop relationships with others likely to be good study partners.
3. Plan for at least 3 hours of study for every hour in class.
4. Ask permission of the college instructor to record lectures. Be sure to explain why (to improve learning).
5. Do not just record lectures. Listen to them afterward and take notes. Compare notes with a study partner and detect differences. Contact other students to resolve note-taking differences or contact the instructor for clarification.
6. Use memory or mnemonic strategies to memorize material.
7. Provide adequate lead time to finish assignments such as book reports, papers, research reviews, etc. Note the due date on a calendar, estimate the amount of time the assignment will take (then multiply times two, seriously), and start work without delay or procrastination.
8. With multiple classes, providing adequate lead time on assignments means working on several assignments at once. Integrate study time so the student can work on multiple assignments simultaneously.
9. Get to know the college technology systems before starting classes. Use the college online course system, online library, browsers, search engines, and other sources to find information. Be ready to supplement study with effective and efficient online searches and communications with other students.
10. College instructors expect assignments to be done exclusively by the individual student. They expect that tests and assignments reflect the student's own performance. Know the college's policy on academic integrity and what constitutes violations (i.e., cheating). Consequences for violations can be very serious, such as immediate dismissal.
11. Understand one's disability and how it affects performance. Meet with DSO personnel the first week of the term, if not before.
12. Rehearse the explanation of one's disability in order to explain to the college instructor the reason for requesting a modification. Deliver DSO documentation to the instructor during the first week of classes.

Analytic Writing

Hamblet (2011) notes that in college, analytic writing is critical, especially when students write essays on their views of topics, including their rationale and justification. Graphic organizers, concept maps, or outlines will be necessary. Students should practice analytic writing assignments in preparation for PSE.

Reading Comprehension Strategies

Requirements for reading are much greater than in high school. Not only are there more pages to read, but comprehension requirements are sky high. Strategies are necessary, such as survey–question–read–recite–review (SQ3R; McCormick & Cooper, 1991). Mnemonic systems for memorization may help (Mastropieri & Scruggs, 1997).

Note Taking

Students should practice taking notes prior to college (Hamblet, 2011). They should know what constitutes information necessary to record and how to do it efficiently. College instructors present information in a variety of different ways. Effective students find out early in a college term how an instructor presents information and the essential elements for which students will be held accountable. Dictaphones or Scribe pens (*www. livescribe.com*) allow a student to write notes while recording a lecture for later playback.

Study Strategies

These strategies may include rewriting or making idea maps of lecture notes, developing mnemonics (e.g., making up a story to memorize long lists of terms), reviewing notes repeatedly, and using chapter questions to review information (Hamblet, 2011). Students should set aside study time each day and follow the schedule. In setting reading assignments, college instructors use a formula of 3 hours of study for every hour of class time.

Organization and Time Management

Effective college students manage their time and organize materials. Unlike in high school, no one imposes these requirements in college (Hamblet, 2011). Students should come to college with a paper or electronic daily schedule and planner. A daily schedule is necessary to record assignment due dates, study sessions, and so forth. A planner captures all the essential information about those events, such as details about the assignments. Schedules and planners must be used frequently throughout the day, such as writing assignments within a few minutes after they are assigned in each class period.

Compensatory Strategies

Students with disabilities should learn compensatory techniques to work around academic weaknesses. These strategies can include technology, cognitive or memory methods, and time management (Hamblet, 2011).

Technology

Effective use of technology is becoming increasingly important in higher education (Izzo, 2014). Critical skills include (1) using word processing, presentation, and database programs; (2) organizing files and folders on a computer; (3) using the Internet (e.g., using search engines and databases, citing sources from the Internet, uploading and downloading files, using the university course system, getting definitions of terms); (4) backing up work on a frequent basis; and (5) using assistive technology (Hamblet, 2011).

Independent Living

Hamblet (2011) identifies survival life skills, including laundry, checkbook, credit card, phone, and conversational skills. From our experience, we would add apartment/dorm safety, food preparation and storage, cooking, dressing, cleaning, hygiene, and interpersonal skills.

One of the authors recently participated in developing admission criteria for a college-based program for students with developmental disabilities. Aside from "hard criteria" set by the university (e.g., high school diploma, minimum GPA, scores on entrance test), additional requirements included:

- High levels of student motivation to learn in a dynamic, fast-paced college environment.
- High levels of support from the parent/guardian and/or family to assist the learner.
- Independent skill levels in regard to physical orientation, moving promptly from one location to the next on a campus (assuming direction from a classmate or global positioning system [GPS]), taking public transportation, and asking for help when necessary.
- Independent skills in regard to safety awareness (identifying emergencies or hazards and responding correctly, avoiding interaction with strangers, following safety rules, etc.).
- Self-advocacy, including willingness to disclose one's disability to the DSO and to course instructors. Training on specific skills (when to approach the instructor, what to say, what not to say) can be provided, given a willingness to participate.
- Absence of aggressiveness, defiance, excessive complaining, running away, self-injury, promiscuousness, stealing, cheating, and reporting information contrary to fact (*www.aggieselevated.com*).

This collection of skills and personal traits is vital for students in preparation for PSE, particularly for 2- and 4-year college environments. But clearly, the list is incomplete. For example, prerequisite academic skills for certain classes and majors are not listed yet are critically important. The student, parents, and transition professional should each assess preparedness well before entering PSE so that missing skills can be targeted. The rating scale in Figure 9.1 is an informal one designed to be completed independently by the student, parent, and teacher. There is no scoring system, but the scale may point out differences in perception (across the student, parent, and teacher) as well as skill levels needing to be targeted in preparation for PSE.

As you read over this list, you may remark that many students start college without being adequately prepared on all items. After all, many of these skills/traits are acquired in adulthood at the time they are needed. We agree. Participating in PSE programs, indeed, is a time of considerable adaptation and learning "on the fly." However, the rating scale provides an opportunity for key stakeholders to work with the student to prepare as much as possible.

EXERCISE 9.3

Use the PSE Preparation Rating Scale as an assignment. Find a student interested in attending a PSE program and his or her parent or family member. Arrange for them fill out the scale separately and independently. Arrange for a teacher to fill out the scale as well. Identify similarities and differences. What did the participants learn from filling out the scale and comparing ratings?

WHAT CHALLENGES MIGHT BE ANTICIPATED IN PSE?

For all its promise, there are formidable challenges awaiting students and their transition teams in PSE. This section briefly identifies and responds to some of the challenges.

Paying for College

Perhaps the greatest challenge when considering PSE is paying for it. Financial assistance can include grants, loans, work–study jobs on campus, and scholarships (Pierangelo & Giuliani, 2004). A prospective student should first fill out a Free Application for Federal Student Aid (FAFSA) because it is required to receive most state-sponsored and college-sponsored assistance. The FAFSA is used by PSE programs to determine the amount of the student's expected family contribution. This is the amount that PSE programs expect the student's family to contribute toward college education. The high school counselor or PSE advisor can direct the student/family to get assistance with the FAFSA application.

Transition teams should note that the HEOA of 2008 established rules allowing students with intellectual disability to access federal financial aid, such as Pell Grants, Federal Supplemental Education Opportunity Grants, and the Federal Work–Study Program. If a student with an intellectual disability is attending a "comprehensive transition program" approved by the HEOA, he or she can apply for financial aid to assist in paying for the costs of attending that program. The Institute for Community Inclusion at the University of Massachusetts Boston maintains a list of currently approved comprehensive transition programs (*www.thinkcollege.net*). For more information, go to *https://studentaid.ed.gov/eligibility/intellectual-disabilities#ctp-programs*. See the end of this chapter for a listing of financial aid opportunities.

Rate the following descriptions of skills according to this scale:

4 = skill mastered or very good   3 = skill is emerging   2 = skill is starting; needs work

1 = skill is absent or very weak   NA = not applicable   DK = don't know

Skill area	Rating
STUDY SKILLS	
1. When I read, I write or dictate notes. Later, I go back and review my notes.	1 2 3 4 NA DK
2. When in class, I take notes *and* record the lecture.	1 2 3 4 NA DK
3. I ask my instructor how to effectively take notes to get the information I need.	1 2 3 4 NA DK
4. I use a Dictaphone or other recording device to take notes during class.	1 2 3 4 NA DK
5. I play back my recorded notes at a later time and memorize important material.	1 2 3 4 NA DK
6. When I study my notes from class sessions, I use strategies to help me memorize long lists and complex concepts.	1 2 3 4 NA DK
7. When I write essays, I can think critically and analyze various topics.	1 2 3 4 NA DK
8. I use graphic organizers, concept maps, or outlines to assist in my writing.	1 2 3 4 NA DK
9. When I read, I use strategies to help me memorize lists or unfamiliar concepts.	1 2 3 4 NA DK
10. I study about 3 hours for every hour of class time.	
TIME MANAGEMENT	
11. I use a daily schedule or planner to record assignment due dates and information.	1 2 3 4 NA DK
12. I refer to my daily schedule and planner frequently each day.	1 2 3 4 NA DK
COMPUTER/COURSE MANAGEMENT SYSTEMS	
13. I use word processing, presentation, and database programs.	1 2 3 4 NA DK
14. I organize my files on a computer.	1 2 3 4 NA DK
15. I use search engines and databases, and cite sources from the Internet.	1 2 3 4 NA DK
16. I upload/download files from the Internet.	1 2 3 4 NA DK
17. I use the university computer and course management systems.	1 2 3 4 NA DK
18. I get definitions of terms and get answers to questions using the Internet.	1 2 3 4 NA DK
19. I know whom to contact if I need answers to computer questions.	1 2 3 4 NA DK
20. I back up my files and I do it frequently.	1 2 3 4 NA DK
SELF-ADVOCACY	
21. I can seek help from my instructor after class or during office hours.	1 2 3 4 NA DK
22. I can describe my disability, learning style, and learning needs to DSO staff.	1 2 3 4 NA DK
23. I can ask instructors to repeat information or give more explanation if needed.	1 2 3 4 NA DK
TEST PREPARATION/TEST TAKING	
24. I use flashcards or quiz apps to help memorize vocabulary terms.	1 2 3 4 NA DK
25. I help organize and attend study groups.	1 2 3 4 NA DK

(continued)

FIGURE 9.1. A PSE Preparation Rating Scale, to be completed by the student, parent, and teacher.

Skill area	Rating
TEST PREPARATION/TEST TAKING *(continued)*	
26. When taking objective tests such as those with multiple-choice questions, I read *all* sample answers before responding.	1 2 3 4 NA DK
27. After reading all multiple choices on a test question, I start by figuring out which choices are *not* correct before marking the correct one.	1 2 3 4 NA DK
28. On a multiple-choice test question, if I can only narrow it down to two or more correct answers, I make my decision based on what we studied in class.	1 2 3 4 NA DK
29. On true–false questions, I understand some statements are *false* on purpose.	1 2 3 4 NA DK
30. On multiple-choice tests, I understand what it means when a choice states something like "both A and B above."	1 2 3 4 NA DK
31. When I finish taking a test, I review all of my answers to make sure I answered every question. I don't rush through the test to be done early.	1 2 3 4 NA DK
INDEPENDENT LIVING	
32. If I am living away from home, I have adequate skills in apartment/dorm safety, food preparation and storage, cooking, dressing, cleaning, and hygiene.	1 2 3 4 NA DK
33. If I am living away from home and I need self-help or domestic advice, I know whom to call and I can follow the advice.	1 2 3 4 NA DK
34. I can identify safety hazards/emergencies and respond to eliminate the danger.	1 2 3 4 NA DK
35. I avoid communications with strangers in all settings and on the Internet.	1 2 3 4 NA DK
36. I effectively use public transportation.	1 2 3 4 NA DK
37. I can use cash, a debit card, or credit card appropriately and within my budget.	1 2 3 4 NA DK
38. I know how to contact a medical professional, how to make an appointment, and how to provide information about my medical insurance when I am sick or injured.	1 2 3 4 NA DK
39. I can describe what medications I take and why they were prescribed.	1 2 3 4 NA DK
40. I can safely take medications as prescribed.	1 2 3 4 NA DK
41. I can tell time and get to class without being late.	1 2 3 4 NA DK
42. I put away a cell phone and electronics when I need to pay attention to instruction.	1 2 3 4 NA DK
Rate the following statements according to this scale:	
4 = excellent 3 = good 2 = fair	
1 = poor NA = not applicable DK = don't know	

Statement	Rating
43. I am motivated to excel in my chosen PSE program.	1 2 3 4 NA DK
44. I have support from my parents and family.	1 2 3 4 NA DK
45. I have physical orientation skills and know my location, or I can ask for help when needed.	1 2 3 4 NA DK
46. I can advocate for myself and disclose my disability to Disability Service Office staff and to course instructors.	1 2 3 4 NA DK
47. I consistently use Disability Service Office accommodations when needed.	1 2 3 4 NA DK
48. I do not engage in any of the following behaviors: aggressiveness, complaining, tantrums, running away, self-injury, promiscuousness, cheating, or stealing.	1 2 3 4 NA DK

FIGURE 9.1. *(continued)*

Disconnection between Eligibility Assessment in College and IDEA Assessment

In order to establish access to courses and services at 2- and 4-year colleges (i.e., higher education), students may need to provide documentation of their disability. However, the evaluations and documentation typically provided by special education services in school districts may differ from what is required in PSEs (Gormley, Hughes, Block, & Lendman, 2005). Special education conducts assessments to identify disabilities according to IDEA (2004). In contrast, higher education follows the mandates of Section 504 of the Rehabilitation Act and ADA consistent with ensuring equal access and reasonable accommodations. But the fifth edition of the *Diagnostic and Statistical Manual of Mental Disorders* (DSM-5; American Psychiatric Association, 2013) used by higher-education DSOs has new definitions of specific learning disability, intellectual and developmental disorder, attention-deficit/hyperactivity disorder, and autism, which should reduce the need for separate evaluations. The student or student's family applying for entry into a PSE should obtain specific information about the requirements for documenting a disability.

Low Expectations

Researchers (Uditsky & Hughson, 2008) found that a significant challenge facing students with ID were low expectations among some secondary and PSE professionals. Low expectations often result in low performance. Professionals at all levels need to be educated to set high but realistic expectations of students with disabilities entering PSE. Otherwise, they get what they expect.

Attitudinal Limitations

Not everyone is abreast with the increasing trend of PSE involvement by students with disabilities. Many parents, educators, and others fail to understand the influx of students with disabilities into PSE programs. Reasons may relate to lack of information, misunderstanding of intent, or discriminatory attitudes. One of the authors has been involved in an incident with a parent who refused to allow her daughter, an incoming college freshman, to share a dorm room—or even be in the same dormitory building—with an incoming freshman with Down syndrome. The incident reminds us that education is needed for everyone to understand the changes taking place in PSE.

Retention in PSE

Becoming involved in a PSE program is one thing; staying involved is another. Only 16% of individuals with disabilities who enter college finish their bachelor's degree, compared to 52% of individuals without disabilities (U.S. Government Accountability Office, 2003). In a sample of 890 2-year college students with disabilities (e.g., sensory loss, mobility impairment, or learning/emotional conditions), nearly 25% dropped out after their first year and 51% left by the end of their third year. In a survey of students with and without disabilities at a 2-year college, Jorgensen, Ferraro, Fichten, and Havel (2009) found that students with disabilities had significantly lower scores on academic self-confidence and social connection. When asked why they dropped out, a large proportion of students with disabilities pointed to their disability or personal health issues. Getzel (2008) reviewed literature to identify characteristics of PSE programs to help young adults with disabilities persist in college. Factors aiding persistence included self-determination and self-management skills, assistive technology, and promotion of career development through internships and other career-related experiences. To increase persistence and retention, Getzel recommended that faculty become more knowledgeable of the characteristics and needs of students with disabilities.

WHAT ARE ACCOMMODATIONS AND UNIVERSAL DESIGN FOR LEARNING?

Accommodations are supports that offer students with disabilities equal access to PSE courses, programs, and activities. *Equal access* means "an opportunity to attain the same level of performance or to enjoy equal benefits and privileges as are available to a similarly situated student without a disability" (Section 504 of the Rehabilitation Act). The topic of accommodations is familiar to most students who receive special education services in the K–12 setting. According to Sharpe, Johnson, Izzo, and Murray (2005), if a student received accommodations in K–12 school programs, he or she is likely to receive the same or similar accommodations in PSE. Sharpe and colleagues identified the most common accommodations in PSE, including (1) extra time for exams, (2) quiet environment for exams, (3) priority course registration, (4) audio recording of lectures, (5) accessible instructional materials (i.e., Braille, audio, large print), and (6) assistive technology (i.e., text-to-speech reading software, magnification devices, amplification systems). Importantly, an accommodation cannot result in a fundamental alteration of the course, program, or activity. Also, accommodations must not pose an undue financial or administrative burden on the PSE program. Lastly, accommodations cannot address a personal need such as an attendant, an individually prescribed device, a reader for personal use or study, or other devices or services of a personal nature (Simon, 2011).

Providing accommodations is a four-step process, with steps 3 and 4 being repeated each semester.

1. The student self-discloses the disability by completing a DSO application form.
2. The DSO requests documentation from an appropriate professional (e.g., an audiologist for a student with hearing impairment) who describes the student's disability and relevant functional limitations.
3. The student and a DSO staff member meet to discuss accommodations. Students should be prepared to explain their disability and how it impacts their education. Summaries of performance (SOPs), IEPs, and/or other material that describe accommodations the student received in K–12 special education services are helpful.

4. The student, DSO, and instructors fulfill their individual obligations. Examples of these obligations include: (a) the student is responsible for notifying instructors of accommodation requests in a timely manner (i.e., at least 5 days in advance); (b) the DSO is responsible for providing exam accommodations according to the instructor's instructions (e.g., students may not refer to the textbook or notes during an exam); and (c) the instructor is responsible for supplying the DSO with instructional material (e.g., handouts, exams) for conversion into accessible formats.

We should note that providing accommodations is a reactive response to equal access. In other words, only when a student submits an accommodation request is equal access achieved.

Conversely, *Universal Design for Learning* (UDL) is a proactive approach to equal access. UDL provides instructors with a framework for selecting teaching strategies and designing course materials that considers the diverse needs of all students, including students with disabilities. This framework includes three principles (Center for Applied Special Technology, 2014):

1. Multiple means of representation, which gives students various ways of acquiring information and knowledge.
2. Multiple means of student action and expression, which provides students with alternative ways of demonstrating what they know.
3. Multiple means of student engagement, which taps into students' interests, thus motivating them to learn.

The National Center on Universal Design for Learning (*www.udlcenter.org*) has examples of UDL in PSE and forums to discuss UDL within the context of transition. A combination of accommodations and UDL is often needed for students with disabilities to succeed in PSE.

SUMMARY

In this chapter, we examined the rationale for PSE and the trend toward increasing the involvement of students with disabilities in postschool educational options. We describe the various PSE options, including colleges and universities, community colleges, vocational/technical schools, and community education. Because the selection of a compatible program is a key ingredient for a student and the transition team, we considered factors important in making the choice. Differences in PSE expectations compared to secondary education were considered, including motivation to learn, increased choice, self-determination, independence, self-advocacy, and self-management (or behavioral control). The chapter addressed the preparation of students with disabilities for PSE. Challenges were considered, including costs of PSE, low expectations, attitudinal problems, and dropping out. The chapter concluded with a description of accommodations and UDL.

REVISITING JOSEFINA

The person-centered planning group had decided that Josefina should consider taking classes to become a child development specialist while remaining available at home to supervise her sisters and niece. Her teacher, Ms. Martin, helped Josefina fill out the college application and FAFSA forms. Josefina was excited that her career was coming together. Ms. Martin had finished her work in the classroom after school and was preparing to leave.

"Excuse me, do you have a minute?" It was Raul, Josefina's father.

"Of course, Mr. Hernandez, come in." Mariana, Josefina's mother, followed.

"Ms. Martin," Mr. Hernandez started. "We appreciate all that you are doing for Josefina. But we cannot go forward with the plan. We think her brother and Vanessa are moving her in the wrong direction. It will be too much for Josefina. She has cerebral palsy and speech problems. If she fails at South Shore, it will hurt her deeply. Sorry, we just wanted to tell you."

Ms. Martin was surprised. Josefina and her family had appeared united on her direction.

"Can we talk about this?" Ms. Martin asked. The parents nodded.

"It sounds like you are concerned this plan will hurt Josefina. Is that what I'm hearing?"

"*Sí.* She would not recover. It was not so hard for her in high school. She had many supporters. South Shore is big and she will not have friends in her classes."

"So you think the risks are too great. You think if she fails, she will have no supports."

"*Sí*, that's exactly it. She will be devastated. And what will we do then?"

"I hear your concerns and I understand what you're saying. If I were in your position, I would have concerns too. I know you want Josefina to have a great life with much fulfillment. But look at Josefina. She has so much promise. She made positive impressions with her high school teachers and she can do the same with college instructors. She creates her own support system. She wants this opportunity so much. Can we deny her the chance to try?"

"You're right, we are afraid," said Mr. Hernandez. "And we do care about her. We don't feel like this is a risk we can take."

"Have you talked to Josefina about this?" Ms. Martin asked.

"No. We wanted to talk to you first," said Mr. Hernandez.

"Mr. and Ms. Hernandez. Josefina sees how much you have done for her. She sees how hard you work for your family. She wants to contribute like you do. She wants to be like you. Let her give back to her family by showing what she can contribute."

"But the risk is too great."

"I really hope you will reconsider, Mr. and Ms. Hernandez."

"I'm sorry."

EXERCISE 9.4

Consider the vignette involving Mr. and Mrs. Hernandez and Ms. Martin above. Let's say the conversation ended on a slightly different note. Let's say Mr. and Mrs. Hernandez agreed to meet again next week, although they were still very reluctant and uncertain about involving Josefina in college classes. Take the role of Ms. Martin. What materials/resources would you prepare for them? What would you say to gently show them that Josefina could take courses toward a license as a child development specialist and be successful by relying on available supports at the college?

EXERCISE 9.5

Schedule an interview with the director of a DSO. Ask questions about the characteristics and organization of the DSO. For example:

- Is the DSO centralized or dispersed across campus?
- What are the demographic data regarding students with disabilities served by the DSO (e.g., numbers and percentages of each type of disability)?
- What accommodations are available to students served by the DSO?
- How is UDL being used?

If you are taking a course on transition, compare results of your interview with results from other students. How was the DSO program staffing, goals, and services similar and different? What conclusions can you draw from your comparison of DSOs?

WEBSITES WITH ADDITIONAL INFORMATION

Think College Standards

www.thinkcollege.net/administrator/components/com_resdb/files/standardsbriefinsert_F2.pdf

Scholarships for individuals with disabilities

www.scholarships.com/financial-aid/college-scholarships/scholarships-by-type/disability-scholarships

www.collegeview.com/articles/article/financial-aid-for-students-with-disabilities

https://heath.gwu.edu/files/downloads/pse_id_final_edition.pdf

www.collegescholarships.org/grants/disabilities.htm

Federal student aid for individuals with ID

https://studentaid.ed.gov/eligibility/intellectual-disabilities

Loans, scholarships, and financial aid for college students with disabilities

www.wrightslaw.com/info/fin.aid.index.htm

CHAPTER 10

Transition to Independent Living

This chapter addresses . . .

- Residential options.
- Research on transition to independent living.
- How students can prepare for independent living.
- Centers for independent living.
- Requirements for Medicaid home- and community-based waivers.

WHAT CHANGES ARE INVOLVED IN THE TRANSITION TO INDEPENDENT LIVING?

Independent living skills are defined as skills or tasks that contribute to the successful functioning of an individual in adulthood (Cronin, 1996). We refer to independent living skills as those necessary to participate meaningfully in residential and community environments. In independent living, residential living arrangements are separate from those in the home of a parent, guardian, foster parent, or other adult who supervises a youth through the developmental years. We realize that some residential living arrangements, such as group homes and specialized facilities, may not involve "independent" living. Nonetheless, we included these living arrangements as they are independent and separate from the residential living that youth experienced during the developmental years.

At the point of transition from school to adult living, many of the supports and routines students traditionally rely upon fade or disappear. Some students with disabilities, especially those with significant disabilities, may have formal supports provided by state agencies to help them develop independent living skills (e.g., services provided in supported apartments or group homes), whereas others may not meet strict eligibility requirements for formal supports and rely on informal and other community supports. Because the supports for independent living are often difficult for students and families to navigate, it is never too early to start the planning process toward this goal.

WHAT ARE RESIDENTIAL LIVING OPTIONS FOR YOUNG ADULTS IN TRANSITION?

There are numerous residential living options for young adults with disabilities, although their availability varies across localities. Also, some options are available only to individuals who meet eligibility criteria. We refer readers to their state agencies for eligibility requirements. We begin by describing residential living options for young adults with disabilities, including (1) apartments, (2) university housing, (3) adult foster care, (4) boarding homes, (5) supported living units, (6) group homes, (7) residential treatment centers (RTCs), and (8) intermediate care facilities (ICFs) (Eisenman & Mancini, 2010; Pierangelo & Giuliani, 2004).

Apartments

Many young adults begin their independent living by renting apartments. Residents pay bills, maintain the facility, and comply with rules specified in contracts established by apartment managers. Support services are usually informal and come from friends and family (e.g., completing a rental contract, fixing a leaky faucet).

University Housing

Increasingly, college students with disabilities are living in university housing. On-campus housing is typically restricted to full-time matriculated students, so dorm living is usually limited to full-time students with disabilities. However, some colleges make exceptions and provide housing to nonmatriculated students, especially if a formal request is made through the university's DSO (Eisenman & Mancini, 2010). Like all college students, residents with disabilities must demonstrate independent self-care, domestic, and safety skills. They must also follow student codes of conduct. Some college students with disabilities choose off-campus supported living arrangements or apartments as alternatives to college dorms.

Adult Foster Care

Adult foster care involves a licensed residence offering family-style home care for individuals who require minimal assistance in activities of daily living such as dressing, bathing, eating, and so forth (Adult Foster Care Services, 2014). Eligibility is based on age of majority (18), diagnosis of disability, and the need for only minimal assistance.

Boarding Homes

Similar to adult foster care in terms of assistance needs, boarding homes are residential facilities offering minimal structure for adults with disabilities. Most boarding homes offer separate sleeping quarters and provide meals and varying degrees of assistance in activities of daily living (Pierangelo & Giuliani, 2004).

Group Homes

Representing a continuum of residential options, group homes are generally environments with up to 16 people in a home-like structure. Group homes are divided into two types: semi-independent, such as supervised apartments, and supervised living arrangements, such as larger group homes (Pierangelo & Giuliani, 2004). Residents in semi-independent arrangements may receive only occasional visits from care providers, whereas those in supervised living who have substantial and intensive needs may receive 24-hour care. The advantage of group homes is that they allow individuals with disabilities to live in typical neighborhoods and participate in community activities. Group homes with adequate supervision and well-trained staff can maintain an individual's level of independence and increase integration into the community. Eligibility varies, but may be based on age of majority (18), diagnosis of disability, and needs for assistance in activities of daily living (Pierangelo & Giuliani, 2004).

Residential Treatment Centers

Representing programs for children and adults with behavioral, mental health, or substance abuse issues, RTCs provide intensive help for individuals requiring 24-hour care. RTCs offer individualized treatment plans, individual and group therapy, psychiatric care, and other forms of therapy. Many programs offer a continuum of care ranging from outpatient therapy to day treatment to RTC. Level of service need is based on a comprehensive evaluation.

Intermediate Care Facilities

Representing programs for individuals requiring significant supports, ICFs provide 24-hour services involving nursing and medical care, habilitation (i.e., training in self-care and other skills), and support. ICFs may be necessary for such individuals, including those who are medically fragile or have significant health conditions. States may divide ICFs into different categories depending on the level of care and size of facility. ICFs are administered by the state's department of health or developmental disability services (names vary across states), and eligibility is restricted to individuals and families covered by Medicaid.

WHAT IS THE CURRENT THINKING ON THE RANGE OF RESIDENTIAL LIVING OPTIONS?

Traditionally, adult residential options for individuals with disabilities, especially for those requiring significant supports, have been limited to "congregate" (i.e., group) living arrangements where the individual had limited choices. Today, however, residential options are expanding and advocates are calling for more choice and awareness about residential options. For example, the American Association on Intellectual and Developmental Disabilities (AAIDD; 2012) issued a joint position statement with The Arc (an advocacy organization for people with IDD) on housing options. AAIDD provides several statements that articulate its position, and we highlight a few here:

• People must have freedom, authority, and support to exercise control over their housing, including choice of where and with whom they live, privacy within their homes, access to flexible supports and services when and where they choose, choice in their daily routines and activities, freedom to come and go as they please, and housing that reflects their personal preferences and styles. Providers should honor individual choices and preferences.

• Housing should afford people with IDD the opportunity to interact with people without disabilities to the fullest extent possible.

• Housing for people with IDD must be coordinated with home- and community-based support systems, including transportation services, and should ensure access to other typical public resources.

• There must be adequate funding of services to support people to live in the community. Funding must be stable and not subject to arbitrary limits or cuts. People with IDD must not be subjected to unnecessary institutionalization or removal from their homes and communities due to state budget cuts.

• Housing for people with disabilities should be within typical neighborhoods and communities, and should reflect the natural proportion of people with disabilities in the general population.

• Public funds must be shifted from restrictive institutional settings to community supports. Institutional settings and large congregate living arrangements are unnecessary and inappropriate for people with IDD, regardless of type or severity of disability (AAIDD, 2012).

The 1999 *Olmstead* decision described in Chapter 3 has been the catalyst for changes in the way we conceptualize and support community living for people with disabilities. In fact, in 2009, the White House commemorated the 10-year anniversary of *Olmstead* by directing the Health and Human Services Secretary and the Housing and Urban Development Secretary to collaborate to improve access to housing, community supports, and independent living arrangements. President Obama reinforced this commitment by stating:

The *Olmstead* ruling was a critical step forward for our nation, articulating one of the most fundamental rights of Americans with disabilities: Having the choice to live independently. . . . I am proud to launch this initiative to reaffirm my Administration's commitment to vigorous enforcement of civil rights for Americans with disabilities and to ensuring the fullest inclusion of all people in the life of our nation. (White House, Office of the Press Secretary, 2009)

As a result of these advocacy and policy efforts, students with disabilities and their families should be aware of the range of community living options currently available. Students and families should be encouraged to explore residential living options throughout the transition process so they can make informed decisions about how they choose to live in their communities.

WHAT ARE RESEARCH FINDINGS ON TRANSITION TO INDEPENDENT LIVING?

As shown in Table 10.1, the percentages of young adults with disabilities living independently increased with amount of time out of high school (Newman et al., 2011). Note the major increase in independent living from 3–5 years to 5–8 years out of high school. The study did not address the reason(s) for the major increase in independent living. We might speculate that the increase is related to a number of variables, including increased maturity and financial stability of individuals with disabilities over time. It is worth noting that Newman and colleagues (2011) also reported that adults with intellectual disability or multiple disabilities were less likely to live independently than those with specific learning disabilities, speech/language impairments, or emotional disturbances.

HOW CAN TRANSITION PROFESSIONALS PREPARE STUDENTS FOR INDEPENDENT LIVING?

Successful transition to independent adult living requires a student to move from the relative support and routines of school life to environments in which young adults typically assume more responsibility for independent living. With careful planning and instruction, transition educators can assist students to reach their independent living goals.

TABLE 10.1. Residential Independent Living Based on Number of Years Since Leaving High School

	Less than 3 years	3 to 5 years	5 to 8 years
Percent of young adults with disabilities living independently	38.9	47.8	70.5

Note. From Newman et al. (2011). Reprinted with permission from SRI International.

TABLE 10.2. Categories of Independent Living Skills Relevant to Transition

• Bathing and washing	• Meal preparation /menu planning
• Bicycle use	• Medications (self-administration and proper
• Bill payment	storage)
• Clothing care	• Menstrual care
• Community safety and awareness	• Money management
• Conflict resolution	• Nail care
• Conversation skills	• Participation in community activities
• Cooking	• Personal safety
• Domestic skills	• Physical fitness
• Dressing/undressing	• Recognizing/responding to safety hazards
• Eating/diet management	• Recreation activity
• E-mail and other electronic	• Responding to landlords and other authority
correspondence	figures
• Emergency reporting: calling 911	• Responding to strangers/avoiding solicitation
• Financial decision making	• Shaving
• Fire safety	• Shopping
• First aid/responding to medical	• Social skills
emergencies	• Sportsmanship
• Food storage	• Stress management
• Friendship (respect, mutuality)	• Telephone skills
• Grocery shopping	• Time management/using a planner
• Health and wellness	• Toileting
• Home safety	• Toothbrushing
• House cleaning	• Transportation
• Hygiene	• Use of deodorant
• Internet use and safety	• Use of manners
• Keeping appointments/being on time	• Vacuuming
• Laundry/folding clothes	• Yard care
• Leisure activity	

Independent living in adulthood requires a wide spectrum of skills. Assessment and transition planning are necessary to identify high-priority skills in most probable adult environments. Transition-related skills may include those shown in Table 10.2. We briefly touch on independent living categories that are particularly critical to transition. These include transportation, self-care, domestic, social, and safety skills.

Transportation Skills

In order to maintain independent living and to participate fully in community living, students with disabilities must learn to navigate their communities using different modes of transportation. Transition professionals can prepare students to use public transportation, obtain a state driver's license, walk to community sites, and utilize other personal transportation options such as a bicycle. Determining which transportation skills to teach depends on a number of student variables, including age, functional skills, and cognitive and motor skills. The determination also depends on availability of transportation modes (public/private transportation) and locations of travel (Moon, Luedtke, & Halloron-Tornquist, 2010). Moon and colleagues (2010) recommended four steps for determining which transportation skills to teach:

1. Conduct direct observations and interviews with the student and family using a mobility checklist. These observations and interviews provide an opportunity to gather data on student skills and priorities.
2. Develop a community resource profile that identifies state, local, and private transportation resources. The profile should list the names and contact information of individuals from transportation emergencies.
3. Obtain parent/guardian permission prior to community instruction. The permission form should include information about goals of instruction, personnel responsible for instruction, emergency contacts, and release of liability.
4. Complete an ecological inventory to identify specific travel routes for teaching pedestrian and personal or public transportation skills. (p. 3)

With rapid technological advances, students requiring significant supports can be taught to independently use public transportation. For example, we worked with a transition educator who used an iPad to develop a picture-based task analysis for teaching bus routes to students with IDD. Similarly, Davis, Stock, Holloway, and Wehmeyer (2010) used a personal digital assistant (PDA)–based software system with GPS to provide visual and auditory prompts to people with intellectual disabilities on a public bus route. The device was programmed with multiple travel routes and instruction sets. Participants were instructed to select a desired travel route. Once the travel route was selected, the PDA displayed a prompt screen with a picture of the specific bus route to take and an audio prompt. The program required the individual to input information at various points during the training; this input changed the screen display to progress through each step of the route. A majority of participants in the study learned their bus route using the PDA system.

Technology can also be used for assisting individuals with personal travel needs. A colleague of ours assisted a college student with severe memory loss by creating Go-Pro videos showing how to navigate routes to classes on a college campus. The student then played the appropriate video while walking from one class to another.

Self-Care Skills

Self-care skills typically include bathing, washing, toileting, grooming, hair and nail care, menstrual care, feeding, and dressing. For students with disabilities, particularly those requiring significant supports, self-care skills may be limited by fine- or gross-motor development, reduced social awareness, inadequate learning opportunities, and/or limited cognitive development (Westling et al., 2015). Because self-care skills are important to maintain health and well-being and to maximize access and involvement in community living and participation, they should be taught in natural contexts. Self-care skills are often taught using a task analysis and an LTM prompts procedure (see Chapters 5 and 8). Transition educators should encourage family involvement in assessment, instruction, and maintenance of these critical skills. In addition, transition educators should advise families about the supports available to students who are eligible for Medicaid home- and community-based waivers described later in this chapter. Certain self-care services may be available through state developmental disabilities agencies.

Domestic Skills

In the process of moving from home living during the developmental years to independent living, domestic skills rapidly emerge as crucial to success. Anyone who has served as an apartment manager, residential assistant, or homeowner knows the importance of having a resident keep the physical facility clean, organized, and safe. Domestic skills include clothing care, food storage, dusting, sweeping, vacuuming, cleaning of household surfaces and appliances, food preparation, cooking, dishwashing, bed making, laundry, disposing of garbage, and making minor household repairs. Young adults with disabilities must be taught to keep ample supplies of different cleaning agents on hand and should understand their use. Bright Hub Education maintains a website for teaching cooking skills to students with disabilities (*www.brighthubeducation.com/special-ed-inclusion-strategies/101233-teaching-cooking-to-persons-with-intellectual-disabilities*). Much like self-care skills, domestic skills are often taught using a task analysis, preferably in natural contexts. Teaching procedures include forward and concurrent chaining (teaching a task according to steps from start to finish), backward chaining (providing assistance on the last task in a sequence and moving backward to the first step), video modeling (showing steps using video demonstration), and video prompting (showing separate steps using video). Teachers will need to develop specific strategies so the youth and young adults with disabilities maintain these skills. These strategies may include involving family members or others who provide support to the student over time.

Social Skills

Important in a variety of contexts, social skills are critical for young adults as they establish independent living. Adolescents spend proportionately more time with peers as they get older and develop interpersonal relationships that are important to self-esteem and social competence (Carter & Hughes, 2005). In various environments, young adults may interact with employers, coworkers, college professors, apartment managers, group home staff, police officers, emergency personnel, or solicitors. The impressions they make on other adults will facilitate or inhibit their status in independent living. To underscore the importance, Elksnin and Elksnin (2001) estimated that deficits in occupational social skills account for almost 90% of job loss among young adults with disabilities. Social skills of youth as they interact with law enforcement authorities can determine the outcomes of police decisions to arrest or release (Kirigin, Braukmann, Atwater, & Wolf, 1982).

Specific social skills important in the transition years include following directions, reporting back after following an instruction, asking if additional tasks must be carried out, making eye contact, responding appropriately to criticism or correction, asking questions for clarification, responding to questions by providing sufficient information, initiating conversation, asking to join in, asking for or offering help, giving critical feedback, saying "no" and dealing with peer pressure, responding assertively (e.g., using "I" statements), and dealing with teasing and bullying (Spence, 2003). Social skills are complex because they require accurate interpretation of subtle, contextual cues originating in the language of others (e.g., idioms and figures of speech) and nonverbal actions (e.g., winks, rolling of eyes). The social response itself must meet specific criteria, such as intermittent eye contact while speaking and listening, standing at an appropriate distance from others, and maintaining certain facial expressions. These contextual cues and responses vary depending on one's cultural background or social group.

Transition educators can teach social skills using modeling, behavioral rehearsal (or role playing), feedback and reinforcement, social perception skills training (i.e., pointing out social cues and context), or social problem solving (Spence, 2003). Like other independent living skills, social skills require considerable practice for the learner. Educators should program multiple practice opportunities. Additionally, learning social skills depends on the familiarity of the person with whom one is interacting. Transition educators may teach students a social skill, but the skill may not be displayed with unfamiliar people or in new locations. Therefore, unfamiliar "interactors" and new locations should be a part of the skill acquisition process.

Safety Skills

For young adults with disabilities, independent living environments can include their residence, place of work, community, and/or public transportation venues. In all of these environments, safety skills are vitally important. Employers surveyed about their perceptions regarding hiring individuals with disabilities identified safety as a key concern (Morgan & Alexander, 2005). Lapses in safety may result in fire, property damage, accidents, or injury. Moreover, safety issues can arise in a variety of situations, such as management of medication, prevention of substance abuse, navigation of the Internet, and responses to telephone or electronic communications from "scammers." For all these circumstances, young adults with disabilities participating in independent living activities may be at risk. However, we would argue that lack of safety skill has nothing to do with the presence of a disability but the absence of adequate training. Transition educators can teach safety skills by using steps of a task analyses, modeling, or role playing (Agran, 1994). We strongly encourage transition professionals to recognize the importance of teaching safety skills as part of all independent living activities.

HOW CAN TRANSITION EDUCATORS PLAN FOR INDEPENDENT LIVING?

Transition educators need to teach a sequence of independent living skills leading to most likely environments. Jameson and McDonnell (2010) recommended that transition programs cumulatively build independent living skills. That is, educators should create transition plans that cumulatively develop each student's capacity to live independently. For example, at the preliminary stages of transition planning, students should be provided with opportunities to engage in basic independent living tasks that can be acquired in a home economics or career technical education course. Later, instruction should shift to more complex independent living skills that will help the student achieve his or her postschool goals.

EXERCISE 10.1

Tara is a 15-year-old with IDD. She has limited experience with financial management and is just beginning to understand the "next-dollar" strategy to purchase items at the school store (i.e., provide the cashier one more dollar than the total amount of purchase). Tara expressed to her teacher that she would like to live in her own apartment when she finishes school. Her parent agrees and supports Tara's desire for independence. Describe how you would develop a transition plan to cumulatively build financial skills that would enable Tara to achieve her goal of living in an apartment.

Transition Assessment and Planning for Independent Living

Specific transition goals should be based on comprehensive assessment of students' independent living skills. This assessment should take into account the preferences, strengths, and interests of each student. To accurately determine students' independent living and community integration needs, transition educators should use competency-based assessments (e.g., Karan, DonAroma, Bruder, & Roberts, 2010). Karan and colleagues (2010) outline several important steps to community assessments for independent living:

1. *Create a vision.* Develop a long-term plan for independent living that identifies preferred residence, employment, and recreation/leisure activities. Also, identify the level of support the student will need to live independently.
2. *Determine and prioritize skills to be assessed.* Develop a series of checklist items that will help the transition team determine training priorities and where to assess the skills.
3. *Familiarize the student with the setting.* This step allows the student to feel more comfortable during the assessment.
4. *Collect baseline data on current levels of skill performance.* Collect data to determine student's current level of functioning in an applied setting.
5. *Develop instruction programs that help the student acquire the expected skill independently.* Once specific independent living skills are identified, transition educators should work with the student and family to develop instruction promoting acquisition, maintenance, and generalization of these skills.

Using assessment and skill-based instruction in natural contexts, transition educators can prepare a student for independent living. Clearly, not all independent living skills can be taught prior to encountering situations. Part of the preparation process should include equipping the student with skills to access assistance when needed. These skills may include contacting family or friends, calling technicians and asking appropriate questions, or finding step-by-step instructions on the Internet. In any event, independent living skills should be considered priorities as students enter the transition years.

WHAT ARE CENTERS FOR INDEPENDENT LIVING?

Centers for independent living (CILs) empower people with disabilities to have more independence and more consumer choice and control. Recently, the Independent Living Research Utilization (2014) reported 403 CILs in the United States. CILs are federally funded through the Rehabilitation Act. Title VII of the Rehabilitation Act outlines the core philosophy of CILs:

- Consumer control of the center regarding decision-making, service delivery, management, and establishment of policy and direction of the center.
- Self-help and self-advocacy.
- Development of peer relationships and peer role models.
- Equal access of individuals with significant disabilities to society and to all services, programs, resources, and facilities, whether public or private and regardless of funding source (29 U.S. Code § 796).

CILs provide specific core services, including peer counseling, independent living skills training, and information and referral (White, Simpson, Gonda, Ravesloot, & Coble, 2010). First, peer counseling provides opportunities for a counselor and an individual with a disability to exchange ideas and develop strategies to overcome barriers to independent living. Second, independent living educators teach skills, such as money management, household maintenance, and employment application. Finally, information and referral services assist the individual with disabilities with community resources, organizations, and services.

Historically, CILs and school-based transition programs have operated independently with little collaboration (Wehmeyer & Gragoudas, 2004). Recently, however, CILs have been expanding their capacity to collaborate with schools on issues related to transition. For example, the New Jersey Statewide Independent Living Council has a tiered program to assist students with identifying career preferences (*www.njsilc.org/content/ student-transition-and-employment-adults-through-cils*). This program is designed so that transition programs and CILs collaborate to provide students with the comprehensive training needed for employment and community living.

EXERCISE 10.2

Contact and interview a CIL professional in your area. What types of supports and services does the professional provide for independent living? Describe ways in which the CIL and your transition program could collaborate to teach students with disabilities the needed independent living skills.

WHAT RESOURCES ARE AVAILABLE FOR INDEPENDENT LIVING?

We describe three different resources for independent living: (1) home- and community- based services (HCBS) waivers, (2) supported living, and (3) personal assistance services (PAS). Transition professionals should make use of these resources when pertinent.

HCBS Waivers

Authorized in 1981 to provide funding to states to expand community-based supports for people with disabilities, HCBS waivers are designed to expand community-based residential and employment options for individuals with disabilities who would traditionally be served in more restrictive settings. Typically, individuals requiring significant supports utilize HCBS waivers. In Table 10.3, we provide a description of the types of core waiver services (Centers for Medicare and Medicaid Services, 2015). HCBS supports include, among other categories, residential and day habilitation, chore services, adult companion services, and personal care. Waivers are designed to support an individual with a disability in home and community living environments. Transition professionals should provide information to students and families about how to access waiver services in their state.

Transition professionals should also be cognizant that in many states, a large number of individuals with disabilities are on waiting lists for HCBS waiver services. In fact, Larson, Salmi, Smith, Anderson, and Hewitt (2013) reported that across 41 states, 73,106 individuals with IDD were on formal waiting lists for residential services. Therefore, transition teams may need to identify other community resources available to students with disabilities. Professionals should also advise families to investigate HCBS application requirements early in the transition process.

EXERCISE 10.3

Research your state developmental disabilities agency's HCBS program. What services are available for independent living? Is there a wait list for services? How long is the estimated wait? If so, are the other independent living supports available?

Supported Living

The concept of supported living emerged as an alternative to group living arrangements for people with disabilities. The supported living paradigm assumes that (1) individuals with disabilities should live in their own homes, (2) housing should be separate from support staff, and (3) supports should be tailored to meet the individualized needs of the person with a disability (Stancliffe & Lakin, 2007). Supported living is generally funded using HCBS funds. Braddock and colleagues (2011) reported that in 2009, supported living spending increased 10% per year from 2006 to 2009. Also, the authors reported that in the same year, 49 states and the District of Columbia provided supported living and personal assistance to 246,882 individuals.

When an individual with a disability resides in a supported living arrangement, a case manager with the state developmental disability agency usually coordinates services. In many cases, this means the state developmental agency contracts or vends with a service provider. Service providers are agencies providing support to people

TABLE 10.3. Core Residential Waiver Service Descriptions

Core Service	Description
Residential habilitation	Refers to individually tailored supports that assist with the acquisition, retention, or improvement in skills related to living in the community. These supports include adaptive skill development, assistance with activities of daily living, community inclusion, transportation, adult educational supports, and social and leisure skill development—all of which assist the participant to reside in the most integrated setting appropriate to his/her needs. Residential habilitation also includes personal care and protective oversight and supervision.
Day habilitation	Refers to a provision of regularly scheduled activities in a nonresidential setting, separate from the participant's private residence or other residential living arrangement, such as assistance with acquisition, retention, or improvement in self-help, socialization, and adaptive skills that enhance social development in performing activities of daily living and community living. Activities and environments are designed to foster the acquisition of skills, building positive social behavior and interpersonal competence and greater independence and personal choice. Services are furnished consistent with the participant's person-centered service plan.
Chore services	Refers to services needed to maintain the home in a clean, sanitary, and safe environment. This service includes heavy household chores such as washing floors, windows, and walls; tacking down loose rugs and tiles; and moving heavy items of furniture in order to provide safe access and egress. These services are provided only when neither the participant nor anyone else in the household is capable of performing or financially providing for them, and where no other relative, caregiver, landlord, community/volunteer agency, or third party payor is capable of or responsible for their provision. In the case of rental property, the responsibility of the landlord, pursuant to the lease agreement, is examined prior to any authorization of service
Adult companion services	Refers to nonmedical care, supervision, and socialization when provided to a functionally impaired adult. Companions may assist or supervise the person with such tasks as meal preparation, laundry, and shopping. The provision of companion services does not entail hands-on nursing care. Providers may also perform light housekeeping tasks that are incidental to the care and supervision of the participant. This service is provided in accordance with a therapeutic goal in the service plan.
Personal care	Refers to a range of assistance to enable waiver participants to accomplish tasks that they would normally do for themselves if they did not have a disability. This assistance may take the form of hands-on assistance (actually performing a task for the person) or cuing to prompt the participant to perform a task. Personal care services may be provided on an episodic or on a continuing basis. Health-related services that are provided may include skilled or nursing care and medication administration to the extent permitted by state law.

From Centers for Medicare and Medicaid Services (2015).

with disabilities. Each provider assures that services align with state policy. Services can include transportation training, leisure activities, self-care activities, home maintenance, grocery shopping and cooking, budgeting, and supported and customized employment, among others.

EXERCISE 10.4

Contact and interview a supported living service provider in your area. Ask the provider to describe a typical supported living arrangement. What are the most common supports provided to individuals residing in supported living? What can transition programs do to help prepare students with disabilities for independent living?

Personal Assistance Services

Some transition-age young adults with disabilities, particularly those requiring significant supports, require additional assistance in activities of daily living. Personal assistants provide services such as reading, communicating, performing manual tasks, bathing, feeding, toileting, and assisting with personal hygiene (National Collaborative on Workforce and Disability for Youth, 2010). PAS are funded through Medicaid. Transition professionals should address what types of daily living supports will be required for a young adult with disabilities. To determine what level of support is necessary, the National Collaborative on Workforce and Disability for Youth recommend that transition professionals address:

- *Personal care needs.* These needs include dressing, grooming, bathing, hygiene, housekeeping, meal preparation, transportation, companionship, and medical assistance, among others.
- *When and for how long assistance will be needed.* Professionals determine the amount of assistance needed each day and when these services will be provided.
- *Personal assistance preferences.* Professionals examine what types of characteristics the personal assistant must possess (gender, age, disability or no disability, language, strength, etc.).
- *Knowledge, skills, and abilities.* Professionals consider personal issues that may arise between the person with the disability and the assistant, such as money management disagreements, need for conflict resolution, time management disagreements, and the development of a romantic/sexual relationship.

The National Collaborative on Workforce and Disability for Youth (2010) suggested that young adults develop specific plans addressing resources, activities, and steps necessary to achieve independent living. Also, the National Collaborative developed an Activities of Daily Living Worksheet that can serve as a tool in determining support needs (see Figure 10.1). The worksheet is divided into different activities (e.g., mobility, menu planning and food preparation). An informant or the young adult completes the worksheet, indicating whether no assistance, partial assistance, or full assistance is required for each skill. The information can help determine the types of PAS needed.

Activity	No assistance	Partial assistance	Full assistance
Mobility—wheelchair (includes pushing a manual wheelchair, clearing a path for the wheelchair, opening doors, daily maintenance of wheelchair)			
Positioning (includes amount of help needed for comfort or to relieve pressure while sitting or sleeping or positioning of pillows or wedges)			
Toileting (includes assistance needed for bowel programming, catheter and/or colostomy cares, and general toileting assistance)			
Transfers (includes moving from one position to another, e.g., moving from bed to a wheelchair or sitting to standing position)			
Medications (includes medications that need to be taken in the morning, evening, during the day, and/or during sleeping hours)			
Meal planning and food preparation			
Menu planning			
Grocery shopping			
Putting food away in cupboards and refrigerator			
Preparing food (cutting, cooking)			
Putting food on plates and table			
Serving food			
Clearing the table			
Putting away leftovers			
Washing dishes/putting dishes in dishwasher			
Laundry			
Sorting clothes			
Putting soap in washing machine			
Putting clothes in washing machine			
Putting clothes in dryer			
Folding clothes			
Ironing clothes			
Putting clothes away			

(continued)

FIGURE 10.1. Activities of Daily Living Worksheet. Adapted from National Collaborative on Workforce and Disability for Youth (2010). Adapted by permission.

Activity	No assistance	Partial assistance	Full assistance
Medical appointments			
Assistance to vehicle			
Accompaniment to appointment			
Help into/out of building or office			
Registering as a patient			
Going to exam room			
Taking notes during exam			
Filling prescriptions			
Transferring onto exam tables/chairs			
Light housekeeping and chores			
Sweeping			
Mopping			
Dusting			
Taking out the garbage			
Making the bed			
Cleaning the windows			
Cleaning the bedroom, kitchen, and bathroom			
Shopping			
Preparing a shopping list			
Assistance into vehicle/nearest public transportation			
Help into/out of store			
Taking items off the shelf			
Carrying the items/pushing the cart			
Handling money			
Loading/unloading purchases into/from vehicle			
Putting items away at home			
Outings/events			
Keeping calendar of events			
Getting directions			
Assistance into a vehicle			
Help at an event			

FIGURE 10.1. (*continued*)

WHAT RESOURCES ARE AVAILABLE FOR RENTING AND HOMEOWNERSHIP?

Previously, we discussed living options for individuals with disabilities who have an HCBS waiver. These waivers are available only for individuals who meet strict eligibility requirements. Many students receiving special education and related services are not eligible. As such, transition professional, students, and families may need to access other types of support designed to help individuals obtain residential living, including (1) housing choice vouchers, (2) Fannie Mae's Community HomeChoice, or (3) individual development accounts (IDAs).

Housing Choice Vouchers

The housing choice voucher program is designed to assist low-income families, people who are elderly, and people with disabilities to obtain housing. The program is administered locally by public housing agencies (go to *HUD.gov*). Eligibility for a housing voucher is based on the total gross income and family size. Typically, this means a family's income cannot exceed 50% of the median income in the county where the individual is seeking housing. Individuals determined eligible for a voucher are asked to locate a residence they plan to occupy. The local public housing agency will subsequently inspect the residence and determine the amount of rent subsidy.

Fannie Mae's Community HomeChoice

Community HomeChoice is designed for individuals with low to moderate income who have disabilities or for families with a young adult with a disability. The program provides flexibility in down payment options, loan to value, and qualifying ratios. To be eligible, the borrower or family member residing with the borrower must have a disability defined by the Fair Housing Act (see website at the end of this chapter). In addition, income for an eligible borrower must not exceed 115% of the area's median income where the property is valued (FannieMae, 2014).

Individual Development Accounts

IDAs are matched savings accounts designed to help individuals with low to moderate incomes. IDAs are offered through established partnerships with banks, credit unions, or nonprofit organizations. For every dollar an individual saves in an IDA, a degree of match is made to the account. For example, an individual may put $25 a month in an IDA for 2 years resulting in $600 savings. If the IDA agency offers a 3:1 match, the individual would receive an additional $1,800 match (World Institute on Disability, n.d.). Most IDAs are used to start a small business, buy a home, or pay for school tuition. In order to utilize an IDA, an individual must be within of 200% of the poverty threshold. Individuals who have an IDA are required to take a financial education class and other training related to asset management. The IDA program can be short term or last several years depending on the individual's goals and saving capacity. See the website at the end of this chapter for more information.

EXERCISE 10.5

SUMMARY

In this chapter, we described strategies that transition educators can use to prepare students for independent living. We also reviewed different ways to support students in obtaining and maintaining independent living. Transition educators should make efforts to elicit input from both the student and family to develop independent living goals, objectives, and priorities. Instruction for independent living skills should cumulatively build throughout the transition years. We described CILs, as well as three different resources for independent living: HCBS waivers, supported living, and PAS. Finally, we reviewed supports designed to help individuals obtain residential living, including housing choice vouchers, Fannie Mae Community HomeChoice, and IDAs.

REVISITING DEMARIUS

Demarius, his grandmother, and Gabriel walked passed an array of treadmills.

"So what do you think of this, Demarius?" Gabriel asked as he panned across the sports academy with his outstretched arm.

"Looks like a lot of people sweating," Demarius muttered.

"Yeah, I guess you could say that. Or you could say that they are getting healthy, extending themselves, trying to stretch their limits and improve their horizons."

"First you're a personal trainer. Now you sound like one of those motivational speakers."

Gabriel smiled. "The people I work with here, they have a dream and they want to reach it. Do you have a dream, Demarius?"

"I don't know."

"Our members, before they start working out in the gym, they have to come to grips with who they are. Be honest with themselves. Are you honest with yourself, Demarius?"

"Maybe."

"It means accepting who you are right now just as you are. You're OK. And then you can look at yourself honestly. You can set realistic goals—not superman fantasies, just reachable goals. And the people here who come to work out, they work hard because the goal is right in front of them. Once they reach that goal, they set another one. Know what I mean?"

"Look, man, I hear what you're saying," Demarius said. "What do you want me to do?"

"I just want you to find your dream. Just strip away all the pain and b------and think about what you want. What do you want for your life?"

"I don't know. I don't even think about that . . . I guess I want my gramma to be happy. And I know she wants me working and thinking about college."

"And what do you want?"

"I don't think about what I want."

"Try thinking about it now. Let's just say 'Demarius is OK as is, right now.' You're OK. Nobody's on your case to be different, to be somebody else. What do you want for yourself?"

"I want to not be afraid. I want to make money so I can do some things myself and do nice things for gramma."

"And how can you do that?"

Demarius paused. He exhaled heavily then looked at Gabriel.

"I guess I need to take charge of myself."

WEBSITES WITH ADDITIONAL INFORMATION

RTCs

www.aacap.org/AACAP/Families_and_Youth/Facts_for_Families/Facts_for_Families_Pages/The_Continuum_Of_Care_For_Children_And_Adolescents_42.aspx

ICFs

www.medicaid.gov/Medicaid-CHIP-Program-Information/By-Topics/Delivery-Systems/Institutional-Care/Intermediate-Care-Facilities-for-Individuals-with-Mental-Retardation-ICFMR.html

Independent Living Skills Curricula

www.nsttac.org/content/transition-curricula

Cooking Skills

www.brighthubeducation.com/special-ed-inclusion-strategies/101233-teaching-cooking-to-persons-with-intellectual-disabilities

Independent Living Center Directory

www.ilru.org/projects/cil-net/cil-center-and-association-directory

Individual Development Accounts Directory

http://cfed.org/programs/idas/directory_search

http://portal.hud.gov/hudportal/HUD?src=/topics/housing_choice_voucher_program_section_8

Medicaid Home and Community Based Waivers

www.medicaid.gov/Medicaid-CHIP-Program-Information/By-Topics/Waivers/Home-and-Community-Based-1915-c-Waivers.html

Fair Housing Act

http://portal.hud.gov/hudportal/HUD?src=/program_offices/fair_housing_equal_opp/FHLaws/yourrights

Corporation for Enterprise Development: Individual Development Accounts

http://cfed.org/programs/idas

CHAPTER 11

The Role of the Family in Transition

This chapter addresses . . .

- The family's role in a youth's transition to adulthood.
- How the child's growing up affects the family.
- The educator's role in assessing family values in the transition process.
- Research on family roles and parent/family contributions in transition planning.
- How to establish rapport and develop working relationships with the family.
- Working with culturally and linguistically diverse families.
- How family values and ideals can strengthen transition from school to adulthood.

WHAT IS THE FAMILY'S ROLE IN A YOUTH'S TRANSITION TO ADULTHOOD?

The daughter of one of the authors discovered a robin's nest in the backyard. For days, she watched as the mother nurtured her four babies. Clearly a budding ornithology researcher, she observed that the mother would bring food to the baby robins and distribute it among the young. In 12–15 days from birth, it was time for the baby robins to begin flying lessons. During flight school, the mother robin nudged each bird to the edge of the nest and waited. During the 2-week fledgling period, a young robin would jump from the nest, use its wings to brace for a landing on the ground, and eventually take flight. The mother robin would fly to a nearby perch and watch. As the young robins began flying to Mom's perch, she would fly farther away as if to say, "Follow me." One of the four babies (whom the daughter named "Lewis") remained in the nest while his siblings learned to fly. Lewis needed extra time, but eventually, Mom nudged him out of the nest as well. The mother robin flew to a perch on the back fence of the yard and waited. Lewis made several attempts to join his mother, but crashed head first into the fence several feet short of the top rail. The mother robin patiently repeated the process until Lewis surmounted the top rail, only to see his mom fly to a more distant destination.

Like the robin that had to monitor four fledgling fliers, parents must attend to a myriad of details, including the needs of (sometimes) multiple children, payment of bills, demands of one or more jobs, upkeep of a residence and vehicle, provision of food and shelter, activities of extended family, and so forth. When such a complex system meets the equally complex process of transitioning a youth with disabilities to adulthood, the probability of a simple and seamless adjustment rapidly diminishes. Parents need support. A team effort is essential, but each team member needs to understand the roles and responsibilities of the other (Everson & Moon, 1987).

AS YOUTH GROW UP, HOW DOES THE PROCESS AFFECT THE FAMILIES?

As the youth gets older, a parent's perception of the child must change. Growth is rapid during the adolescent years, requiring all family members to frequently adjust their lens to view the youth in a new light (Collins, 2014). This process may be particularly difficult for families with a youth who has a disability. As stated by Dwyer, Grigal, and Fialka (2010):

> Where once family members played the role of guardian, overseer, protector, and decision maker, they must learn to step back and support their child in taking more control. This may mean watching their child make new and different and potentially less optimal choices, and watching him/her stumble and learn to recover. (p. 208)

Frequently adjusting one's perception and behavior, particularly when it involves relinquishing control, is challenging for parents of a youth with a disability (Cavendish, Montague, Enders, & Dietz, 2014). Giving up control means giving away one's authority, supervision, and guardianship. Some parents and other family members harbor doubts on whether youth, with or without a disability, can assume total responsibility. Moreover, when youth do make less than optimal decisions (and they will), some parents and family members question their decision to relinquish authority. They may engage in the "should have game." For example:

> "I should never have given my child the authority to make that decision."
> "I should have made that decision for her."

Some parents respond by moving back to a position of authority. Rather than allow the youth to make a mistake again, they reestablish their control. Although this may be necessary in extreme cases (e.g., when the youth is abusing alcohol), we recommend that the occasion be viewed as a learning opportunity in which parents can debrief with a child. That is, as objectively and unemotionally as possible, identify answers to these questions:

- What went wrong?
- What were the alternatives?
- What were the consequences for all the alternatives?
- What decision should be made in future circumstances?

Although parents and families could use assistance from an external source as they navigate these changing family dynamics, they may not seek it out for fear of exposing vulnerability. If they do seek assistance, parents and families need a receptive educator who can assure them that their challenges and fears are part of a normal process.

A Family Systems Perspective

Family systems theory focuses on events impacting a family as a whole rather than on individual members (Fingerman & Bermann, 2000). The theory posits that one must focus on each family and its behavior, family members' beliefs about each other, conflicts, separateness and connectedness, roles and boundaries, and adaptation to stress (Robin & Foster, 1989). Using a family systems approach, Witt, Riley, and Coiro (2003) studied families with children with disabilities. They found a positive correlation between children's functional limitations and family stressors.

The family systems perspective posits that families resist change in order to maintain a steady state of *homeostasis* (Fingerman & Bermann, 2000). Faced with the transition from school to adulthood for a family member with a disability, the family must deal with a major change. Each individual may react differently. It is important to understand that, from an educator's perspective, only the changes involving the youth in transition may be known. Observing behavior change from only one perspective may not reveal the changes that other family members are experiencing.

For example, one of the authors recalls Tory, an 18-year-old with a specific learning disability and emotional disturbance who received a certificate of completion from high school and struggled to find a job. Tory went to the VR office for assistance, but after several months, the VR counselor referred Tory to a university employment clinic (i.e., a program in partnership with VR to place transition-age young adults into jobs), saying that Tory was unable to hold employment because of family conflict. Tory's family situation was characterized by poverty and maladaptive behavior. His parents survived largely on public assistance. Neither his mother nor father worked, and his father lived at home only intermittently. The mother had bipolar disorder with mixed features (American Psychiatric Association, 2013). The father was reportedly an alcoholic. An older brother lived independently, working as a car mechanic, and provided financial support. Two younger sisters lived at home. During his transition from school to adulthood, Tory was helped by the clinic to find a job at a restaurant. However, clinicians found out that Mom and Dad were taking Tory's paycheck to use for food, alcohol, and cigarettes. Both were relying on Tory for cash. The older brother wanted to be the sole provider for the family and asked Tory to stay home to protect their mother from the father's abusive behavior. Tory's behavior at his job became inconsistent. His problems with employment were related to his uncertainty about how to behave, given his family's persistent conflicts.

Although complex family systems may not be their direct responsibility, transition professionals can assist in making referral to appropriate services and supporting the student. For transition professionals, the family systems approach helps them understand behavior patterns of youth during the transition process. Although no research has targeted this topic, we offer the following guidelines from our experience:

- Reactions to a youth's transition depend on the individual family's beliefs and values.
- Transition means major disruption to homeostasis, and family members struggle to redefine their roles and responsibilities.
- During transition, families will use their belief systems to interpret what is happening. In doing so, they may behave inconsistently, and in some cases, display behaviors that run counter to goals on the youth's ITP.
- If families approach them, transition professionals should understand their roles as supporters and information sources. They can offer advice, teach skills, provide counseling, and make referrals.

In Table 11.1, we present some of the changing roles of parents and other family members during transition of a youth with a disability.

Letting Go, Pulling Back

One of the authors recalls a psychologist describing a parent's behavior during the transition of a youth with a disability as "pushing her out the door with one hand while pulling her back with the other." Parents often desire to see their youth become

TABLE 11.1. Changes in Parent and Family Member Roles as Youth Transition to Adulthood

Former role	Transition role
Doer.	Observer.
Performer of tasks.	One who waits for the youth to perform tasks.
Advocate for the child.	One who helps observe the youth self-advocate.
Problem solver.	Consultant who remains available should the youth ask for help in solving a problem.
Choice maker.	One who allows youth to make choices.
One who does more.	One who does less.

independent, but as they watch them grow and flourish, they also resist it (Robin & Foster, 1989). Some parents interpret independence as the end of their roles as nurturers and caregivers. It signals that they, as parents, must search for new roles, which, in turn, raises their uncertainty and anxiety.

Transition professionals who understand that parents and other family members undergo this process can establish themselves in key roles as supporters and guides. Parents and other family members may react to their changing roles by engaging in various behaviors directed toward the professional (e.g., aggressiveness, self-blame, withdrawal) (Robin & Foster, 1989). Professionals must refrain from defensiveness, judgment, criticism, or rejection of the youth in transition (Egan, 2010). Instead, professionals must understand the changing roles and frustrations of parents/family members. It is imperative that transition professionals remain objective, neutral, and focused on the student's successful transition outcome (Test et al., 2006). If professionals are consistently receptive, open, and inviting, parents and other family members may eventually come to them for support and/or information. Developing a partnership with the parents and other family members during transition is ideal, and an open attitude is a key ingredient.

Transition May Change the Educator's Role

As educators reflect on what transition means to families (disrupter of homeostasis, changer of roles and responsibilities), it is important to understand that the same process may affect educators. Many transition educators develop close relationships with their students. Much like families, transition disrupts the educator's homeostasis with the student and forces the educator to redefine his or her roles and responsibilities. Once teachers, transition educators must now become mentors and consultants. Once prompters and doers, educators must stand back and wait for the student to initiate action (Dogoe & Banda, 2009).

WHAT CAN PARENTS AND OTHER FAMILY MEMBERS CONTRIBUTE AS PARTNERS IN TRANSITION?

Parents and other family members are critical to successful transition (Lindstrom et al., 2007; Test et al., 2009). They can become active team players and take on roles that educators cannot. At home they can reinforce skills taught at school. They can enable self-determination, teach independent living skills, assist youth in making contacts with adult agency personnel, help with applying for services or PSE programs, assist in transportation, and use the family network to look for job opportunities. Although this latter role can be instrumental, it is often overlooked. If an educator administers a transition assessment to identify job preferences, parents and other family members can take the next step by searching for preferred jobs through contacts with extended family, community contacts, coworkers, churchgoers, friends, club members, and others (Morgan & Schultz, 2012). The family network can leverage considerable influence in finding jobs for youth with disabilities.

Research on Family Roles

We find it useful to examine research on family roles and parent/family contributions in transition planning. Lindstrom and colleagues (2007) conducted multiple case studies on family variables impacting employment of 13 young adults ages 21–27 with specific learning disabilities. They focused on family structure variables such as parents' education, occupation, and socioeconomic status (SES). Qualitative data from 59 interviews were coded and analyzed for themes. Participants with higher SES had widely divergent employment outcomes (ranging from unemployment to full-time jobs), but the sample was small, thus limiting inference to the population. Two themes emerged for low-SES participants: (1) Young adults were often expected to make ongoing contributions to the family through work, and (2) young adults often sought to "be different from their parents" (p. 357). These themes should be considered when planning transition with families of low SES. Lindstrom and colleagues also found that family process variables influenced career development and outcomes. Participants with families characterized as "advocates" fared better in employment than participants whose families were less involved, regardless of SES. Participants whose families were characterized as "protectors" or "less involved" had lower wages and often lived at home instead of on their own (p. 356).

Research on Parent/Family Contributions

Landmark and colleagues (2010) found that family involvement was the third most evidence-based practice in transition, trailing only paid work experience and employment preparation. Correlational research revealed that young adults with specific learning disabilities and intellectual disabilities whose parents were moderately or highly involved in transition planning worked more hours, earned more money, maintained jobs longer, and lived more independently than those whose parents were less involved (Heal, Gonzalez, Rusch, Copher, & DeStefano, 1990; Schalock, Holl, Elliott, & Ross, 1992). In some cases, moderately and highly involved parents were active in assisting the youth with a disability in employment placement and in career decision making.

Wagner, Newman, Cameto, Javitz, and Valdes (2012) used the NLTS-2 database to study parent involvement in transition planning meetings. Findings from interviews with up to 6,860 parents and students included the following:

- A large majority of parents (87–90%, depending on age of the youth) reported attending their child's most recent IEP meeting.
- Parents whose annual household income was at least $25,000 were more likely to attend IEP/transition planning meetings than parents with lower incomes.
- About 70% of parents reported their level of involvement in the IEP meeting was "about the right amount" (p. 147), but parents of about 28% of students reported desiring more involvement in IEP/transition planning decisions.
- Youth whose parents were actively supportive of their education at home were more likely to play active roles in transition planning.

- When parents had high expectations for their youth pursuing PSE, the youth was a more active participant in the meeting.
- Satisfaction with the IEP/transition planning meeting was significantly higher among parents of 11- to 14-year-old youth than parents of 15- to 19-year-old youth, which authors attributed to burnout after years of dealing with special education.
- Lower rates of attendance, satisfaction, and active participation were reported by nonwhite parents than white parents.

More research is needed on family roles and contributions to transition planning. Targeted research on these topics would help educators understand how to best engage family members in transition efforts.

WHAT ISSUES ARISE WHEN FAMILIES PARTICIPATE IN TRANSITION PLANNING?

From the findings above, it appears that parents view themselves as involved in their children's planning. Many want *more* involvement, although family income affects degree of involvement. Satisfaction with transition planning decreases as children get older. Because involvement of parents and families is critical to transition success, educators need to investigate further to learn how they can facilitate this participation. Researchers have examined parent concerns about transition planning (e.g., Dukes & Lamar-Dukes, 2009; Rueda, Monzo, Shapiro, Gomez, & Blacher, 2005). These research findings and our recommendations for improvement are shown in Table 11.2.

TABLE 11.2. Research on What Transition Educators Can Do to Enable Increased Parent/Family Involvement

Finding	Recommendation
More than one-third of surveyed parents did not know the term *transition planning* (Landmark, Zhang, & Montoya, 2007).	Explain terms to students, parents, and family.
Professionals moved too fast when explaining terms, test scores, etc. (Dukes & Lamar-Dukes, 2009).	Slow down and explain things to students, parents, and family.
Parents felt like outsiders (Hetherington et al., 2010).	Make parents feel welcome and encourage them to communicate their expertise of the youth and actively participate.
Adequate information was not provided to parents (Rueda et al., 2005).	Insist that information is provided in understandable "dosages." Encourage parents to find advocates to attend meetings alongside them, or schedule premeetings for additional explanation and preparation.

One theme that runs through the findings from existing research is that educators may sometimes behave in a stereotyped way that does not convey sensitivity to the needs of parents and other family members (e.g., Dukes & Lamar-Dukes, 2009; Greene, 2011; Rueda et al., 2005). Although educators may have busy workloads, they should be sensitive to parent/family needs and understand the critical nature of developing a transition partnership. As Flexer and colleagues (2013) stated, "The sensitivity and willingness to suspend typical expectations and the openness to valuing the contributions of each family member, regardless of how different, are . . . the skills needed to be effective with all families" (p. 59). Beyond sensitivity, educators need to remain as open as possible to the needs of family members, including those who are ethnically, culturally, or linguistically diverse or from a different SES, gender or sexual orientation, nationality, or religion.

Working with Culturally/Linguistically Diverse Families

Most families, including many culturally/linguistically diverse families, have preconceived notions about educators. Many parents themselves had negative experiences in school (Pérez Carreón, Drake, & Calabrese Barton, 2005). Transition educators must counter negative attitudes and strive to establish partnerships. We offer three guidelines in working with culturally/linguistically diverse families. First, of course, not everyone of a particular culture, ethnicity, or language shares the same characteristics. Diversity exists within any particular culture, ethnicity, or language. As Greene (2011) stated, "When education professionals and practitioners make any of these assumptions, this can potentially lead to labeling and stereotyping, which limits their ability to respect the diverse practices of others and to rely on these individuals as a helpful resource" (p. 3). The focus should be on the needs, preferences, and characteristics of the individual family.

Second, many parents and other family members, regardless of background, are not educators themselves and do not speak "educator language." These parents and other family members do not understand the behaviors common to educators and may misinterpret certain actions. In Table 11.3, we address "inadvertent educator behaviors" and how to avoid them in establishing partnerships.

Third, some families from certain cultural/linguistic backgrounds do not share the values expressed in the IDEA legislation (2004) that transition should be a results-oriented, goal-directed process leading to postschool independence. For example, Rueda and colleagues (2005) conducted focus groups of 16 Latina mothers of youth with disabilities to understand their views of transition-related issues. The researchers concluded that these mothers' values focused on the home as the sanctuary of the family, as a place of shelter, and as the destination after graduating from high school. The values of these mothers were clearly different from those underpinning the IDEA and from the transition educator's view of youth with disabilities entering adulthood (striving toward goals related to employment, PSE, and independent living). When parents seek to maintain the youth at home after school, transition educators must balance requirements of legislation mandates with the need to fulfill parent and family aspirations.

TABLE 11.3. "Inadvertent Educator Behaviors" and How to Avoid Them

What educators sometimes do	What educators can do to develop partnerships with parents/families
Start the meeting with formal introductions.	Introduce all participants, but take a couple of additional minutes to get to know parents and other family members.
After introductions, recite the student's present levels of performance leading to transition goals.	Ask the student/parent/family about their vision of the future. Find common themes and similar points of view among family and educators.
Systematically read reports from each transition professional.	Ask the student to explore in depth goals and desires and how they relate to family beliefs. Note how they are similar to the educators' views.
Cite formal and informal transition assessment test scores (standard scores, grade-equivalence scores, etc.).	Ask all team members prior to the meeting to cite the tests administered (no abbreviations) and to explain test scores, providing examples.
Name the student's measurable postsecondary goals and annual goals.	Rushing into the future and setting goals can be very foreign to members of some cultures. Break down goals into small, time-limited steps.
Describe the student's goals as consensus decisions by the professionals without context.	Describe what the goals will mean to the student and family. Describe implications for family life and what supports will be available.
Move immediately ahead after family contributions to discussion.	Summarize using a phrase such as "What I hear you saying is . . ." Ask for verification.
Ask for questions only at the end of the meeting.	Break the meeting into short segments and ask for questions after each segment.
Stare at the paperwork.	Make eye contact with parents and other family members.
Look at your watch or the clock on the wall.	Set a relaxed pace in which the important factor is understanding, not daily schedule.

On the surface, this conflict can appear dichotomous: Either one side or the other must acquiesce. Because "staying home" does not meet the results-oriented postschool outcome requirements of a school district and the IDEA (2004), the transition team may pressure the parents/family in attempts to sway them to their point of view and the letter of the law. Instead, transition professionals are encouraged to negotiate with parents/family members by first finding common visions and processes. Opportunities are often hiding behind problems. Acceptable compromises may be available to transition teams willing to examine the needs of the family and consider creative ideas. For example, parents/family may accept innovative employment goals (e.g., family businesses or Web-based commercial enterprises) or PSE goals (e.g., online courses at community colleges or internships/apprenticeships) that do not compromise family values and interests in having the youth stay home. Greene (2011) offered recommendations for practice when interacting with diverse families of youth who have disabilities in the transition planning process.

- Ask for, listen to, and respect parents' perspectives and what they have to say about their child with a disability.
- Encourage parents to share their hopes and dreams for their child's future, even if they are different from the transition team's beliefs. Support parents' hopes and dreams as much as possible and incorporate them to craft transition goals reflective of a positive future for the child and the family.
- Be sensitive to the survival needs of families by scheduling meetings at a time and place that is convenient for all team members. Parents may hold jobs that require them to be present each day in order to get paid and maintain employment.
- Take the time necessary to build trust, rapport, and credibility with immigrant families of youth with disabilities to help ease potential fears of deportation.
- Keep an open mind because families may have different concepts of individualism, independence, and the importance of family (p. 7).

EXERCISE 11.1

If you were (are) a parent, what attributes and values would you like an educator to know about you? What attributes and values would you rather keep private? How should educators approach you to establish trust, rapport, and credibility?

EXERCISE 11.2

Respond to the following scenarios:

Jamal is a 15-year-old adolescent of the Wallace family. Jamal and his family are African American. Jamal, his mother (Ms. Wallace), and two younger siblings (Isabella and Macy) arrive for the IEP/transition planning meeting. After working with you (his teacher), Jamal is ready to conduct the meeting and describe his transition plan, which focuses on a business career. This plan will require that he perform well in math and language arts classes (not his personal strengths), develop study skills, and increase attendance. Jamal has been classified as having emotional disturbance. Upon arrival, Ms. Wallace says, "Jamal just needs to stay out of trouble. Every boy in our neighborhood ends up in jail. And Jamal is no exception. He could go that way. So I just want him to stay out of trouble." How do you proceed?

Sofia Aurelio is 17 years old; she and her family are Hispanic. Sofia has been classified as having autism. She lacks social and communication skills, but excels in math and computer skills. She has expressed interest in working toward a career in Web design and database management. She has taken courses in Web development. Mr. and Mrs. Aurelio have not been involved in Sofia's education. As her parents arrive for the IEP/transition planning meeting, Sofia describes her plan with occasional help from the teacher (you) and other transition team members. On several occasions, you ask the parents if they have questions, but they remain silent throughout the meeting. Near the end, you ask again if they have questions. Mr. Aurelio shakes his head without speaking and Mrs. Aurelio looks at the floor. What should you do? How do you proceed?

Sixteen-year-old Alyssa Smith has been classified with intellectual disability. Her mother, Ms. Smith, arrives 20 minutes late for the IEP/transition planning meeting. (Both are white.) Alyssa performs at low levels in academic skills but enjoys socializing with peers and teachers. She has expressed intevrest in working as a receptionist for a local business and taking classes at the community college. Alyssa is prepared to conduct the meeting and describe her plan. As Alyssa begins, Ms. Smith starts to cry. You (the teacher) offer tissue and ask what you can do to comfort her. Ms. Smith says, "Nothing." Ms. Smith continues to cry. Alyssa stops describing her plans. What should you do? How do you proceed?

WHAT IS QUALITY OF LIFE FOR FAMILIES?

Interacting with any family whose life view differs from that of educators requires flexible thinking. A worthwhile exercise for the educator is to draw back from the situation and consider quality of life. The World Health Organization (1997) defined *quality of life* as "an individual's perception of their position in life in the context of the culture and value systems in which they live, and in relation to their goals, expectations, standards, and concerns" (p. 1). Theoretically, many young adults with disabilities achieve a high quality of life by gaining meaningful employment, creating a career path through PSE, and living independently to the extent possible. In some family situations, however, a young adult with a disability could experience a high quality of life by staying home after high school—without being employed or involved in PSE. The ingredients for a high quality of life are determined by the young adult and his or her family. Only the young adult and his or her family members are in positions to evaluate quality of life; others may make judgments but be unaware of the unique set of ingredients that go into the equation. As educators, we have the responsibility to carry out transition planning as mandated by federal law (IDEA, 2004). Nevertheless, we sometimes have competing responsibilities to recognize family values that are different from our own, respect different qualities of life, and plan accordingly. The decisions we make will reflect our own values and professional practices.

EXERCISE 11.3

Respond to the following questions:

- How would you describe your quality of life?
- What factors impact your quality of life?
- To what extent do you think you evaluate the quality of life of others based on your own values?
- How do you reconcile differences in values?
- How do you decide which values to uphold?
- If competing values are part of the mix in establishing transition goals for a particular student and his or her family, which vway do you go?

HOW SHOULD EDUCATORS ASSESS FAMILY VALUES AS A PART OF TRANSITION PLANNING?

Clearly, one guide that emerges from working with families is the importance of understanding their values as a part of the transition assessment and planning process (Rueda et al., 2005). The more we know about a particular family's values, the better we can assist youth with disabilities in determining their futures in a way that is compatible with those values. Considerable research has addressed family values and how they affect career choice (e.g., Super, 1957; Whiston & Keller, 2004). Of note here are Whiston and Keller's (2004) findings that numerous contextual family factors are related to career choice, including SES, gender, transmission of parent values to children, presence of one or both parents, parent involvement in child development and school activities, and high versus low parent expectations, among many others.

HOW CAN EDUCATORS DEVELOP PARTNERSHIPS WITH FAMILIES?

Developing partnerships with families is essential to successful postschool outcomes (Greene, 2011). Nonetheless, the process can be time-consuming and labor intensive. We recognize from our own experience the effort level necessary to establish functional and effective partnerships with parents. We offer these recommendations to transition educators:

1. Contact parents on days when their youth has had positive achievements at school or in the community. Make a "call from school" a positive event instead of a sign of a problem. At the beginning of the school year, describe your plan to parents and ask them when the best time might be to call to avoid busy work schedules or other conflicts.

2. Before the school year begins, meet parents and family members at the school or community location. Tell the parents, "I want to get to know you and find out what you want for your [son or daughter]." Keep things informal and pleasant for the family.

3. Take time to get to know parents and their families. Find common interests and experiences to boost conversation.

4. Schedule meetings at times that do not conflict with parent work schedules or child care needs. Understand that parents may interpret messages differently. When an educator says to a parent, "I want to schedule an appointment with you, your son, and the VR counselor," a parent may hear, "You want me to take off work and find a child sitter."

5. Teach parents to understand education terminology, processes, and outcomes. Generally, parents are interested in learning about transition services. One study showed that, once trained and prompted to make contacts, many parents acted constructively to seek out transition services (Young, Morgan, Callow-Heusser, & Lindstrom, 2014).

6. Step back from negotiations to reflect on whether you, as an educator, are imposing your values on the family and youth in transition.

7. Flexer and colleagues (2013) noted that assistive technology for youth with disabilities should be presented cautiously to parents and other family members. Although educators value assistive technology for providing access to curricula and environments, parents may view it as a device requiring periodic repair. In turn, this may mean time off work, transportation, and needs for child care.

SUMMARY

As a youth with a disability grows, parents and other family members must constantly adjust their perceptions and behaviors. In this chapter, we described family systems theory as a useful philosophy for focusing on individual families to understand their beliefs about each other, their conflicts, and their patterns of separateness and connectedness, cohesion, and adaptation to stress. Families may resist change in order to maintainhomeostasis. Because transition involves a major change for the youth, behaviors of parents and family members may appear inconsistent. Parents and other family members need a transition educator who is receptive, open, and inviting. And just as parents and family must change their behaviors toward the youth with a disability, so must an educator. Transition educators who have become accustomed to playing roles of prompters and doers must now stand back, at times, and wait for the youth to initiate action.

Successful postschool outcomes depend on the involvement of parents and other family members. They play roles that educators cannot play, such as enabling self-determination, teaching independent living skills, assisting youth in making contacts with adult agency personnel, and using the family network to look for job opportunities. Researchers have shown that the majority of parents report attending IEP/transition planning meetings, although far fewer parents of low SES attend. Satisfaction with the IEP/transition planning process was reported as lower for parents of older adolescents than for younger adolescents. Meeting attendance, satisfaction, and active participation were lower for nonwhite parents than white parents. To some degree, these findings may relate to certain "inadvertent educator behaviors" that must be avoided. Three guidelines were offered for working with culturally/linguistically diverse families. Additionally, several implications for practice were offered for interacting with diverse families of youth who have disabilities in the transition planning process. When considering different values and beliefs about becoming an adult, such as staying home versus becoming independent, a useful perspective is to consider one's perception of quality of life. To better understand a family's perception of quality of life, family assessment is recommended. Once the transition educator assesses perceptions among a particular family's members, the educator can work to develop a shared vision for transition planning. Several recommendations were offered for establishing functional and effective partnerships with parents and other family members.

REVISITING JOSEFINA

Mateo knocked on the door of his parent's home. He held his 6-month-old daughter, Paola.

"*Hola*, Mateo," Mariana said as she opened the door. "Paola, my baby. Let me hold my granddaughter."

"*Hola*, Mom," said Mateo as he passed his baby to her grandmother. "*¿Cómo estás?*"

"I'm fine now that you brought me my little Paola!"

"Here, she's all yours, at least for a few minutes. How is everyone?"

"Great. How is your job at the auto parts place?"

"*Muy bien*. Can't complain. I might get a raise soon."

"Great. You have been working so hard, Mateo. You should get a raise. Come in, come in. I'll pour some coffee."

"Momma," Mateo sighed, "I need to talk to you about Josefina."

Mariana paused, holding the baby still. "Is something wrong?"

"No. I'm just confused. I thought we said in her meeting that she could sit the children and still become a child development specialist. And I thought in order to do that she had to take classes at South Shore Community College. Then she tells me that you and Dad went to her teacher at Ignacio and told her that she can't take classes after all. Momma, what is going on?"

"I talked to Raul and we had a change of heart. That's all."

"That's all? A change of heart? Momma, it's Josefina's future we're talking about."

"Mateo, it is our family we are talking about. Listen, I can't do everything at home. I need Josefina here to help me with the kids. Like little Paola. I need her help."

"Momma, Josefina has a great opportunity. You can't take that away from her."

"Like I said, it is our family we are talking about. We must stay together."

"We have a better chance of staying together if we are happy, and Josefina wants to take classes at the college. Let her have her dream, Momma."

"What if she takes classes, gets a job, and moves out?" His mother paused. "That would not make anyone happy. That's what you did!"

"Momma, I am a grown man."

"And she will soon be a grown woman. If everyone moves away, we will not have a family."

"Is that what this is about? Do you think we are going to leave you? Momma, I have my own family, but I didn't go away. Look, today I am visiting and bringing my daughter to you. We grow up and have our own lives, but we always stay connected to you. Josefina will be the same way. She is making herself better, but she will never lose connection to you. People can make themselves better as individuals and it makes the family better. As individuals, we can grow up, get stronger, smarter, happier—all that makes the family better."

"Mateo, I understand what you're saying. I see that you are grown and you still visit me. I know you still care. But I get worried. I get worried about change. We're changing as a family. Josefina is changing. I don't like change. It worries me that the family will change."

"Momma," Mateo started slowly. "Listen to me. I have changed. Josefina has changed. Look at little Paola. She is different today than yesterday. Everyone changes. Every individual in the family changes. The family itself changes. Change is part of life. But we still have each other. Sometimes we need family to resist change. Sometimes we have family to celebrate change. When everything changes, we will still have family."

EXERCISE 11.5

Review the recommendations in this chapter for increasing parent/family involvement in meetings and developing partnerships. Interview a transition educator and ask questions about one or two specific recommendations on how to increase involvement. How did the educator respond? Describe what you learned.

Review the list of "inadvertent educator behaviors." Interview a transition educator and ask questions about the effects of these behaviors. That is, ask, "Have you seen situations in which educators engaged in this behavior? What damage did this behavior do? What are the potential consequences of doing this?" Describe what you learned.

Let's return to Tory's case. What would you recommend to improve Tory's employment outlook? What would you recommend for his parents and family? What would you say to his brother to enlist his cooperation?

WEBSITES WITH ADDITIONAL INFORMATION

PACER Center: Parent Information Center for Families of Children and Youth with All Disabilities

www.pacer.org

Family Advocacy and Support Training Project

www.fastfamilysupport.org

Support for Families

www.supportforfamilies.org/internetguide/transition.html

Resources for Families of Youth Who Manage the Health Care Needs of Children

www.chop.edu/service/transition-to-adulthood/resources-for-patients-and-families.html

Child Welfare Information Gateway

www.childwelfare.gov/outofhome/independent

Utah Parent Center Transition to Adult Life

www.utahparentcenter.org/resources/transitiontoadult

College Options for People with Intellectual Disabilities

www.thinkcollege.net

CHAPTER 12

Interdisciplinary and Interagency Collaboration

This chapter addresses . . .

- The importance of interdisciplinary and interagency collaboration.
- Barriers sometimes encountered in collaboration and potential solutions.
- Research on effective collaboration strategies.
- Roles and functions of professionals representing various disciplines and agencies in the collaboration process.
- Community and state transition teams.
- The dimensions necessary for establishing an infrastructure for collaboration.

WHAT IS COLLABORATION?

Helen Keller said, "Alone we can do so little. Together we can do so much" (*www.psychologytoday.com/blog/here-there-and-everywhere/201205/25-quotes-collaboration*). Working together across professional disciplines and adult service agencies is essential to creating successful postschool outcomes for youth in transition. *Interdisciplinary collaboration* refers to relationships between two or more professional disciplines but not necessarily different agencies (Foster-Fishman, Berkowitz, Lounsbury, Jacobson, & Allen, 2001). Special and general educators, career technical educators, and school counselors may work together from different disciplines, but still work for the same "agency" (e.g., a school district). Steere and colleagues (2007) defined *interagency collaboration* as "key people from school personnel, family members, businesses, and human service agencies working together to promote successful post-school outcomes" (p. 115). As Test and colleagues (2006) noted, *interagency* is a term describing the relationships between representatives of two or more organizations (p. 145). Used here, *organizations* refer broadly to families, schools, and other groups.

Because transition is complex and involves school personnel, agencies, businesses, and community groups, interdisciplinary and interagency collaboration is instrumental to the process. As we illustrate in this chapter, it is only when transition professionals actively work together that they can produce successful transition outcomes for youth with disabilities.

Note that although representatives of different agencies may interact, they do not necessarily *collaborate*. Agency representatives can submit reports and attend meetings without collaborating in an active and ongoing way. Test and colleagues (2006) emphasized that "collaboration demands coordination and communication among multiple team members who may represent differing agencies and organizations" (p. 146). To be collaborative, Test and colleagues stated, a transition team must articulate common goals; share common values; agree on operating structures; share roles, responsibilities, and resources; and understand their shared accountability for success and failure. In this light, collaboration is a purposeful operation requiring intensive coordination, shared leadership, ongoing commitment, and active involvement of all team members. Beyond team membership, collaboration is a systemic process leading to successful transition to postschool outcomes for all youth with disabilities in a school, district, or state.

WHAT ARE THE BARRIERS TO COLLABORATION?

At the outset, we should note that many professionals initially find interdisciplinary and interagency collaboration uncomfortable. Interacting and developing relationships with professionals from different disciplines, philosophical orientations, and skill sets can be unsettling and challenging (Hurlburt et al., 2014). Based on our professional experience, we offer four possible explanations for the discomfort. First, educators may feel they are singularly responsible for a youth's transition and therefore fear that collaboration will reveal their own weaknesses or inadequacies in transition planning. Second, considerable differences in philosophies, language, and procedures across disciplines can cause professionals to hesitate in developing relationships with others or in delegating responsibilities to them. Third, biases against other disciplines or in favor of one's own profession can stifle collaboration. Fourth, and perhaps most importantly, we find that many transition professionals have very limited collaboration skills. Consider the transition teacher's responsibility. To facilitate transition, teachers are often charged with developing relationships with VR counselors, ASPs, employers, college-level DSO representatives, social workers, mental health therapists, and others. Yet, coordination of professional activity is a relatively new skill for teachers (Benitez, Morningstar, & Frey, 2009). Many do not receive adequate training in fostering collaboration skills in their teacher preparation programs (Blalock et al., 2003). There are few, if any, opportunities in already overflowing teacher education curricula for trainees to develop relationships with professionals from other disciplines or agencies. So we understand that interdisciplinary and interagency collaboration takes transition teachers into new territory.

Many professionals from different disciplines and agencies are uncertain of what to do when they must collaborate with others outside their field. For example, Agran, Cain, and Cavin (2002) conducted separate but "mirror-image" surveys with 54 special educators and 62 VR counselors to identify transition barriers. About half of the VR counselors reported they had never been asked to attend a transition services IEP meeting, even though they had transition-age youth on their caseloads. Of those who had attended transition planning meetings, 62% indicated they had not played an integral role. Many VR respondents indicated they had not received information on the youth in transition prior to the meeting and felt they had nothing to offer. About half of special education respondents indicated they rarely invited VR counselors to IEP meetings for transition-age youth. (Note that this study predated the 2004 reauthorization of the IDEA.)

The majority of special educator respondents indicated they did not know how to engage VR counselors in discussion targeted to achieving employment for youth in transition (Agran et al., 2002). Furthermore, they acknowledged they did not provide information prior to the meeting to inform VR counselors of individual needs. Information from an individual's educational file cannot, of course, be distributed without prior signed release from the parent/guardian. Finally, some special educators and VR counselors felt intimidated because they did not understand terms and abbreviations used by the other profession. Given these data, barriers begin to take on better definition and scope. Perhaps potential solutions begin to take form as well. In Table 12.1, we present some of the barriers and potential solutions (adapted from Morgan, Schultz, & Woolstenhulme, 2011).

HOW IMPORTANT IS COLLABORATION?

The IDEA (2004) noted the importance of collaboration by describing transition services as a coordinated set of activities to facilitate movement from school to postschool, "including postsecondary education, vocational education, integrated employment (including supported employment), continuing and adult education, adult services, independent living, or community participation" (34 CFR 300.43[a]). With this cue from federal legislation, transition professionals—many of whom have little or no formal training—face the need to become effective collaborators.

HOW DO DISCIPLINES AND AGENCIES COLLABORATE IN TRANSITION?

A starting point for developing effective collaboration is to understand the roles and responsibilities of each agency and discipline. One task is to identify the categories of professionals that, in many states and locales, support youth in transition by

TABLE 12.1. Barriers and Potential Solutions to Reducing Collaboration Problems between Special Education and VR

Barrier	Potential facilitators
VR counselors are not being invited to transition planning meetings or provided with information on a youth's needs that would allow them to prepare as active participants.	If acceptable given school district policies, educators may seek a parent/guardian's signature releasing limited information (e.g., current IEP goals, relevant assessment results) to the VR counselor prior to the meeting. Educators may want to send a note to the VR counselor about how the meeting will be conducted (i.e., whether the youth or teacher will direct the meeting), who will be present, and what transition outcome may be sought.
Once at the meeting, VR counselors are not being actively engaged as participating team members.	The educator may want to provide the VR counselor with a list of questions to ask at the meeting. Although these questions may evolve into different ones at the meeting, they will provide the VR counselor with a starting point for active engagement. At the beginning of the meeting, the educator or the youth needs to introduce all team members and make each one feel comfortable and respected.
Special educators and VR counselors speak different languages.	In transition planning meetings and in conversations, avoid acronyms; spell out each term and explain what it means. Respect the listener's need and desire to understand.
Special educators and VR counselors do not have a single meeting opportunity where they can engage each other in meaningful dialogue.	Combine conferences and meetings across disciplines. Arrange social opportunities and "transition fairs" with invitations to both professions. On days of IEP meetings, provide VR counselors with private space to meet with teachers, students, or parents; review records (with signed release); and make adequate preparation.

Note. From Morgan, Schultz, and Woolstenhulme (2011). Adapted with permission from the authors.

participating on transition teams. Table 12.2 shows these professional categories, with their roles and responsibilities, and partners with whom they may collaborate. We include a column of "primary collaborators" in Table 12.2 to show the probable partners for professionals. One caveat: Collaboration must be directed toward achieving goals for the student, not merely seen as an opportunity for professionals to develop relationships with others. The transition teacher should encourage collaborations but make it clear that professionals must work together for the purpose of bringing a youth closer to a successful postschool outcome.

Collaboration begins with an attitude of receptivity. To get started, professionals representing different disciplines and agencies need to be open to working with each other; "check egos at the door"; communicate as clearly as possible, including avoidance of all abbreviations and terms used within one's discipline or agency; and focus on the goal, which is the successful postschool outcome for youth in transition.

TABLE 12.2. Categories of Professionals, Their Roles and Responsibilities, and Others with Whom They May Collaborate in Transition Efforts

Profession	Roles and responsibilities	Primary Collaborators
Special education teachers	Develop, manage, and evaluate the student's IEP; coordinate transition services. Ensure that collaborative activities are goal-directed and designed to benefit the student.	All collaborators
General education teachers	Evaluate performance of students in the general education courses.	All collaborators
VR counselors	Conduct assessments with students, make decisions on VR eligibility, provide guidance and counseling regarding job prospects, arrange accommodations or assistive technology, and make job placement.	Special educators, career technical educators, school counselors, employers, ASPs
School counselors	Provide career counseling guidance and referral to students. Work with other educators to develop a student's course of study.	VR, special educators, general educators, career technical educators
Career technical educators	Suggest career technical education courses, assess student vocational performance, provide career education, and explore student preferences and interests.	Special educators, VR, 2- and 4-year colleges and technical schools, school counselors, employers
Counselors/ advisors from 2- and 4-year colleges and technical schools	Assist with student application process and financial aid; provide information on accommodations, assistive technology, and accessibility; provide advisement and counseling.	VR, special educators, general educators, career technical educators, school counselors
Speech and language, occupational, and physical therapists	Provide therapy to students designed to strengthen certain functions and modalities, such as speech, language, communication, mobility, sensorimotor function, or motor skills.	Special and general educators, VR
Health and medical specialists	Offer diagnosis and treatment of chronic health impairments and other conditions	Special educators, VR, social workers
Mental health specialists	Provide counseling and treatment services, work with families, and refer to appropriate programs.	Special educators, VR, social workers
Social workers	Assist with mental health, transportation, housing, financial, and other matters.	VR, special educators, general educators, school counselors, mental health specialists

(continued)

TABLE 12.2. *(continued)*

Profession	Roles and responsibilities	Primary Collaborators
Independent living specialists	Provide information for self-advocacy and understanding one's rights; provide training programs dealing with money management, sexuality, leisure activities, socialization, etc.	VR, special educators, ASPs
Adult service providers (ASPs)	Conduct assessments, provide counseling, develop and place youth on jobs.	VR, special educators, employers
Employers	Provide information on job shadowing and community-based instruction at work sites. Assist with job interview skills by working with students in schools. Work with teachers and youth to arrange supported or customized employment.	VR, special educators, career technical educators, general educators

WHAT ARE THE SKILLS REQUIRED TO BUILD COLLABORATION?

Developing a relationship with a professional from a different discipline and philosophical background is a task similar to accepting a new child into a classroom. Let's say a 7-year-old has just arrived at a new classroom after his family moved to the city. The teacher must understand the initial discomfort of the child, recognize the child's motivation (to be accepted by peers), and focus on the task at hand (the subject matter). Furthermore, the teacher must respect the new child's background, establish a positive and goal-directed environment, and make the child's roles and responsibilities clear to everyone. If the teacher makes an effort up front, the assimilation will likely be successful. Although we do not want to oversimplify the task of collaboration, we believe that educators can develop the skill sets needed to function as excellent collaborators and coordinators.

Collaboration should be goal-directed. Professionals from various disciplines and agencies can learn to work together if they share a common goal: for example, the successful transition from school to adulthood for a particular youth. But professionals must also learn the requisite skills (Noonan, McCall, Zheng, & Gaumer Erickson, 2012). Researchers (Foster-Fishman et al., 2001) conducted an analysis of 80 articles and chapters on community coalitions to identify the essential competencies that comprise the skill of collaboration. They divided the competencies into four skill areas: member, relational, organizational, and programmatic. Examples of key skills are listed below:

- *Member*: skills related to conflict resolution and understanding perspectives of other members, communicating effectively, creating and building effective programs, understanding target community, maintaining a positive attitude and commitment to targeted issues and program, showing respect for different perspectives, viewing others as legitimate and capable.
- *Relational*: being cooperative, trusting, open and honest; developing a shared

vision; sharing power; making decisions with input from others; minimizing status differences among members; valuing diversity; developing positive external relationships.
- *Organizational*: being an effective leader, managing resources, being task-oriented, clarifying staff roles and responsibilities, establishing effective communication systems, using timely and frequent information sharing, seeking continuous improvement.
- *Programmatic*: setting clear, focused objectives and goals; identifying intermediate goals; providing innovative services. (pp. 244–245)

Noonan and colleagues (2012) described successful collaboration in transition as requiring (1) key individuals who work together representing education and adult services, (2) monthly interagency planning meetings, (3) cross-agency training opportunities, and (4) use of a variety of collaboration and team building practices (p. 143). Other transition researchers (Johnson, Zorn, Yung Tam, Lamontagne, & Johnson, 2003) noted additional factors: (1) commitment, (2) communication, (3) strong leadership from key decision makers, (4) understanding the culture of other agencies, (5) engaging in preplanning as an interagency group, (6) providing adequate resources for collaboration, and (7) minimizing turf issues (p. 201). Wehman (1998) suggested the importance of established and functional state- and local-level interagency groups to provide an infrastructure supporting transition. Collectively, these factors comprise an integrated framework that may increase the probability of effective collaboration. In Figure 12.1, we illustrate these factors. We find the configuration of these interagency collaboration factors impressive and suggest that readers examine the status of their own collaboration networks in the exercise below. In doing so, some readers will rate their interagency

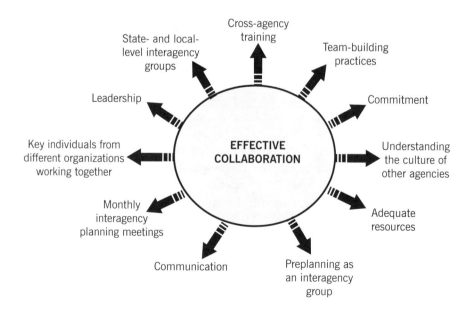

FIGURE 12.1. Interagency factors contributing to effective collaboration.

collaboration as high and others as low, but we assume that all readers will find factors that can potentially be improved.

EXERCISE 12.1

Using the rating scale and items below, rate the adequacy of school, district, or state interagency collaboration in your area (1 = poor, 2 = satisfactory, 3 = good). Ask a colleague to rate collaboration independently, then share your ratings. Examine the ratings for strengths and weaknesses.

1. Key individuals who represent education and adult services	1	2	3
2. Monthly interagency planning meetings	1	2	3
3. Cross-agency training opportunities	1	2	3
4. Variety of collaboration and team-building practices	1	2	3
5. Commitment to the collaboration process	1	2	3
6. Communication across disciplines and agencies	1	2	3
7. Strong leadership from key decision makers	1	2	3
8. Understanding the culture of other agencies	1	2	3
9. Preplanning as an interagency group	1	2	3
10. Adequate resources for collaboration	1	2	3
11. Minimization of turf issues	1	2	3
12. Established and functional state- and local-level interagency groups	1	2	3

WHAT IS THE RESEARCH EVIDENCE ON EFFECTIVE INTERAGENCY COLLABORATION IN TRANSITION?

Considerable research has analyzed interagency collaboration in transition (e.g., Aspel, Bettis, Quinn, Test, & Wood, 1999; Noonan, Gaumer Erickson, & Morningstar, 2013; Noonan, Morningstar, & Gaumer Erickson, 2008). For example, Noonan and colleagues (2008) identified school districts considered to be high performing in their transition programs. Focus group members in high-performing districts noted that a local transition coordinator was necessary—someone who was knowledgeable about multiple agencies, eligibility requirements, and funding—and who could network among all service providers and team members. The coordinator must be aware of scheduling issues in working with team members. For example, VR counselors may book up their calendar with counseling appointments several weeks in advance. On the other hand, educators cannot schedule appointments until after school hours. Therefore, creative scheduling, such as reserving a certain afternoon each month for transition IEP meetings, is needed.

High-performing districts made follow-up contacts during the transition period, such as calling students/families at least every 2 months for the first 6 months, then tapering the schedule (Noonan et al., 2008). Follow-up contacts were similar to those required of states to gather evaluation data on IDEA Indicator 14. Administrators in high-performing districts supported transition by paying substitutes so that educators could attend joint training with professionals from other disciplines and agencies. Participants in joint training included educators, VR counselors, adult agency representatives, families, and related-services professionals. Advantages to joint training included building relationships and gaining knowledge about other disciplines and agencies (Noonan et al., 2008).

Noonan and colleagues (2013) configured community transition teams for purposes of studying levels of collaboration. Participants included community transition team members consisting of 41 educators and 28 adult agency staff from one state. Communities ranged in size from less than 10,000 to over 50,000 in population. Participants received training in how to develop community transition teams. Sixteen teams were formed, each consisting of a school administrator, secondary special education/transition specialist, a VR representative, and three other members chosen based on individual needs of the community. That is, each team included representatives from different professional disciplines. The teams focused on activities to improve collaboration skills, including goal setting, action planning and education on adult agency services, as well as strategy development to address difficulties experienced in the collaborative process. Goal setting and action planning involved input from each discipline. After training, effectiveness was measured, based on responses to a 15-item transition collaboration survey. The survey included indicators of high-quality collaboration (Noonan et al., 2008). Results were compared to a pretraining survey of the participants. Researchers found that school staff rated all indicators higher after training, whereas adult agency staff rated 13 of 15 indicators higher. No data were provided on how the community transition team facilitated transition activities within schools or student outcomes, and it should be noted that these variables would have been difficult to isolate. In future studies, researchers may want to investigate the connection between team activities and transition outcomes.

WHAT ARE COMMUNITY AND STATE TRANSITION TEAMS?

Community transition teams consist of professionals from various disciplines and local agencies, as well as students and parents, who share resources, hold informational fairs, and influence policy (deFur & Patton, 1999, as cited in Noonan et al., 2013). Community teams can assist in creating interagency collaboration, sharing of information, and preventing duplication of efforts and services. Teams can identify local needs, plan and implement new programs, and evaluate efforts. Researchers (Aspel et al., 1999; Benz, Johnson, Mikkelsen, & Lindstrom, 1995; Malloy, Cheney, & Cormier, 1998) found that community teams were effective in increasing collaboration and postschool outcomes.

Malloy and colleagues (1998) evaluated the effects of a community transition team. Project RENEW (Rehabilitation, Empowerment, Natural Supports, Education, and Work) served 17 youth ages 16–22 with diagnoses consistent with serious mental illness, only two of whom were employed and only five of whom had finished high school. The project provided comprehensive case coordination to strengthen the students' prospects for employment, ongoing education, social–emotional adjustment, and community experience. The office for the project was located at a community technical college. Each youth participant was assigned a career and education specialist who coordinated services to accomplish personal goals (e.g., high school completion, employment, PSE). The community transition team consisted of representatives from community mental health, VR, the National Alliance for the Mentally Ill (NAMI), the school district, the community technical college, public agencies, and participants themselves. Collaboration included (1) gaining consensus on goals, (2) developing positive relationships among team members and youth, and (3) working to obtain resources. The team held monthly meetings to discuss person-centered planning efforts for individual youth. Each team member carried out assignments to assist individual youth. During an 8-month period, 16 of 17 youth secured competitive jobs and 13 maintained employment. Employed youth worked an average of 26 hours. Of 12 youth who had not finished high school, seven graduated or received their GED during the 8-month period. Fifty percent of the project's graduates enrolled in PSE programs. Project RENEW demonstrated the effects of focused interagency collaboration efforts in a community transition team.

State transition teams consist of state-level policymakers (e.g., special education, VR, career technical education, social service agencies) and representatives from higher education, school districts, parent organizations, and self-advocacy groups. Purposes of state transition teams include (1) providing expertise, (2) acquiring external funding (e.g., grants, foundations), (3) gaining local input, (4) providing ongoing support and training, and (5) disseminating information (Noonan et al., 2012). State teams are strategically positioned to assist community transition teams and to serve as a model for interagency collaboration.

Noonan and colleagues (2012) analyzed the collaboration efforts of a state-level interagency team. A mixed-methods study used social network and focus group procedures to determine the extent to which collaboration changed among team members. Results indicated that involvement on the team improved partnerships, cooperation, sharing of information and resources, joint leadership planning, and joint training. Specifically, members visited each others' agencies and became knowledgeable about their activities. At annual retreats, the state group reviewed data from multiple agencies, set priorities based on analysis of data, and developed action plans to target areas of need. Joint training was arranged for educators, VR, and the Department of Corrections staff working together. According to Noonan and colleagues, "During this time of decreased resources and growing workloads, it is important to understand that participating in the state transition team created stronger ties between individual agencies and a denser overall network" (p. 152).

Not all states have transition teams, and existing teams vary in their level of activity. Most teams are unfunded and instead function on a voluntary basis. As noted by Noonan and colleagues (2012), it is likely that state and community transition teams working together can improve performance on Indicators 13 and 14, although research is needed.

UTAH'S TRANSITION ACTION TEAM

One example of a state transition team is the Utah Transition Action Team (UTAT), which started as an interagency resource to local transition teams and IEP/transition planning teams. With over 50 active members, UTAT consists of representatives from higher education, state offices of education and rehabilitation, school districts, regional VR offices, state service agencies, community rehabilitation providers (CRPs), the Utah Parent Center, CILs, the Utah Disability Law Center, advocacy groups, and self-advocates. UTAT adopts the position that, through comprehensive assessment of barriers, diligent problem solving, and implementation of measurable objectives, the team can produce improved postschool outcomes. Targeted outcomes include (1) PSE opportunities in integrated environments (2- and 4-year colleges, internships, apprenticeships, and community education courses); (2) employment leading to career pathways (part- and full-time work in inclusive job settings); and (3) independent living (academic and functional skills, social and problem-solving skills, self-determination in decision making).

UTAT stakeholders focus their energies on five objectives: (1) increased collaboration with parents to strengthen their involvement in all phases of transition from school to adulthood; (2) heightened partnership with PSE programs across the state to promote educational opportunities for young adults with disabilities; (3) closer alliance between special education and VR to identify and reduce barriers to communication; (4) stronger affiliation with employers to provide their perspective on employment for young adults with disabilities; and (5) increased awareness of community resources for young adults with disabilities. Members often comment that UTAT offers a forum for the sharing of information that was previously unavailable.

UTAT holds quarterly meetings and an annual symposium. Unlike typical conferences with "breakout sessions," the UTAT symposium usually arranges daylong topical "brainstorming" groups in which participants identify barriers, issues, and resources; then develop action plans. Recent brainstorming topics included:

- Early academic and related skills in preparation for college entry
- Teaching self-advocacy and disclosure of disability in preparation for college
- Self-determination: guidance and instruction during the high school years
- Setting up inclusive "college experience" programs at institutions of higher education
- Interagency collaboration leading to college course taking: special education and school counseling, disability services in higher education, and VR
- College planning from the family perspective
- Vocational, technical, and community education
- Integrated, entry-level employment in community settings

Following a keynote speaker's presentation to the entire audience in the morning, participants select topic groups and go to separate meeting rooms. Two facilitators assist the group in developing action plans throughout the day. After two 90-minute sessions, groups report their action plans to the audience. Quarterly meetings serve as opportunities to report updated actions. A website allows participants to meet throughout the year and share resources. The symposium, which is held each summer with 80–100 participants, presents opportunities for stakeholders to get actively involved in seeking solutions to transition problems.

EXERCISE 12.2

Contact local education or state education agency representatives (special educators), transition educators, or state or regional VR representatives in your area. Are there community and/or state transition teams in your area? If so, what are their functions? How often do they meet? If a meeting is planned in the near future, ask if you can attend as a guest interested in learning more about interagency collaboration.

HOW IS COLLABORATION ESTABLISHED AS AN EXPECTATION IN TRANSITION PRACTICE?

In this chapter, we considered research on what constitutes effective collaboration. We discussed key ingredients. But how can collaboration be framed so that it becomes an expected practice? What infrastructure must exist to establish and sustain collaboration? Thomson, Perry, and Miller (2007) described the infrastructure for collaboration, and Noonan and colleagues (2013) related it to transition. Five "key dimensions" were described: (1) governance, (2) administration, (3) mutuality, (4) norms, and (5) organizational autonomy (Noonan et al., 2013, p. 102).

Governance and Administration

For interdisciplinary and interagency collaboration to thrive, it must be clear who is in charge, how decisions are made, and what the rules are for gaining consensus. Whether it is a state or community transition team or an individual youth's transition team, these issues are critical. Without them, dissension may arise or effort may dissipate. As much as possible, all collaborators should have a voice and share leadership. Differing ideas should be voiced, heard by all, respected, and considered. When professionals from different disciplines get together in the same space, differences should be expected. However, a proactive plan must be established for settling differences.

Mutuality and Norms

We have made the point that the goal of all collaboration is successful postschool outcomes for the youth in transition. But in pursuit of the outcome, the process requires mutual respect, an understanding of differences, and an ability to celebrate diversity (Thomson et al., 2007). This process starts with the youth in transition, whose vision for the future should be respected and supported by all. Collaborators should think twice about turf wars and petty posturing when it comes to generating group synergy on behalf of a youth in transition.

Organized Autonomy

Collaborators must understand that transition takes a team effort and each player plays a different position. Participants must remain autonomous because they are the only ones who can play certain roles. But it is the organization of autonomous players that makes the team successful in its collaboration effort.

CREATING A COMFORT ZONE

Although coordination and management of professionals from different disciplines and agencies can be uncomfortable, we encourage all transition stakeholders to view this as a highly rewarding and enriching activity. Working with a diverse array of professionals is a rare opportunity and exposes educators to new perspectives and knowledge. We have been fortunate to know many transition professionals who are excellent collaborators and respected by members of diverse professions. More important, through collaboration, these professionals are effective in producing successful transition outcomes—which means they are also respected by young adults with disabilities and their families.

Collaboration, we believe, can evolve from being a cause for discomfort to a source of strength in a youth's transition. Table 12.3 presents effective strategies to enhance collaboration.

SUMMARY

In this chapter, we described what collaboration means to a transition team, distinguished between interdisciplinary and interagency collaboration, and noted the barriers and their potential solutions. We divided collaboration competencies into four skill areas (member, relational, organizational, and programmatic) and discussed their component skills. The importance of collaboration was traced to federal legislation and effective transition outcomes. We described specific roles and functions of

---

TABLE 12.3. Effective Strategies to Enhance Interagency Collaboration

1. Build relationships.
2. Conduct interdisciplinary and interagency presentations to schools and adult agencies.
3. Hold conferences attended by professionals of various disciplines.
4. Create public service announcements and "success stories" about transition showing school and adult agency staff working together.
5. Develop flexible scheduling to accommodate professionals from other disciplines.
6. Arrange joint training of school and adult agency staff.
7. Develop and maintain transition councils.
8. Hold transition fairs and invite professionals of various disciplines, parents, and students.

various organizations and disciplines and cited research on interagency collaboration that has identified effective strategies. We detailed the actions of high-performing districts to understand best practices. Research on community and state transition teams is described. Finally, we discussed establishing collaboration as an expected practice in the field of transition.

REVISITING KENLEY

The first few months after Ashton left for college were trying times for the Schneider family. Ashton struggled in a college math class and devoted considerable time to getting a passing grade. Kenley was heartbroken to see his brother leave for college. His daily existence at home seemed empty and hollow. Ashton, or as Kenley called him, "Brother," had left to pursue his dream. Also, Mr. Schneider developed health problems that limited his activity at home and work. But with a shift in the family came changes in roles. Mrs. Schneider took a more active role in assisting Kenley and working with his teacher, Mr. White, and the VR counselor, Ms. Schmidt. And Ashton helped from a distance, checking on his brother and calling around town about job openings. The phone calls with Kenley were difficult for Ashton, who still struggled with his decision to leave his brother for college. Also, Kenley had always struggled with phone conversations because they required reading subtle social cues in voice tone that were hard for him to detect. And now it seemed his brother was in a foreign and faraway place.

But Ashton's absence was also producing a positive shift in Kenley's behavior. Kenley had to do chores at home that Ashton and Mr. Schneider had done previously. He saw himself helping out with family affairs like his brother had done. Kenley realized that he could accomplish tasks at home, such as mowing the lawn and shoveling snow "like Brother." When he was placed in a community job sample at Reicker's farm implement, Kenley began to perform tasks with confidence. Mr. White and Ms. Schmidt talked to Mr. Reicker about the prospect of a part-time job.

"Maybe. Let's see how he does first."

Kenley showed good skills in keeping inventory of tractor and implement parts by updating the computer files and reporting to Mr. Reicker when orders of new parts were necessary.

Ashton sighed as he took out his phone. Time for a phone call to the family. He dialed his family's home number. To Ashton's surprise, Kenley answered.

"Hi, Kenley."

"Hi, Brother. Oh, Brother! You know what? I'm doing stuff at Reicker's, Brother."

"You're at Reicker's?"

"Yes. It's just school. Not a job."

"Oh, I see."

"I'm doing stuff on the computer for Mr. Reicker."

"That's cool."

"Cool. Yeah. I might have a job there some day. I might do it."

"Really? Seriously? A job?"

"Yes, Brother. A job. I might do it, Brother."

EXERCISE 12.3

Interview a local professional who works in transition and has participated in interagency collaboration. Likely candidates for an interview are transition teachers, VR counselors, career technical educators, or school counselors. If these people are unavailable, interview a school district special education director. Ask about the person's experience in interagency collaboration. What made the collaboration effective? Ineffective? What barriers have been encountered? What, in the interviewee's opinion, would reduce those barriers?

WEBSITES WITH ADDITIONAL INFORMATION

Interagency Collaboration Annotated Bibliography

http://nsttac.org/content/interagency-collaboration-annotated-bibliography

Interagency Collaboration and Transition

www.pacer.org/tatra/resources/inter.asp

National Center for Secondary Education and Transition: Putting Interagency Agreements into Action

www.ncset.org/publications/viewdesc.asp?id=1689

Association for University Centers on Disability: Collaborative Interagency, Interdisciplinary Approach to Transition: Executive Summary

www.ncset.org/publications/viewdesc.asp?id=1689

Key Considerations for Implementing Interagency Collaborative Mechanisms

www.gao.gov/assets/650/648934.pdf

The Seven Norms of Collaborative Work

http://theadaptiveschool.weebly.com/7-norms-of-collaborative-work.html

CHAPTER 13

Accessing Supports in Transition

with SCOTT KUPFERMAN and HEATHER WEESE

This chapter addresses . . .

- Supports that youth may need during transition.
- The role of the transition educator as a support coordinator.
- Types, definitions, and examples of supports.
- Self-advocacy.
- Assistive technology.

WHAT SUPPORTS ARE NEEDED IN TRANSITION?

As youth with disabilities enter adulthood, they may require numerous supports in employment, PSE, and independent living. These supports may consist of people who provide assistance and deliver services (natural supports), resources, and assistive technology. Additionally, and perhaps most importantly, youth must develop "self-supports." In Figure 13.1, we illustrate the types of supports described in this chapter.

Throughout this book, we have stressed the importance of young adults learning skills to a level of independence. However, all young adults need supports in some

Scott Kupferman, PhD, CRC, is Assistant Professor in the College of Education at the University of Colorado, Colorado Springs. Heather Weese, MS, is Clinical Instructor in the Department of Special Education and Rehabilitation at Utah State University.

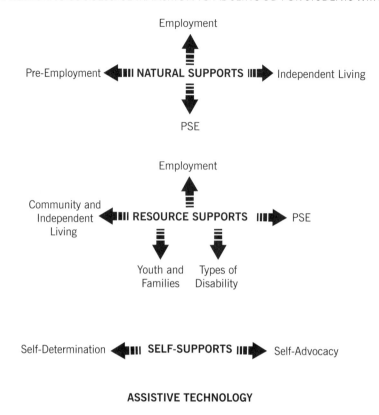

FIGURE 13.1. Types of support needed in transition.

areas. The important distinction is knowing which skills should be performed independently and which supports are needed for other activities. This chapter focuses on identifying and accessing supports.

Because supports are of paramount importance to the transition process, the transition educator plays a key role as support coordinator. Educators who understand their role as support coordinators can be essential to facilitating youth transitions to successful postschool outcomes.

WHAT ARE NATURAL SUPPORTS?

Natural supports are those typically available from other people in an environment. These supports can come from a variety of sources, including family members, classmates, coworkers, neighbors, peer tutors, education coaches, mental health therapists, health care providers, social workers, and others. Generally, these are professional, paraprofessional, or unpaid individuals who deliver services to the youth in transition. Professionals and paraeducators are necessary supporters for youth with disabilities because they offer specialized, targeted services. For example, a mental health counselor conducts assessments and provides therapy to assist youth in psychological, social, and emotional adjustment in transition to adulthood. For both professionals and paraeducators, specialized training is necessary.

Transition educators must ensure that staff members who provide support are adequately trained and supervised. In a qualitative research study involving observations of classroom activities and interviews, Giangreco and colleagues (1997) found that paraeducators who were responsible for supporting students who required significant supports sometimes performed tasks for the students rather than pause and allow students to perform tasks independently. From our observations, staff members who are paid to perform services for students with disabilities sometimes feel compelled to be "doing something." They have difficulty simply observing as a youth with disabilities learns to perform a task independently because the staff appears to be "doing nothing." Assuming a student in transition has received instruction in how to perform the steps of a task, merely observing the youth attempt independent performance while providing no extra prompts is entirely adequate (Crockett & Hardman, 2010).

For example, Matias is a senior who takes the city bus with his paraeducator (Vivian) to perform various tasks in the community. He has been working on these tasks in the classroom, and now must demonstrate that his new skills have "generalized" to the community. One of his tasks is to check the balance of his checking account at an ATM machine. Vivian has provided instruction in the classroom and Matias has performed the task independently. Now, in a community location, she tells Matias, "Do this on your own. If you need help, you can ask me, but then you'll have to do it again independently." Matias inserts his card in the ATM slot. Vivian simply watches to make sure Matias performs all steps in sequence. Matias looks at Vivian on a couple of occasions, but she says nothing and focuses her attention on the task. Matias eventually completes all the steps on his own. Vivian then gives him a high five.

All supporters, paid or not, need to understand that learning is not accomplished until the learner performs a task independently—that is, with no prompts. In turn, transition educators need to teach staff to avoid prompting unless it is absolutely necessary. Assuming a student can perform a task independently, the best support may appear to be no support at all.

When supports are needed, they can be provided to youth in transition in a variety of environmental contexts. We examine pre-employment, community education, employment, PSE, and independent living supports.

Pre-Employment Supports

The process of finding employment for a youth in transition usually involves:

1. The youth identifying job preferences.
2. The youth and supporters examining the local job market to find similar employment possibilities.
3. The youth and supporters going through the process of researching possible positions and applying for them (or in the case of customized employment, negotiating with an employer for a job).
4. The youth acquiring the job.

For youth with and without disabilities (and all job seekers), supports are often needed in the process of finding employment. To whom do we turn when we are seeking employment? Key support systems are friends and family.

The Friends and Family Support Network

When we seek employment, we often contact friends, family, coworkers, neighbors, churchgoers, and club/organization members. If we do not find someone who knows of a preferred job, we ask people to pass the word to others they know. The friends and family support network works relatively well in generating job leads. Yet, as Murphy and colleagues (1994) noted, in the case of youth with disabilities, "individuals, family members, friends, and associates have often been left out of the process and released of any role in finding employment with the job seeker" (p. 21). Transition educators can teach youth to use their friends and family network by (1) making a list of supportive individuals, (2) noting contact information for each person on the list, (3) contacting each person to inquire about job leads, and (4) writing or recording notes. The notes need to be updated frequently. The youth should follow up on job leads by contacting employers.

On a related topic, social media contacts can often assist the youth in locating employment (Duersch, 2013). With support, youth who are seeking jobs can use social media to announce their intentions for employment and to connect with potential employers.

Importantly, without consent from the parent/guardian, educators may not be able to influence the friends and family network directly due to the confidential nature of the youth's educational records. Thus, educators must first obtain parent/guardian consent before supporting students to explore their networks. See the Friends and Family Support Network Form in Figure 13.2. Youth and families can use this form to make contacts regarding a preferred job and to track leads.

Preferred job: _____
Friends and family to contact:

Name	Phone	E-mail	Notes
_____	_____	_____	_____
_____	_____	_____	_____
_____	_____	_____	_____
_____	_____	_____	_____
_____	_____	_____	_____

FIGURE 13.2. A Friends and Family Support Network Form.

Community Education Supports

The process of finding a community education class for a young adult can follow the same process described above. If a young adult is interested in a community education class but is unlikely to sign up independently, this support can be valuable. Friends and family are often aware of community education offerings. The youth and supporters can refer to local library, hospital, county, or adult education sources for information about community education courses. Transition professionals can also provide community education supports.

Employment Supports

When transition professionals set up situational assessments or community-based employment training for a youth in transition, they may want to work with employers to tap into an important support system available in most job sites: coworkers. Business and industry have long relied on coworkers to teach the steps involved in performing a specific job and to solve problems. McDonnell (2010) described three steps to fostering natural supports from coworkers:

1. Establish a working relationship with the supervisor.
2. Support the youth's participation in typical orientation and employee training activities.
3. With the supervisor's approval, train coworkers to support the youth. The transition professional should encourage the coworkers and supervisor to communicate directly with the youth, not through the professional.

Achieving "Natural" Supports

Transition professionals should use support systems that are compatible with the particular work environment (Murphy et al., 1994). Support of the youth with a disability should be as natural to the workplace as possible. Initially, supervisors and coworkers may be hesitant to interact directly with the youth if they think it is the transition educator's role. Transition educators should encourage all workers to communicate directly with the youth, not through the transition professional.

PSE Supports

Because transition educators may assist youth with disabilities in planning for PSE involvement, an understanding of PSE supports is important. In PSE programs, youth may be supported in a variety of ways. Education coaches (similar to peer tutors, but at a college level) and DSO counselors are two sources of support. The role of the DSO was described in Chapter 9. Education coaches are often college students who play roles of (1) helping students adjust to the pace of a class; (2) encouraging appropriate classroom behavior; or (3) teaching organizational, study, and time management skills (Paiewonsky & Roach Ostergard, 2010). Transition educators who work with college-bound students with developmental disabilities can ask that DSO program staff explore the prospect of education coaches. Some college students may seek to be education coaches if they are pursuing a teaching career and need "independent study" credits. Others may want to be education coaches if they are involved in "service learning" courses. Transition educators should be aware that the role of the education coach is strictly related to increasing study and other skills, not to teaching content. Additionally, coaches usually do not attend classes alongside students and never attend in place of students.

Independent Living Supports

Supports can be provided in supervised apartments (with the resident supported through periodic visits from ASP staff), college dormitories (with the resident supported by residential assistants), or group homes. Transition educators may provide information on the independent living support needs for youth in transition to adulthood. Educators can also inform independent living supporters regarding the needs of youth with disabilities, such as individuals' strengths and weaknesses, skills to be taught, and health conditions.

WHAT ARE INFORMATION RESOURCE SUPPORTS?

Information resources include websites, webinars, presentations, printed documents (e.g., brochures), and media. These resources are geared to (1) youth or families, (2) employment, (3) PSE, (4) community and independent living, or (5) types of disabilities. They are available on a local, state, or national level. See the website list of national resources in Table 13.1. The challenge for transition teachers and other team members is to organize and maintain a list of currently available resources so that all stakeholders have ready access. Available resources depend on one's locale, funding, and staffing. A useful starting point to find information resources is one's local CIL, which provides information and referral regarding resources to individuals with disabilities. See the CIL websites at the end of this chapter.

EXERCISE 13.1

Create or locate a list of locally available transition-related resources with (1) name of resource, (2) description of services provided, and (3) contact information. Contact individuals directly to verify the availability of services.

WHAT ARE SELF-SUPPORTS?

If *self-determination* is conceptualized as volitional actions necessary for maintaining or improving quality of life (Wehmeyer, 2005), then *self-supports* are the products or outcomes of those actions. Self-supports are a repertoire of skills allowing youth to adapt to new situations, advocate for themselves, access new environments, and create

TABLE 13.1. Resources Available to Youth with Disabilities and Their Families

Youth and family services

Family Resource Network	*www.familyresourcenetwork.org/?gclid=CP-HvOWly78CFac7MgodqB4A3A*
HEATH Resource Center at the National Youth Transitions Center	*http://heath.gwu.edu*
Transition Coalition	*http://transitioncoalition.org/transition/index.php*
Parent Training and Information Center	*www.pacer.org*

Employment services

U.S. Department of Labor	*www.dol.gov/dol/topic/disability*
National Organization on Disability	*http://nod.org*
Job Accommodation Network	*https://askjan.org*

PSE: See Chapter 9

Types of disability

Autism Speaks	*www.autismspeaks.org*
Learning disabilities	*www.ldonline.org*
Intellectual disability	*www.thearc.org* *http://aaidd.org*
Traumatic brain injury	*www.traumaticbraininjury.com*

Community services

Centers for independent living	*www.ncil.org/about/aboutil* *www.ilru.org/projects/cil-net/cil-center-and-association-directory*

General information

U.S. Government website providing information on disability programs and services	*www.disability.gov*
National Secondary Transition Technical Assistance Center	*http://nsttac.org*
Teaching Self-Advocacy	*http://teachingselfadvocacy.wordpress.com*

new opportunities. Youth with disabilities must be taught skills that facilitate self-determination during the transition period so they are not solely dependent on externally provided supports in adulthood. Wehmeyer, Agran, and colleagues (1998) noted, "Students need to learn how to be as independent as possible, but they also need to learn how to gain access to resources that are available in their community that provide supports, instead of waiting on someone else to gain access to that resource for them" (p. 66).

We discuss a set of skills related to self-determination that lead to self-support: self-advocacy skills. These skills are critical in numerous environments that youth will access as adults.

Self-Advocacy Skills

Advocating for oneself involves a complex set of skills that develop throughout adulthood. Few of us enter adulthood with well-tuned self-advocacy skills. But youth with disabilities must have the rudiments of self-advocacy skills as they enter adulthood because there will be occasions to use them. Researchers have identified component skills and situational contexts for self-advocacy. Grigal and Hart (2010) cited three component skills of self-advocacy for college students with intellectual disability: (1) identifying and describing one's disability, (2) naming one's needed supports/accommodations, and (3) asking for accommodations.

Many times, students are reluctant to talk about their disability (Eisenman & Mancini, 2010). However, the subcomponents that comprise the skill of disclosing one's disability can be taught to students with disabilities. These subcomponents include (1) understanding the rationale and justification for discussing the disability (i.e., getting what one needs to perform well); (2) rehearsal, practice, and feedback in the disclosing of this information; and (3) knowing when, where, and with whom to disclose.

Beyond these skills, additional ones are also necessary. For example, Eisenman and Mancini (2010) suggested that critical PSE self-advocacy skills consist of understanding one's learning style and providing a rationale for needed accommodations. In searching for employment, Luecking (2009) described self-advocacy skills as including the ability to:

- Summarize interests and preferences.
- Name preferred geographical locations for work.
- Identify a preferred schedule and why.
- Describe situations to avoid and why.
- Note any job accommodations needed.

Teaching Self-Advocacy

Other than research on self-determination curricula (see Chapter 7), there is limited research on how to teach self-advocacy skills to youth with disabilities (Balcazar, Fawcett, & Seekins, 1990). Grigal and Hart (2010) suggested components of the teaching process. Actual lesson plans for teaching self-advocacy depend on a youth's communication skills, functional capacity, and environmental context within which the skills are taught. Here are the rudiments suggested by Grigal and Hart for teaching self-advocacy to youth with disabilities:

1. Provide a rationale. Youth need to understand why it is important that they learn to advocate for themselves. Transition educators should convey the message that "you can go more places, find more opportunities, and get what you want when you advocate for yourself."

2. Note that everyone has strengths and weaknesses. Educators should self-describe strengths and weaknesses. Have students describe their own strengths and weaknesses. Describe abilities and disabilities. Even famous people have disabilities. (For numerous examples, see *www.disabled-world.com/artman/publish/article_0060.shtml*.)

3. Educators should convey that there is no shame in describing one's disability. It simply means that one needs assistance in accomplishing some things.

4. Students should take turns describing their abilities and disabilities. Example: "I am a good athlete and can play most sports. I also have a learning disability in math, so I have problems with numbers. So I have strengths and weaknesses, like everybody else."

5. Describe accommodations. Transition educators can communicate that, when people have disabilities, they simply need assistance in some matters. Assistance comes in the form of people, resources, and services (define and describe reasonable accommodations). Show examples of how to ask for reasonable accommodations and allow students to practice. Example: "I need extra time to count, add, and subtract numbers."

6. Distinguish the right time and place. Describing one's disability and needed accommodations requires carefully distinguishing the correct time and place to do so. Students should describe disabilities in private meetings with a DSO counselor, a college instructor, or an employer. There are many other situations in which descriptions are contraindicated (e.g., to unfamiliar persons, to large gatherings, on social media). To facilitate distinctions, provide several examples and nonexamples.

7. Use a script. Barnard-Brak, Lechtenberger, and Yan (2010) conducted interviews with college students who had disabilities. All interviewed students reported they used a prelearned script to describe their disability and needed accommodations. From their reports, using a script reduced anxiety and increased confidence. Using such a script, students with no vocal language could work with a support person to create a recorded message.

8. After describing one's disability and needed accommodations, express appreciation for the person's understanding. To avoid being shunned or outcast for talking about disability, say "Thanks for understanding." The student might add, "It is hard for me to talk about this, and it might be hard for you to hear. So I really appreciate and respect you for listening."

Practicing Self-Advocacy Skills

For students to learn to self-advocate, they need opportunities to practice and receive feedback from transition teachers. Unfortunately, there are few practice opportunities until a student enters employment, PSE, or independent living (Izzo & Lamb, 2002). Transition educators need to brainstorm ways to strategically develop practice opportunities for self-advocacy skills. These may include mock interviews with employers or DSO staff at colleges, or scripted conversations with high school faculty, peer tutors, or others.

EXERCISE 13.2

Create a lesson on how you would teach students to self-disclosure their disability. Select the characteristics and ages of students you are teaching and the context. Then, list the steps in the teaching process and the practice activities of the students (similar to those illustrated above).

Assertiveness Training

Before we leave self-advocacy, we want to point out that learning self-advocacy skills involves use of assertive behaviors. Assertiveness training has a long history in psychology (Alberti & Emmons, 1970). Key components of assertiveness training include:

- Using "I" statements, such as "I will work very hard on this job. What I need is. . . . "
- Making eye contact with the person during at least 50% of a conversation.
- If talking to a group, making eye contact periodically with each person.
- Speaking with socially acceptable voice volume (not too loud, not too soft).
- Distinguishing between assertiveness, passiveness, and aggressiveness. Assertive statements are those that convey the message that a person is standing up for his or her rights.

Teaching students to be assertive will move them along the path to developing self-advocacy skills. Transition teachers who teach self-assertion will equip students with important skills to support themselves as they enter adulthood. For more information, see Nangle, Erdley, Carpenter, and Newman (2002).

WHAT IS ASSISTIVE TECHNOLOGY?

From eyeglasses to iPads, we all rely upon technology to learn, work, and socialize. When technology is specifically designed to help people with disabilities, it is called *assistive technology*. The IDEA (2004) defines assistive technology as "any item, piece of equipment or product system, whether acquired commercially off the shelf, modified, or customized, that is used to increase, maintain, or improve the functional capabilities of children with disabilities" (Authority 20 U.S.C. 1401[1]). This broad definition leads to an equally broad range of possibilities. Able Data (2014) identified nearly 40,000 types of assistive technology devices in 20 categories. For practical purposes, eight common categories are highlighted below.

1. *Computer access*. People with a variety of disabilities use assistive technology. For example, a person with a physical disability may use speech recognition software to navigate a computer and input content into a word processor. A person who is blind may use screen reading software to navigate a computer and have content read aloud. Other examples include touch screens, screen magnification software, large monitor, head-operated pointers, and adaptive keyboards.

2. *Daily living*. Assistive technology within this category relates to devices that aid in cooking, eating, clothing, self-care, and other home and personal activities. For example, people with physical disabilities often use grab bars and a shower chair within bathroom settings and accessible eating utensils and plates when eating.

3. *Environmental access*. Within this category, assistive technology reduces or removes physical barriers for people with a variety of disabilities. A common example is an environmental control unit, which allows an individual with a physical disability to turn on lights, lock doors, control heating/cooling, etc. Other examples include wheelchair ramps, flashing smoke alarms, ergonomic workstations, automatic door openers, and lowered counters.

4. *Hearing*. People who are deaf or hard of hearing often use assistive technology. Examples include personal amplification systems, video relay systems, text telephones, and closed captions.

5. *Learning*. People with specific learning disabilities, cognitive disabilities, and developmental and intellectual disabilities often use assistive technology. Examples include word prediction software, text-to-speech software, personal organization devices, and mind-mapping software.

6. *Mobility*. People with physical disabilities use mobility-related assistive technology, including wheelchairs, scooters, walkers, transfer aids, stair lifts, and accessible vehicles.

7. *Speech/language*. People with speech and language disabilities are the primary users of assistive technology. An example is an augmentative and alternative communication (AAC) device. A basic AAC device is a set of static pictures that an individual can point to in order to communicate. More complex AAC devices have computerized speech output and a dynamic vocabulary list.

8. *Vision*. People who are blind or have low vision often use assistive technology. Examples include text-to-speech devices, optical character recognition scanners, Braille devices, talking watches/clocks/calculators, tactile image makers, and large button phones.

Historical and Legislative Background of Assistive Technology

One way to acclimate youth with disabilities to the notion of assistive technology is to start with a history lesson. The earliest documented use of assistive technology is traced to a collection of Indian hymns written around 1700 B.C.E. These hymns described a prosthetic iron leg used by a wounded warrior, allowing him to return to the battlefield

(Griffith, 1889, p. 203). Modern-day assistive technology began in the late 1980s and early 1990s. Electronics, specifically microprocessors, have spurred much of the development. Students who are blind, for example, can scan printed materials and have the text read aloud via screen reading software. Those who are deaf can communicate in sign language with others remotely using a video relay system. Students with speech and language disabilities can communicate through the use of an AAC device. Those with physical disabilities can control a computer through speech and eye movements. Additional examples are plentiful and emerging on a daily basis.

The availability of assistive technology has been driven, in large part, by federal legislation. Notable is the Technology Related Assistance for Individuals with Disabilities Act (Tech Act) of 1988. This was the first federal legislation directly related to assistive technology. The reauthorizations (Assistive Technology Act, 1998, 2004) required interagency coordination of assistive technology to avoid gaps of availability during the transition process. The Tech Act also required states to offer assistive technology-related outreach to students and families, as well as professional development for educators and other professionals. In addition to the Tech Act, the IDEA of 1990, 1997, and 2004 specifically defined assistive technology devices and services and required that assistive technology be considered as a core component of students' IEPs. Other relevant legislation included the Rehabilitation Act of 1973, Americans with Disabilities Act of 1990, Elementary and Secondary Education Act of 2002, Telecommunications Act of 1996, and Carl D. Perkins Vocational and Technical Education Act of 1998.

Quality Indicators for Assistive Technology

When it comes to assistive technology, transition educators have an important yet challenging task. They must answer the question: "Why is it important?" Providing assistive technology is considered to be an evidence-based practice that can make a difference between success and failure for transition-age students (Webb, Patterson, Syverud, & Seabrooks-Blackmore, 2008). Furthermore, Bouck, Maeda, and Flanagan (2011) found that students who used assistive technology in secondary school had more positive postsecondary outcomes in terms of a paid job, higher wages, and participation in PSE. Why is providing assistive technology a challenge? Transition educators must think beyond the classroom by considering where assistive technology will be used (e.g., work, college, apartment), who will pay for it when it is no longer provided by special education funding (e.g., VR, private insurance), and who will maintain it (e.g., CILs, vendors). To assist transition educators, the Quality Indicators for Assistive Technology (2012) coalition identified six quality indicators that should guide the consideration of assistive technology during the transition planning process (see Table 13.2). The main takeaway point from these indicators is that assistive technology should be an integrated component of the transition planning process rather than an isolated event.

Assistive Technology Teams

Transition educators are not alone in navigating the assistive technology process. Rather, they are members of assistive technology teams who evaluate, select, and support the

TABLE 13.2. Quality Indicators to Guide the Consideration of Incorporating Assistive Technology during the Transition Process

1. Transition plans address assistive technology needs of the student, including roles and training needs of team members, subsequent steps in assistive technology use, and follow-up after transition takes place.

2. Transition planning empowers the student using assistive technology to participate in the transition planning at a level appropriate to age and ability.

3. Advocacy related to assistive technology use is recognized as critical and planned for by the teams involved in transition.

4. Assistive technology requirements in the receiving environment are identified during the transition planning process.

5. Transition planning for students using assistive technology proceeds according to an individualized timeline.

6. Transition plans address specific equipment, training, and funding issues such as transfer or acquisition of assistive technology, manuals, and support documents.

Note. Adapted from Quality Indicators for Assistive Technology (2012). Adapted by permission.

use of assistive technology. Team members often include the student, family members, assistive technology specialist, transition educator, VR counselor, school administrator, occupational therapist, and/or speech–language pathologist. Members may assume multiple roles and contribute their area of expertise. For example, transition educators might teach students when and how to disclose their needs and self-advocate for appropriate assistive technology devices and services in PSE, employment, and community settings. Transition educators might also create and coordinate a plan to fund assistive technology throughout the transition process.

Funding for Assistive Technology

The most common question about assistive technology during the transition process is, "Who pays for it?" Schools are no longer the primary funding source for purchasing assistive technology. Transition educators, along with other members of assistive technology teams, must explore alternatives. Assistive technology programs (see *www.ataporg.org*) are available in every state and offer information about funding options, assistive technology loan programs to bridge the gap between funding sources during transition, and alternative funding options (e.g., low-interest loans, interest buy-downs) when no other source is available. In addition to these state assistive technology programs, VR often pays for assistive technology, particularly when it assists students in attaining their employment or PSE goals. If the assistive technology relates to students' health and daily functioning needs, insurance such as SSDI, Medicaid, and private insurance are potential funding sources. Lastly, CILs and other community organizations may offer funding for specific types of assistive technology, such as transportation-related vehicle modifications. For any of the aforementioned funding sources, the availability and amount of funding are dependent upon why the assistive technology is needed, where it will be used, the age of the student, and the financial resources of the family. See websites at the end of this chapter for assistive technology resources.

CASE EXAMPLES: YOUTH IN TRANSITION
WHO USE ASSISTIVE TECHNOLOGY

Bryson

Bryson is 20-year-old male who attended a local university and lived at home with his parents. He experienced a traumatic brain injury from a car accident when he was 17 years old. Following the accident, Bryson suffered from severe brain swelling (intracranial edema) and loss of eyesight. The edema resulted in loss of word recall (vocabulary) and expressive language. Bryson had to relearn language, vocabulary, and expressive communication. After attending speech and language therapy sessions, his vocabulary started to return and he began to verbally express himself more proficiently. Bryson is now enrolled and taking courses at a university working toward his bachelor's degree. Due to his severe vision loss, Bryson struggled to see the screen of his computer and smartphone. Both of these devices were necessary for him to access course assignments, PowerPoint presentations, social media, and so forth. The limited ability to access presentation software, Web browsers, word-processing programs, and Internet search engines led him to express great interest in learning to manipulate the settings on his computer to make them usable. Bryson's assistive technology specialist at the university DSO decided (1) to manipulate the computer settings to make them more accessible to him and (2) to teach him to use speech-to-text software.

A team at the local university researched the best way to manipulate the computer settings based on Bryson's visual needs. He was taught how to make the desired changes on his computer so he could independently manipulate the settings in the future. Some of the simple adaptions included enlarging the size of the icons on the desktop, organizing the icons by placing them in a certain order, enlarging the mouse pointer, setting up the magnifying tool, making separate user profiles for Bryson and his parents, and setting up icons for easy access to his favorite Internet links. After the initial training, he was given step-by-step instructions on how to make these changes. Bryson was also given a copy of Dragon Naturally Speaking. This speech recognition software allowed him to locate documents, search the Internet, and use e-mail quickly and accurately by using his voice.

Additionally, Bryson needed a way to make his smartphone more accessible for school and everyday life. His phone was a device he carried everywhere. He desired to broaden his vocabulary outside of speech therapy sessions. At the university, he needed a way to easily access his class schedule, track class assignments, and find websites. The specialist installed several applications on his smartphone. Bryson and his parents were trained on the applications. Some of the apps included one published by the university to assist him with accessing his school schedule, locations, professors, assignments, and so forth. He also used a dictionary app to assist with word recall and memory. Bryson had a voice recorder, magnifier, and text-to-speech app to assist with daily living tasks, schedules, homework, and social interaction.

Angela

Angela is a 19-year-old female diagnosed with autism who attended post–high school classes, lived at home, and was preparing for a future job. She needed assistive technology at school, home, and community settings to increase her independence in a variety of areas. Angela had completed the fourth-grade curriculum in several core areas; however, her reading comprehension was at a second-grade level. In order to be more successful at school, additional time receiving reading instruction and testing comprehension was needed. A main focus during Angela's school day included instruction in job skills, daily living skills, and social skills. Because she was preparing to move away from home, she also needed to perform many daily living tasks independently, such as grocery shopping, cooking, cleaning, laundry, and dressing.

Angela had an iPad with an application allowing job, daily living, and social skills to be task-analyzed into simple, step-by-step procedures. The application allowed an instructor to take photos of each step, add text, and voice-record the instructions for each step. Angela's teacher encouraged the use of the comprehension questions to help her generalize and increase her comprehension skills. The step-by-step instructions with the actual photos of her completing each step assisted Angela in her efforts to gain increasing independence in completing these tasks with higher rates of accuracy.

Zachary

Zachary is a 21-year-old who loves music, snacks, and going for walks in his wheelchair. He was born with hydrocephalus, epilepsy, and cognitive impairment. He could walk about 50 yards at a time with a walker and a gait-support belt as long as a trained escort assisted him. Zachary completed a post–high school program, and was now attending a vocational training program at a local community college while receiving assistance from VR. He had assistive technology needs in various settings, including his home and the vocational training center. However, he had not developed verbal communication in previous educational programming. Instead, he had used communication devices such as talking boards and the PECS. Based on a referral from VR, an assistive technology team and Zachary worked at home and at the vocational training center to implement a communication board that was about 24 inches by 36 inches with a series of tangible symbols attached with Velcro. The items on the board were objects that Zachary could physically grab, remove from the board, and give to an individual to express a need. The symbols included a water bottle to communicate the need for a drink, a shoe to communicate he wanted to stand up, a fan to communicate he was hot, a swatch of fleece material to communicate he was cold, a snack box to communicate he was hungry, and a handheld music player to communicate his desire to listen to music. Zachary used a similar system at school, although the tangible symbols were different.

EXERCISE 13.3

The preceding case examples may be incomplete in their applications of assistive technology. What else would you recommend for Bryson, Angela, and/or Zachary to increase, maintain, or improve the functional capabilities of these young adults?

SUMMARY

In this chapter, we examined support systems needed in the transition to adulthood, including people who deliver services (natural supports), resources, self-supports, and assistive technology. Natural supports were divided into pre-employment, employment, PSE, and independent living areas. Resource supports were described in relation to youth or families, employment, PSE, community and independent living levels, and types of disabilities. Self-supports were described as those that allow youth to adapt to new situations, advocate for themselves, access new environments, and create new opportunities. Various component skills and procedures that transition teachers might use to teach the necessary skill of self-advocacy were described. Assistive technology was defined and divided into eight categories. Legislative background, quality indicators, teams, and funding sources for assistive technology were described.

REVISITING JOSEFINA

Josefina, her parents, and Ms. Martin went to South Shore Community College to meet the staff at the DSO. The DSO director provided a tour of the campus. Josefina met some of the instructors of her future classes. After a long day, the family returned home. Mariana, Josefina's mother, walked into Josefina's room.

"Josefina, you must be tired after going all around that college campus."

"Not really," Josefina responded. She looked at her mother. "I'm so excited."

"I can understand your excitement. You're going to take college classes."

"Sí."

"Josefina," her mother started. "This is a very big step for you. I still can't believe it."

"What are you thinking, Momma?"

"I'm just trying to think about all of this. You have graduated from high school. Now you will be going to college. My goodness. It is so much to think about."

"It's OK, Momma."

"But you don't see this like I do. I remember when you were a baby. We were so worried about you, your father and I. We took you to so many doctors. Some of them told us not to think too far into the future. One of them said 'Take one day at a time.' I was so afraid I would lose you. I would hold you and listen to you breathe. I was grateful each day when you would wake up, even if you woke up crying. I just wanted you to still be alive. But now that's changed. You're all grown up. Now you're going to college. Even though I was so worried about you when you were little, I could still take care of you. I could still be your momma. I knew what I needed to do. Now I don't know. Now what will I do?"

"Momma, look at me," Josefina started. She reached up from her wheelchair and held her mother's face. "You will always be my momma."

EXERCISE 13.4

Suppose that you are teaching a class of 10 students with moderate intellectual disabilities. These students are 16–17 years of age and are characterized as passive and possessing low self-esteem. In interactions with authority (e.g., teachers, principal), they typically avoid making eye contact. When asked about disclosing their disability in order to gain future accommodations, they respond, "What disability?" A couple of students say, "I know I have a disability, but what does it matter if I say something about it? Nothing is going to happen." How would you go about teaching self-advocacy and self-disclosure of disability? Where would you start? What supports would you need to teach the lessons? How could you arrange practice opportunities?

WEBSITES WITH ADDITIONAL INFORMATION

Assertiveness Training Resources

Lesson plans for teaching self-determination *www.uaa.alaska.edu/centerforhumandevelopment/ selfdetermination/upload/Lesson-Plan-1-13.pdf.*

What can I do if I want to be assertive?

www.ed.gov.nl.ca/edu/k12/safeandcaring/students/assertive.html

The 411 on disability disclosure

www.ncwd-youth.info/411-on-disability-disclosure

Assistive Technology Resources

Rehabilitation Engineering and Assistive Technology Society of North America (RESNA)

www.resna.org

Assistive Technology Industry Association (ATIA)

www.atia.org

AbleData

www.abledata.com

EnableMart

www.enablemart.com

Assistive Technology Partners

www.assistivetechnologypartners.org

Centers for Independent Living

www.virtualcil.net/cils

www.ncil.org

CHAPTER 14

Future Pathways

Opportunities and Challenges

This chapter addresses . . .

- Future challenges and needs of transition services.
- Potential future directions for transition services, education, research, and technology

WHAT IS THE FUTURE OF TRANSITION SERVICES FOR YOUTH WITH DISABILITIES?

In the Preface we commented on how, over the last 50 years, things had changed in the field of transition, but the changes had not matched the expectations of many stakeholders. Initiatives had gained strength, then stalled. Legislation had passed, but in some cases its impact was limited. The only certainty was that youth continue to make the transition from school to adulthood.

Nonetheless, we write this chapter with great optimism because we see solid evidence of improvement in future transition services. More than just trends and inclinations, momentum is mounting that has force, assertion, and power unlike anything we have seen in our careers. The momentum has already survived the worst economic downturn—the recession of 2008–2012—in nearly a century. And still, the transition field forges onward with impressive vigor. We examine that momentum in this chapter.

Changes in Transition Education

Clearly, secondary school reform in the United States is in full swing and significant changes are imminent. As of this writing, 37 states have established definitions of *college* and *career readiness* (American Institutes of Research, 2014). Definitions are being used by states to guide numerous school reform activities, including strategic planning to address achievement gaps and increase college readiness, high school reform and 12th-grade redesign, PSE placement, and data collection. The Common Core State Standards Initiative has developed "anchor standards" on college and career readiness for reading (literature, informational text, foundation skills), writing, speaking and listening, English language arts, history/social studies, and science (see website at end of this chapter).

Consistent with the college and career readiness definitions, the National Association of State Boards of Education, National Association of Secondary School Principals, National High School Center, and Center for Comprehensive School Reform and Improvement have collaborated with plans to redesign high schools. According to the NSTTAC (2012b), the redesign effort prepares schools to recognize the urgency of change, uses data to make decisions, and develops engaging work for students. The push is to equip schools with the infrastructure, technology, and resources to prepare all students to display 21st-century knowledge and skills. For example, the National Association of Secondary School Principals' *Breaking Ranks I and II* publications called for collaborative leadership, personalization of school environments, and curriculum instruction and assessment to improve school performance (see website at end of this chapter). The National High School Center described eight elements of high school improvement, including (1) rigorous curriculum and instruction, (2) teacher effectiveness and professional growth, (3) stakeholder engagement, (4) organization and structure, (5) assessment and accountability, (6) student and family involvement, (7) effective leadership, and (8) sustainability (see website at end of this chapter).

The National High School Center and the NSTTAC produced an annotated bibliography of high-quality transition research practices and their relationship to the National High School Center's eight elements of redesign (see website at end of this chapter). According to the NSTTAC:

> In an attempt to identify intersections between high school redesign and improvement efforts in secondary transition for students with disabilities, NSTTAC identified commonalities in these sets of recommendations. The most common intersections with the predictors of in-school and post-school success included those related to family and student supports and instructional innovations regarding the specific researched programs from the National High School Center's *Eight Elements*. Personalizing the school learning environment, specifically related to personal adult advocates and teachers conveying a sense of caring from National Association of Secondary School Principals' *Breaking Ranks* recommendations align with some of the predictors of in-school success. (2012b, p. 5)

The policy implications of these efforts bear on the entire scope of education, from teacher preparation standards and elementary and secondary curricula to preparation of youth with disabilities for adulthood. It should be emphasized that the college and career readiness initiative is not separate from education for students with disabilities. The momentum involves transition education for all students, not exclusively for students *without* disabilities.

21st-Century Skills

The Partnership for 21st-Century Skills is a national organization intent on building collaborations among leaders in education, business, community, and government to prepare students for the global economy (see website at end of this chapter). As the organization's website states:

> Every child in the U.S. needs 21st century knowledge and skills to succeed as effective citizens, workers and leaders. This can be accomplished by fusing the 3Rs and 4Cs. There is a profound gap between the knowledge and skills most students learn in school and the knowledge and skills they need in typical 21st century communities and workplaces. To successfully face rigorous higher education coursework, career challenges and a globally competitive workforce, U.S. schools must align classroom environments with real world environments by fusing the 3Rs and 4Cs:
>
> - The 3Rs include: English, reading or language arts; mathematics; science; foreign languages; civics; government; economics; arts; history; and geography.
> - The 4Cs include: critical thinking and problem solving; communication; collaboration; and creativity and innovation.

Izzo (2014) described critical 21st-century skills for youth in transition, including those related to (1) life and career; (2) learning and innovation, information, media, and technology; and (3) core subjects. The author described EnvisionIT, a Web-based curriculum to teach literacy in information technology, reading, writing, and financial skills. The EnvisionIT curriculum, based on the results of research (Izzo, Yurick, Nagaraja, & Novak, 2010), focuses on information technology skills for students with specific learning disabilities in grades 8 through 12. See website at the end of this chapter.

Changes in PSE

Continued growth of PSE programs for youth with developmental disabilities is a virtual certainty. New initiatives may include credentials, certificates, and access to college majors. Educational programs for faculty overseeing work of college students with disabilities (e.g., Debrand & Salzberg, 2005) should see increased use.

We are confident the success of college students with developmental disabilities will send ripples through elementary and secondary school curricula, personal expectations of youth with dreams of going to college, visions of families, and teacher preparation programs in higher education. People with developmental disabilities who believe in themselves should nudge open the doors to new PSE opportunities.

Changes in Transition to Employment

Although data trends in recent years show no increases in integrated employment for youth with developmental disabilities (Butterworth et al., 2014), there is reason for optimism. For example, the Employment First initiative (APSE, 2015) called for employment to be the first priority and preferred outcome for people with disabilities. According to the Office of Disability Employment Policy, U. S. Department of Labor:

> Employment First is a concept to facilitate the full inclusion of people with the most significant disabilities in the workplace and community. Under the Employment First approach, community-based, integrated employment is the first option for employment services for youth and adults with significant disabilities. (*www.dol.gov/odep/topics/EmploymentFirst.htm*)

According to the APSE, the characteristics of the movement include (1) measureable increases in employment of citizens with developmental disabilities within the general workforce, earning minimum wage or higher with benefits; (2) greater opportunities for citizens with disabilities to pursue self-employment; (3) employment as the first and preferred option for citizens with disabilities; and (4) adults with disabilities employed within the general workforce, regardless of the severity of disability and assistance required (see website at end of this chapter). To date, 32 states have enacted formal policy action related to Employment First.

The Office of Disability Employment Policy established an Employment First Leadership Mentor Program (see website at the end of this chapter) that allows states to receive funding to develop and implement strategic plans and on-site, customized technical assistance from national subject-matter experts to help them achieve their goals. In addition, state representatives can discuss their progress with representatives from other states through regularly scheduled community-of-practice teleconference calls.

Changes in Transition to Independent Living

Advances in technology and peer support networks are driving forces in independent living for people with disabilities. The National Council on Independent Living (Independent Living Research Utilization Center, 2014) represents thousands of organizations and individuals, including individuals with disabilities, CILs, Statewide Independent Living Councils, and other organizations that advocate for the human and civil rights of people with disabilities throughout the United States. The focus is on training of independent living skills for youth with disabilities, leading to self-determination, independence, and self-sufficiency.

WHAT MIGHT FUTURE LEGISLATION BRING?

There are several legislative bills being considered in the U.S. Congress that may have significant impact on individuals with disabilities and their families. Rather than review each one and speculate about passage, we will allow the legislative process to run its course. See websites for national disability legislation updates at the end of this chapter. Generally, themes that run throughout bills proposing new legislation include:

- Collaboration across multiple agencies.
- Self-determination.

- Accountability (i.e., demonstrated effectiveness in producing improved outcomes).
- Sustainability (i.e., ability to sustain improvement over time after federal funding ceases).

Legislation seems particularly focused on bringing agencies and organizations together to produce increased collaboration in providing services. Regarding PSE collaboration, Grigal and Hart (2010) write:

> To succeed, those supporting these initiatives will have to cease viewing this as a special education initiative and start defining it in a manner that takes into account the perspective of the system from which change is sought. For K–12 school systems and higher education to collaborate in this change in a meaningful way, the process itself needs to provide outcomes valued by both systems while simultaneously engaging the larger adult service systems. (p. 297)

WHAT CHALLENGES LIE AHEAD?

In 2010, the National Council on Disability report on the workforce infrastructure supporting people with disabilities in the United States reminded us of major challenges at our doorstep—mainly:

> The elderly population of the United States is large and growing rapidly. Since disability rates increase with age, population aging will bring substantial increases in the number of people with disabilities and will have a significant impact on the nation's human service and support needs. Second, improvements in child survival rates mean that more children are born today with birth defects and developmental disabilities than ever before, and many of them will require access to a host of human services and supports throughout their lives. At the same time, large numbers of baby boomers are reaching retirement age, which means that many fewer human service workers will be available. These trends threaten both the availability and quality of future services for people with disabilities. (p. 1)

According to a report from the U.S. Census (2012), 18.7% of people in the United States reported having a disability, including 51.8% of people age 65 or older. With increasing numbers of individuals with disabilities, demands for special education teachers and human service workers will increase. But salaries for teachers and service providers are not keeping pace, creating a disincentive for talented young adults to pursue careers in these fields. Future demands are likely to exceed supply unless powerful incentives are established for entering teaching and human service fields.

The National Council on Disability (2010) report stated, "People with disabilities occupy a strategic place in America's ability to compete. Either their talents and ambitions will be developed into a resource for our society, or they will remain on the margins, battling for shrinking resources" (p. 2). It seems like this is a prime time for disability advocates to develop creative systems of support (e.g., family and community support networks), claim their rightful place as contributing community citizens, and launch a campaign for higher salaries for teachers and service providers.

WHAT ARE THE FUTURE SYSTEMIC NEEDS IN TRANSITION TO ADULTHOOD?

The future needs of youth in transition are numerous. We have touched on several throughout this book. As we close this chapter, we focus on four broad areas of need: (1) a functional, integrated system of services; (2) education for all stakeholders; (3) research; and (4) technology.

A Functional, Integrated System

As we described in Chapter 4, Certo and colleagues (2008) advocated for a transition services integration model (TSIM) as youth with significant intellectual disabilities enter the last 2 years of high school. According to TSIM, responsibility for service would shift in high school from solely school districts to multiple sources, including VR,, state developmental disability providers, and/or other providers as needed. Payment for services would come from multiple sources. Such a system would offer "seamless transition" to meaningful, community-based work outcomes. As the authors stated, "the day after graduation [would be] no different than the day before . . . as the ongoing support to sustain employment and community integration [would remain]" (Certo et al., 2008, p. 89).

We agree that an integrated and seamless system of transition services needs to be available to youth with significant intellectual disabilities, and indeed, to all youth with disabilities. Systems of integrated service delivery could be arranged across school districts, VR, state agencies for individuals with developmental disabilities, PSE programs, and CILs. Based on their backgrounds in working with students, transition professionals could develop a detailed summary of performance file to accompany youth moving into adult services. To function adequately, youth and families would be encouraged to actively participate. Service agencies would be compelled to collaborate in the interests of the youth, shedding concerns about "territory and ego." Self-determination, self-advocacy, family support networks, and interdisciplinary/interagency collaboration would be imperative to drive the transition system. Such a system would require strong administration, management, and a commitment to successful outcomes.

The seamless transition notion seems idealistic and the stuff of dreams, yet the data demonstrating success are already documented. In an application of the TSIM model (Luecking & Certo, 2003), 261 of 293 youth (89%) with significant intellectual disabilities exited school seamlessly with ongoing supports provided by hybrid agencies, and 177 (60%) exited school with employment at the prevailing wage for a mean of 14 hours per week. Similar demonstrations of successful transition to PSE are available (go to *www. thinkcollege.org*).

We understand that implementing an integrated, multiagency system of support is a mammoth and expensive undertaking. Although we respect the enormity of the effort, the limitations of shrinking budgets, and the burden of systemic change, we must conclude that the benefits far outweigh the costs.

Education of All Stakeholders in Transition

Given the heavy emphasis on results-oriented education, postschool outcomes, and college and career readiness, today's educators need to have a comprehensive knowledge of transition services. With interdisciplinary and interagency collaboration a virtual necessity for youth to make successful transitions to adulthood, all educators need to be well versed in this area. Yet, collaboration skills are new and unique to many educators. Understanding how to plan and prepare for students' transitions involves a skill repertoire that many educators do not have and assume will be delegated to some expert. Significant changes in the current practices involved in transition preparedness are required. Morningstar and Clark (2003) wrote:

> It is professionally unacceptable that we live in a society that demands some demonstration of competence through training . . . of certain workers (e.g., accountants, real estate brokers, hair stylists, plumbers, security guards, general contractors, to name a few), while at the same time permitting professionals who have little or no specific training or demonstrated competence to perform a wide range of tasks and roles in delivering transition education and services to students with disabilities. (p. 227)

Research in Transition

Transition research must inform practice. Transition outcome research, similar to the NLTS-2, must be ongoing in order to inform the field of education about the efficacy of its efforts. But transition researchers must step to the plate. Carter and colleagues (2013) reviewed every article published from 1978 through 2012 in *Career Development and Transition for Exceptional Individuals*, the transition journal of the Council for Exceptional Children, to examine methodological trends in research. Over time, increases were found in data-based articles (from about 20% of all publications in the late 1970s to 70–80% in 2010–2012). However, articles describing experimental designs with adequate research controls still constituted a small minority of recently published studies. High-quality research in transition, including research on the effects of interventions, is needed.

Technology

We reviewed some of the recent assistive technology applications in transition and predict that the future will see increased emphasis. Clearly, assistive technology holds promise as a source of support for youth to overcome, cope with, or at least temper the effects of disabilities. Advances in recent years have been impressive, and we expect the future rate of progress to be exponential. On a related note, we look forward to technology-based delivery of training to service providers in transition. Research-based practices, innovative systems, and collaboration opportunities should be available to professionals from various fields who can learn together in webinars and similar forums.

CONCLUSION

A strong transition system requires multiple elements that function in an interconnected whole to support youth in movement from school to adulthood. Four essential requirements are (1) a functional and integrated system of services such as the TSIM (Certo et al., 2008), (2) effective education for all stakeholders, (3) high-quality research to produce a basis of evidence for practice, and (4) technology. Changes in transition education, such as the College and Career Ready Standards and high school reform, are likely to yield impressive results. New PSE initiatives may include credentials, certificates, and access to college majors for youth with developmental disabilities. Faculty members overseeing the work of college students with disabilities need training in how to provide accommodations and individualized instruction. Changes in transition to employment have considerable momentum, given the Employment First and WIOA initiatives. The future of transition to employment should be one resulting in a diverse, integrated workforce: young adults with disabilities working alongside their nondisabled peers. Changes in transition to independent living will be dominated by advances in technology and peer support networks. Clearly, the future will be full of change, excitement, and apprehension, much like transition itself.

EXERCISE 14.1

Please respond to the following questions:

- Ideally, what would you like to see for the future of transition from special education to adulthood for youth with disabilities?
- What do you see as necessary to achieve that ideal?
- What challenges will be most formidable?
- What challenges, not mentioned in this book, must also be considered?
- What resources and supports can be rallied to meet the challenges?

WEBSITES WITH ADDITIONAL INFORMATION

Common Core Standards Initiative

www.corestandards.org

National Association of Secondary School Principals *"Breaking Ranks" I and II*

www.nassp.org/school-improvement/breaking-ranks-ii-and-high-school-reform

National High School Center

www.betterhighschools.org/pubs/documents/EightElementsMappingFramework.pdf

Special Education in High School Redesign: Annotated Bibliography

www.betterhighschools.org/pubs/documents/NHSC_SpecialEdBibliography.pdf

Partnership for 21st Century Skills

www.p21.org

Association for People Supporting Employment First

www.apse.org/employment-first/statement

Office of Disability Employment Policy Employment First Mentor Program

www.dol.gov/odep/media/newsroom/employmentfirststates.htm

Transition Coalition

http://transitioncoalition.org/transition

National Center for Secondary Education and Transition

www.ncset.org

National Disability Rights Network

www.ndrn.org/advocacy/legislative.html

EnvisionIT Technology: Enhancing Transition through Technology

http://nisonger.osu.edu/transition/envisionit.htm

Websites for National Disability Legislation Updates

www.aucd.org/template/page.cfm?id=164
www.easterseals.com/get-involved/advocacy
www.autismspeaks.org/advocacy

References

Able Data. (2014). Resources. Retrieved from *www.abledata.com/abledata.cfm?pageid=19326&ksectionid=19326*.

Adult Foster Care Services. (2014). Adult foster care. Retrieved from *https://dhs.sd.gov/dd/adultfc.aspx*.

Affleck, J. Q., Lowenbraun, S., & Archer, A. (1980). *Teaching the mildly handicapped in the regular classroom* (2nd ed.). New York: Macmillan.

Agran, M. (Ed.). (1994). *Promoting health and safety skills for independent living.* Baltimore: Brookes.

Agran, M., Blanchard, C., Wehmeyer, M. L., & Hughes, C. (2001). Teaching students to self-regulate their behavior: The differential effects of student- vs. teacher-delivered reinforcement. *Research in Developmental Disabilities, 22*, 319–332.

Agran, M., Cain, H., & Cavin, M. (2002). Enhancing the involvement of rehabilitation counselors in the transition process. *Career Development for Exceptional Individuals, 25*, 141–154.

Agran, M., Sinclair, T., Alper, S., Cavin, M., Wehmeyer, M. L., & Hughes, C. (2005). Using self-monitoring to increase following-direction skills of students with moderate to severe disabilities in general education. *Education and Training in Developmental Disabilities, 40*, 3–13.

Agran, M., Wehmeyer, M. L., Cavin, M., & Palmer, S. (2008). Promoting student active classroom participation skills through instruction to promote self-regulated learning and self-determination. *Career Development and Transition for Exceptional Individuals, 31*, 106–114.

Alberti, R. E., & Emmons, M. L. (1970). *Your perfect right: A guide to assertive behavior.* Oxford, UK: Impact.

American Association on Intellectual and Developmental Disabilities. (2012). Housing: Joint position statement of AAIDD and ARC. Retrieved from *http://aaidd.org/news-policy/policy/position-statements/housing#.VCw8u1YQ_Kl*.

American Council on Education. (2011). *Implementing the Common Core State Standards: An action agenda for higher education.* Washington, DC: Author.

American Institutes of Research. (2014). *Definitions of college and career readiness: An analysis by state.* Washington, DC: Author.

American Occupational Therapy Association. (2014). Occupational therapy: Improving function while controlling costs. Retrieved from *www.aota.org/en/About-Occupational-Therapy/Professionals.aspx*.

American Psychiatric Association. (2013). *Diagnostic and statistical manual of mental disorders* (5th ed.). Arlington, VA: Author.

Americans with Disabilities Act of 1990, 42 U.S.C § 12102 et seq.

Americans with Disabilities Act, 28 C.F.R. § 35 (2009).

Americans with Disabilities Act Amendments Act of 2008, Public Law 110-325.

Aspel, N., Bettis, G., Quinn, P., Test, D. W., & Wood, W. M. (1999). A collaborative process for planning transition services for all students with disabilities. *Career Development for Exceptional Individuals, 22*, 21–42.

Assistive Technology Act of 1998. (1998). Public Law 105-394. 112 Stat. 3627.

Assistive Technology Act of 2004. (2004). Public Law 108-364. 118 Stat. 1707.

Association of People Supporting Employment First. (2015). Employment first across the nation. Retrieved from *www.apse.org/wp-content/uploads/2014/10/EmploymentFirst_Infographic.pdf*.

Baer, R., Flexer, R., & Dennis, L. (2007). Examining the career paths and transition services of students with disabilities exiting high school. *Education and Training of Developmental Disabilities, 42*, 317–329.

Bailey, J. S. (1981). Wanted: A rational search for the limiting condition of habilitation in the retarded. *Analysis and Intervention in Developmental Disabilities, 1*, 45–52.

Balcazar, F. E., Fawcett, S. B., & Seekins, T. (1990). Teaching people with disabilities to recruit help to attain personal goals. *Rehabilitation Psychology, 36*, 31–41.

Barnard-Brak, L., Lechtenberger, D., & Yan, W. Y. (2010). Accommodation strategies of college students with disabilities. *Qualitative Report, 15*, 411–429.

Barr, V. M., Hartman, R. C., & Spillane, S. A. (1995). *Getting ready for college: High school students with learning disabilities*. Washington, DC: HEATH Resource Center.

Bates, P. E., Cuvo, T., Miner, C. A., & Korabek, C. A. (1999). Simulated and community-based instruction involving persons with mild and moderate mental retardation. *Research in Developmental Disabilities, 22*, 95–115.

Benitez, D. T., Morningstar, M. E., & Frey, B. B. (2009). A multistate survey of special education teachers' perceptions of their transition competencies. *Career Development for Exceptional Individuals, 32*, 6–16.

Bennett, R. K. (2006). *Bennett Mechanical Comprehension Test*. San Antonio, TX: Pearson.

Benz, M. R., Johnson, D., Mikkelsen, K., & Lindstrom, L. (1995). Improving collaboration between schools and vocational rehabilitation: Stakeholder identified barriers and strategies. *Career Development for Exceptional Individuals, 18*, 133–144.

Benz, M. R., Lindstrom, L., & Yovanoff, P. (2000). Improving graduation and employment outcomes of students with disabilities: Predictive factors and student perspectives. *Exceptional Children, 66*(4), 509–529.

Blalock, G., Kochhar-Bryant, C. A., Test, D. W., Kohler, P., White, W., Lehmann, J., et al. (2003). The need for comprehensive personnel preparation in transition and career development: A position paper of the Division on Career Development and Transition. *Career Development for Exceptional Individuals, 26*, 207–226.

Bondy, A., & Frost, L. (2001). The Picture Exchange Communication System. *Behavior Modification, 25*, 725–744.

Bouck, E. C., Maeda, Y., & Flanagan, S. M. (2011). Assistive technology and students with high-incidence disabilities: Understanding the relationship through the NLTS2. *Remedial and Special Education, 33*(5), 298–308.

Braddock, D., Hemp, R., Rizzolo, M. C., Haffer, L., Shea Tanis, E., & Wu, J. (2011). *The state of the states in developmental disabilities 2011*. Boulder: University of Colorado.

Brigance, A. H. (1999). *Brigance Diagnostic Comprehensive Inventory of Basic Skills—Revised*. North Billerica, MA: Curriculum Associates.

Brinckerhoff, L. C., McGuire, J. M., & Shaw, S. F. (2002). *Postsecondary education and transition for students with learning disabilities* (2nd ed.). Austin, TX: PRO-ED.

Brooke, V., Inge, K. J., Armstrong, A. J., & Wehman, P. (1997). *Supported employment handbook: A customer driven approach for persons with significant disabilities.* Richmond: Rehabilitation Research and Training Center on Supported Employment, Virginia Commonwealth University.

Browder, D. M., & Spooner, F. (2011). *Teaching students with moderate and severe disabilities.* New York: Guilford Press.

Bullis, M., Moran, T., Benz, M. R., Todis, B, & Johnson, M. D. (2002). Description and evaluation of the ARIES Project: Achieving rehabilitation, individualized education, and employment success for adolescents with emotional disturbance. *Career Development for Exceptional Individuals, 25,* 41–58.

Butterworth, J., Smith, F. A., Hall, A. C., Migliore, A., Winsor, J., & Domin, D. (2014). *State data: The national report on employment services and outcomes.* Boston: Institute for Community Inclusion, University of Massachusetts Boston.

Butterworth, J., Steere, D., & Whitney-Thomas, J. (1997). Person-centered planning. In R. Shalock (Ed.), *Quality of life: Applications with persons with mental retardation* (Vol. 2, pp. 5–23). Washington, DC: American Association on Mental Retardation.

Carrow-Woolfolk, E. (1999). *Comprehensive Assessment of Spoken Language.* Bloomington, MN: Pearson.

Carter, E. W., Brock, M. E., Bottema-Beutel, K., Bartholomew, A., Boehm, T. L. & Cease-Cook, J. (2013). Methodological trends in secondary education and transition research: Looking backward and moving forward. *Career Development and Transition for Exceptional Individuals, 36,* 15–24.

Carter, E. W., Chambers, C. R., & Hughes, C. (2004). Parent and sibling perspectives on the transition to adulthood. *Education and Training in Developmental Disabilities, 39,* 79–94.

Carter, E. W., Ditchman, N., Sun, Y., Trainor, A. A., Swedeen, B., & Owens, L. (2010). Summer employment and community experiences of transition-age youth with severe disabilities. *Exceptional Children, 76,* 194–212.

Carter, E. W., & Hughes, C. (2005). Increasing social interaction among adolescents with intellectual disabilities and their general education peers: Effective interventions. *Research and Practice for Persons with Severe Disabilities, 30,* 179–193.

Carter, E. W., Lane, K. L., Pierson, M. R., & Glaeser, B. (2006). Self-determination skills and opportunities of transition-age youth with emotional disturbance and learning disabilities. *Exceptional Children, 72,* 333–346.

Cavendish, W., Montague, M., Enders, C., & Dietz, S. (2014). Mothers' and adolescents' perceptions of family environment and adolescent social–emotional functioning. *Journal of Child and Family Studies, 23,* 52–66.

Center for Applied Special Technology. (2014). About Universal Design for Learning. Retrieved from *www.cast.org/udl.*

Centers for Disease Control and Prevention. (2009). National Health Interview Survey. Retrieved from *www.cdc.gov/nchs/nhis/nhis_2009_data_release.htm.*

Centers for Disease Control and Prevention. (2012). Youth suicide. Retrieved from *www.cdc.gov/violenceprevention/ub/youth_suicide.html.*

Centers for Medicare and Medicaid Services. (2015). Application for a §1915(c) home and community-based waiver [version 3.5]: Instructions, technical guide, and review criteria. Retrieved from *www.medicaid.gov/Medicaid-CHIP-Program-Information/By-Topics/Waivers/Downloads/Technical-Guidance.pdf.*

Certo, N. J., Luecking, R. G., Murphy, S., Brown, L. Courey, S., & Belanger, D. (2008). Seamless transition and long-term support for individuals with intellectual disabilities. *Research and Practice for Persons with Severe Disabilities, 33,* 85–95.

Certo, N. J., Mautz, D., Pumpian, I., Sax, C., Smalley, K., Wade, H. A., et al. (2003). Review and discussion of a model for seamless transition to adulthood. *Education and Training in Developmental Disabilities, 38*(1), 3–17.

Certo, N. J., Pumpian, I., Fisher, D., Storey, K., & Smalley, K. (1997). Focusing on the point of transition. *Education and Treatment of Children, 20*(1), 68–84.

Chadsey-Rusch, J., & Gonzalez, P. (1996). Analysis of directions, responses, and consequences involving persons with mental retardation in employment and vocational training settings. *American Journal of Mental Retardation, 100,* 481–492.

Chadsey-Rusch, J., Karlan, G. R., Riva, M. T., & Rusch, F. R. (1984). Competitive employment: Teaching conversational skills to adults who are mentally retarded. *Mental Retardation, 22,* 218–225.

Cihak, D. F., Alberto, P. A., Kessler, K. B., & Taber, T. A. (2004). An investigation of instructional scheduling arrangements for community-based instruction. *Research in Developmental Disabilities, 25,* 67–88.

Cimera, R. E., Burgess, S., & Bedesem, P. L. (2014). Does providing transition services by age 14 produce better vocational outcomes for students with intellectual disability? *Research and Practice for Persons with Severe Disabilities, 39,* 47–54.

Collins, W. A. (2014). Parents' cognitions and developmental changes in relationships during adolescence. In I. E. Sigel, A. V. McGillicuddy-DeLisi, & J. J. Goodnow (Eds.), *Parent belief systems: The psychological consequences for children* (2nd ed., pp. 175–198). New York: Psychology Press.

Conti-Ramsdem G., & Botting, N. (2008). Emotional health in adolescents with and without a history of specific language impairment (SLI). *Journal of Child Psychology and Psychiatry, 49,* 516–525.

Cook, A. M., & Hussey, S. M. (2002). *Assistive technologies: Principles and practice* (2nd ed.). St. Louis, MO: Mosby.

Cook, B. G., Smith, G. J., & Tankersley, M. (2012). Evidence-based practices. In K. R. Harris, S. Graham, & T. Urdan (Eds.), *APA educational psychology handbook: Vol. 1. Theories, constructs, and critical issues* (pp. 495–528). Washington, DC: American Psychological Association.

Cory, R. C. (2011). Disability service offices for students with disabilities: A campus resource. *New Directions for Higher Education, 154,* 27–35.

Crockett, M. A., & Hardman, M. L. (2010). The role of secondary education in transition. In J. McDonnell & M. L. Hardman (Eds.), *Successful transition programs: Pathways for students with intellectual and developmental disabilities* (pp. 43–60). Thousand Oaks, CA: Sage.

Cronin, M. E. (1996). Life skills curricula for students with learning disabilities. *Journal of Learning Disabilities, 29,* 53–68.

Data Resource Center for Child and Adolescent Health. (2012). 2009–2010 national survey of children with special health care needs. Retrieved from *www.chilhealthdata.org/learn/NS-CSHCN.*

Davis, D. K., Stock, S, E., Holloway, S., & Wehmeyer, M. L. (2010). Evaluating a GPS-based transportation device to support independent bus travel with intellectual disability. *Intellectual and Developmental Disabilities, 48,* 454–463.

Dawis, R. V., & Lofquist, L. H. (1984). *A psychological theory of work adjustment: An individual difference model and its application.* Minneapolis: University of Minnesota.

Debrand, C. C., & Salzberg, C. L. (2005). A validated curriculum to provide training to faculty regarding students with disabilities in higher education. *Journal of Postsecondary Education and Disability, 18,* 49–62.

deFur, S. H., & Patton, J. R. (Eds.). (1999). *Transition and school-based services: Interdisciplinary perspectives for enhancing the transition process.* Austin, TX: PRO-ED.

Demchak, M., & Greenfield, R. G. (2003). *Transition portfolios for students with disabilities.* Thousand Oaks, CA: Corwin Press.

Deno, S. L. (2003). Developments in curriculum-based measurement. *Journal of Special Education, 37,* 184–192.

Dockery, D. J. (2012). School dropout indicators, trends, and interventions for school counselors. *Journal of School Counseling, 10*(12), 1–33.

Dogoe, M., & Banda, D. R. (2009). Review of recent research using constant time delay to teach chained tasks to persons with developmental disabilities. *Education and Training in Developmental Disabilities, 44,* 177–186.

Duersch, J. (2013). *A comparison of social media job search versus traditional job search methods on employment of students with moderate to severe disabilities*. Unpublished master's thesis, Utah State University, Logan, UT.

Dukes, C., & Lamar-Dukes, P. (2009). Diversity: What we know, need to know, and what we need to do. *Research and Practice for Persons with Severe Disabilities, 34*, 71–75.

Dwyer, A., Grigal, M., & Fialka, J. (2010). Student and family perspectives. In M. Grigal & D. Hart, *Think college!: Postsecondary education options for students with intellectual disabilities* (pp. 189–227). Baltimore: Brookes.

Eckert, S. P. (2000). Teaching the social skill of accepting criticism to adults with developmental disabilities. *Education and Training in Mental Retardation and Developmental Disabilities, 35*, 16–24.

Eckes, S. E., & Ochoa, T. A. (2005). Students with disabilities: Transitioning from high school to higher education. *American Secondary Education, 33*, 6–20.

Education for All Handicapped Children Act of 1975, Public Law 94-142, November 28, 1975.

Egan, G. (2010). *The skilled helper: A problem management and opportunity development approach to helping* (10th ed). Belmont, CA: Brookes/Cole.

Eisenman, L., & Mancini, K. (2010). College perspectives and issues. In M. Grigal & D. Hart, *Think college!: Postsecondary education options for students with intellectual disabilities* (pp. 161–188). Baltimore: Brookes.

Elksnin, N., & Elksnin, L. K. (2001). Adolescents with disabilities: The need for occupational social skills. *Exceptionality: A Special Education Journal, 9*, 91–105.

Ellerd, D., & Morgan, R. L. (2013). Employment assessment. In K. Storey & D. Hunter (Eds.), *The road ahead: Transition to adult life for persons with disabilities* (pp. 59–84). Amsterdam: IOS Press.

Enderle, J., & Severson, S. (2003). Enderle–Severson Transition Rating Scales. Retrieved from *www.estr.net*.

Everson, J. M., & Moon, M. S. (1987). Transition services for young adults with severe disabilities: Defining professional and parental roles and responsibilities. *Research and Practice for Persons with Severe Disabilities, 12*, 87–95.

Everson, J. M., & Ried, D. H. (1999). *Person-centered planning and outcome management: Maximizing organizational effectiveness in supporting quality lifestyles among people with disabilities*. Morganton, NC: Habilitative Management Consultants.

Falls, J., & Unruh, D. (2010). Frequently asked questions: Revised Part B Indicator 14 post-school outcomes. Retrieved from *http://psocenter.org/content_page_assets/content_page_19/ind14_faq_rev_may2010.pdf*.

FannieMae. (2014). MyCommunityMortgage: Additional eligibility and underwriting requirements for community solutions and community homechoice. Retrieved from *www.fanniemae.com/content/guide/selling/b5/6/04.html#Community.20HomeChoice.3A.20Income.20Limits*.

Field, S., & Hoffman, A. (1996). *Steps to self-determination: A curriculum to help adolescents learn to achieve their goals*. Austin, TX: PRO-ED.

Fingerman, K. L., & Bermann, E. (2000). Applications of family systems theory to the study of adulthood. *International Journal of Aging and Human Development, 51*, 5–29.

Flexer, R. W., Baer, R. M., Luft, P., & Simmons, T. J. (2013). *Transition planning for secondary students with disabilities* (4th ed.). Boston: Pearson.

Forest, M., & Pearpoint, J. (1992). Putting all kids on the MAP. *Educational Leadership, 50*, 26–31.

Foster-Fishman, P. G., Berkowitz, S. L., Lounsbury, D. W., Jacobson, S., & Allen, N. A. (2001). Building collaborative capacity in community coalitions: A review and integrative framework. *American Journal of Community Psychology, 29*, 241–261.

Frey, G. C., Buchanan, A. M., Rosser Sandt, D. D., & Taylor, S. J. (2005). "I'd rather watch TV": An examination of physical activity in adults with mental retardation. *Mental Retardation, 43*, 241–254.

Gaumer Erickson, A. S., Clark, G. M., & Patton, J. R. (2013). *Informal assessments for transition planning* (2nd ed.). Austin, TX: PRO-ED.

Getzel, E. E. (2008). Addressing the persistence and retention of students with disabilities in higher education: Incorporating key strategies and supports on campus. *Exceptionality, 16,* 207–219.

Giangreco, M. F., Edelman, S. W., Luiselli, T. E., & MacFarland, S. Z. C. (1997). Helping or hovering?: Effects of instructional assistant proximity on students with disabilities. *Exceptional Children, 64,* 7–18.

Gormley, S., Hughes, C., Block, L., & Lendman, C. (2005). Eligibility assessment requirements at the postsecondary level for students with learning disabilities: A disconnect with secondary schools? *Journal of Postsecondary Education and Disability, 18,* 63–70.

Gould, M. S., Greenberg, T., Velting, D. M., & Shaffer, D. (2003). Youth suicide risk and preventive interventions: A review of the past 10 years. *Journal of the American Academy of Child and Adolescent Psychiatry, 42,* 386–405.

Government Accounting Office. (2012). *Students with disabilities: Better federal coordination could lessen challenges in the transition from high school.* Washington, DC: Author.

Graph Paper Press. (2014). Ready, set, action!: Create a video portfolio with new theme auditorium. Retrieved from *http://graphpaperpress.com/blog/ready-set-action-create-a-video-portfolio-with-new-theme-auditorium.*

Greene, G. (2011). *Transition planning for culturally and linguistically diverse youth.* Baltimore: Brookes.

Griffin, C., Hammis, D., & Geary, T. (2007). *The job developer's handbook: Practical tactics for customized employment.* Baltimore: Brookes.

Griffin, C., Hammis, D., Geary, T., & Sullivan, M. (2008). Customized employment: Where we are; where we're headed. *Journal of Vocational Rehabilitation, 28,* 135–139.

Griffith, R. T. (1889). *The hymns of the Rigveda* (Vol. 1). Benares, India: Lazarus.

Grigal, M., & Hart, D. (2010). *Think college!: Postsecondary education options for students with intellectual disabilities.* Baltimore: Brookes.

Grigal, M., Hart, D., Smith, F. A., Domin, D., & Sulewski, J. (2013). *Think College National Coordinating Center: Annual report on the transition and postsecondary programs for students with intellectual disabilities.* Boston: Institute for Community Inclusion, University of Massachusetts Boston.

Grigal, M., Hart, D., & Weir, C. (2012). A survey of postsecondary education programs for students with intellectual disabilities in the United States. *Journal of Policy and Practice in Intellectual Disabilities, 9,* 223–233.

Grigal, M., & Neubert, D. A. (2004). Parents' in-school values and post-school expectations for transition-aged youth with disabilities. *Career Development of Exceptional Individuals, 27,* 65–85.

Grigal, M., Neubert, D. A., & Moon, M. S. (2002). Postsecondary options for students with significant disabilities. *Teaching Exceptional Children, 35*(2), 68–73.

Grossman, H. J. (Ed.). (1983). *Classification in mental retardation.* Washington, DC: American Association on Mental Deficiency.

Guess, D., Mulligan-Ault, M., Roberts, S., Struth, J., Siegel-Causey, E., Thompson, B., et al. (1988). Implications of biobehavioral states for the education and treatment of students with the most profoundly handicapping conditions. *Journal of the Association for Persons with Severe Handicaps, 13,* 163–174.

Halpern, A. S. (1985). Transition: A look at the foundations. *Exceptional Children, 51,* 479–486.

Hamblet, E. C. (2011). *Seven steps for success: High school to college transition strategies for students with disabilities.* Arlington, VA: Council for Exceptional Children.

Hardman, M. L., & Dawson, S. A. (2010). Historical and legislative foundations. In J. McDonnell & M. L. Hardman (Eds.), *Successful transition programs: Pathways for students with intellectual and developmental disabilities* (pp. 3–24). Thousand Oaks, CA: Sage.

Hasazi, S. B., Gordon, L. R., & Roe, C. A. (1985). Factors associated with the employment status of handicapped youth exiting high school from 1979 to 1983. *Exceptional Children, 51,* 455–469.

Heal, L. W., Gonzalez, P., Rusch, F. R., Copher, J. I., & DeStefano, L. (1990). A comparison of successful and unsuccessful placements of youths with mental handicaps into competitive employment. *Exceptionality, 1*, 181–195.

Hendricks, D. R., & Wehman, P. (2009). Transition from school to adulthood for youth with autism spectrum disorders: Review and recommendations. *Focus on Autism and Other Developmental Disabilities, 24*, 77–88.

Hensley, G., & Buck, D. P. (Eds.). (1968). *Cooperative agreements between special education and rehabilitation services in the West: Selected papers from a conference on cooperative agreements.* Boulder, CO: Western Interstate Commission for Higher Education.

Hetherington, S. A., Durant-Johnes, L., Johnson, K., Nolan, K., Smith, E., Taylor-Brown, S., et al. (2010). The lived experiences of adolescents with disabilities and their parents in transition planning. *Focus on Autism and Other Developmental Disabilities, 25*, 163–172.

Higher Education Consortium on Learning Disabilities. (1996). *Unlocking the doors: How to enter postsecondary education from high school—a manual for students with learning disabilities.* Minneapolis, MN: Learning Disabilities Association.

Higher Education Opportunity Act of 2008, Public Law 110-315.

Hoff, D. (2013). Employment First resource list. Boston: Institute for Community Inclusion. Retrieved from *www.apse.org/wp-content/uploads/docs/Employment%20First%2012-13%20 %28SELN%20version%29.pdf.*

Hogansen, J. M., Powers, K., Geenen, S., Gil-Kashiwabara, E., & Powers, L. (2008). Transition goals and experiences of females with disabilities: Youth, parents, and professionals. *Exceptional Children, 74*, 215–234.

Holland, J. L. (1996). Exploring careers with a typology: What we have learned and some new directions. *American Psychologist, 51*, 397–406.

Holland, J. L., Powell, A. M., & Fritzsche, B. A. (1997). *The self-directed search (SDS): Professional user's guide.* Lutz, FL: Psychological Assessment Resources.

Hubbard, D. (2009). *The failure of risk management: Why it's broken and how to fix it.* Hoboken, NJ: Wiley.

Hughes, C., & Carter, E. W. (2012). *The new transition handbook: Strategies high school teachers use that work!* Baltimore: Brookes.

Hughes, C., Copeland, S., Agran, M., Wehmeyer, M., Rodi, M. S., & Presley, J. (2002). Using self-monitoring to improve performance in general education high school classes. *Education and Training in Mental Retardation and Developmental Disabilities, 37*, 262–272.

Hurlburt, M., Aarons, G. A., Fettes, D., Willging, C., Gunderson, L., & Chaffin, M. J. (2014). Interagency collaborative team model for capacity building to scale-up evidence-based practice. *Children and Youth Services Review, 39*, 160–168.

Independent Living Research Utilization Center. (2014). *ILRU directory of centers for independent living (CILS) and associations.* Houston, TX: Independent Living Research Utilization Center. Retrieved from *www.ilru.org/projects/cil-net/cil-center-and-association-directory.*

Individuals with Disabilities Education Act (IDEA), Public Law 99-457 (1990).

Individuals with Disabilities Education Act, Public Law 105-17, 101st Congress (1997). 20 U.S.C. § 1440 et seq.

Individuals with Disabilities Education Improvement Act, Public Law 108-446, H.R. 1350, 108th Congress (2004). 20 U.S.C. § 1440 et seq.

Izzo, M. (2014, June). *Twenty-first century curricula: Preparing students for Common Core standards, college, and careers.* Paper presented at the 2014 Utah Multi-Tiered Systems of Supports Conference, Layton, UT.

Izzo, M., & Kochhar-Bryant, C. (2006). Implementing the SOP for effective transition: Two case studies. *Career Development for Exceptional Individuals, 29*, 100–107.

Izzo, M., & Lamb, M. (2002). *Self-determination and career development: Skills for successful transitions to postsecondary education and employment.* A white paper for the Oost-School Outcomes Network of the National Center on Secondary Education and transition (NCSET) at the University of Hawaii at Manoa. Available at *www.ncset.hawaii.edu/publications.*

Izzo, M., Yurick, A., Nagaraja, H. N., & Novak, J. A. (2010). Effects of a 21st-century curriculum on students' information technology and transition skills. *Career Development of Exceptional Individuals, 33,* 95–105.

Jameson, J. M., & McDonnell, J. (2010). Home and community living. In J. McDonnell & M. Hardman (Eds.), *Successful transition programs: Pathways for students with intellectual and developmental disabilities* (pp. 203–216). Thousand Oaks, CA: Sage.

Javitz, H., Wagner, M., & Newman, L. (2008). *Analysis of potential bias in the wave 4 respondents to the National Longitudinal Transition Study–2* (NLTS-2). Menlo Park, CA: SRI International.

Johnson, L. J., Zorn, D., Yung Tam, B. K., Lamontagne, M., & Johnson, S. A. (2003). Stakeholders' views of factors that impact successful interagency collaboration. *Exceptional Children, 69,* 195–209.

Johnston, J. M., & Pennypacker, H. S. (1993). *Strategies and tactics of behavioral research* (2nd ed.). Hillsdale, NJ: Erlbaum.

Jorgensen, S., Ferraro, V., Fichten, C., & Havel, A. (2009). *Predicting college retention and dropout: Sex and disability.* ERIC Reproduction Service No. ED505873.

Karan, O., DonAroma, P., Bruder, M., & Roberts, L. A. (2010). Transitional assessments model for students with severe and/or multiple disabilities: Competency-based community assessment. *Intellectual and Developmental Disabilities, 48,* 387–392.

Kessler, R., Foster, C., Saunders, W., & Stang, P. (2009). Social consequences of psychiatric disorders: I. Educational attainment. *American Journal of Psychiatry, 152,* 1026–1032.

Kirigin, K. A., Braukmann, C. J., Atwater, J. D., & Wolf, M. M. (1982). An evaluation of teaching-family (Achievement Place) group homes for juvenile offenders. *Journal of Applied Behavior Analysis, 15,* 1–16.

Knapp-Lee, L. J. (1995). Use of the COPSystem in career assessment. *Journal of Career Assessment, 3,* 411–128.

Kochhar-Bryant, C., Bassett, D. S., & Webb, K. W. (2009). *Transition to postsecondary education for students with disabilities.* Thousand Oaks, CA: Corwin Press.

Kohler, P. (1996). *Taxonomy for transition programming: Linking research and practice.* Champaign: Transition Research Institute, University of Illinois at Urbana–Champaign.

Kohler, P. (1998). Transition Planning Inventory (TPI). *Diagnostique, 24,* 249–256.

Korabek, C. A., Reid, D. H., & Ivancic, M. T. (1981). Improving needed food intake of profoundly handicapped children through effective supervision of institutional staff performance. *Applied Research in Mental Retardation, 2,* 69–88.

Kratochwill, T. R., Hitchcock, J. H., Horner, R. H., Levin, J. R., Odom, S. L., Rindskopf, D. M., et al. (2013). Single-base intervention research design standards. *Remedial and Special Education, 34,* 26–38.

Lagomarcino, T. R., & Rusch, F. R. (1988). Competitive employment: Overview and analysis of research focus. In V. B. Van Hasselt, P. S. Strain, & M. Hersen (Eds.), *Handbook of developmental and physical disabilities* (pp. 150–158). New York: Elsevier.

Landesman-Dwyer, S., & Sackett, G. P. (1978). Behavioral changes in nonambulatory, profoundly mentally retarded individuals. In C. E. Meyers (Ed.), *Quality of life in severely and profoundly mentally retarded people: Research foundations for improvement* (pp. 55–144). Washington, DC: American Association on Mental Deficiency.

Landmark, L. J., Ju, S., & Zhang, D. (2010). Substantiated best practices in transition: Fifteen plus years later. *Career Development for Exceptional Individuals, 33,* 163–176.

Landmark, L. J., Zhang, D., & Montoya, L. (2007). Culturally diverse parents' experiences in their children's transition: Knowledge and involvement. *Career Development for Exceptional Individuals, 30,* 68–79.

Larson, S., Salmi, P., Smith, D., Anderson, L., & Hewitt, A. (2013). *Residential services for persons with intellectual or developmental disabilities: Status and trends through 2011.* Minneapolis, MN: Institute on Community Integration. Retrieved from *http://rtc.umn.edu/risp/docs/risp2011.pdf.*

Lengnick-Hall, M. L., Gaunt, P. M., & Brooks, A. R. (2001). Why employers don't hire people with disabilities: A survey of the literature. Retrieved from *www.cprf.org/whyemployersdonthire.htm.*

Lindstrom, L., Doren, B., Metheny, J., Johnson, P., & Zane, C. (2007). Transition to employment: Role of the family in career development. *Exceptional Children, 73*, 348–366.

Lohrman-O'Rourke, S., & Gomez, O. (2001). Integrating preference assessment within the transition process to create meaningful school-to-life outcomes. *Exceptionality, 9*, 157–174.

Luecking, R. G. (2009). *The way to work: How to facilitate work experiences for youth in transition.* Baltimore: Brookes.

Luecking, R. G., & Certo, N. (2003). Integrating service systems at the point of transition for youth with significant support needs: A model that works. *American Rehabilitation, 27*, 2–9.

Malloy, J. M., Cheney, D., & Cormier, G. M. (1990). Interagency collaboration and the transition to adulthood for students with emotional or behavioral disabilities. *Education and Treatment of Children, 21*, 303–320.

Mank, D., Cioffi, A., Yovanoff, P., & Taylor, S. J. (2003). Supported employment outcomes across a decade: Is there evidence of improvement in the quality of implementation? *Mental Retardation, 41*, 188–197.

Martella, R. C., & Marchand-Martella, N. E. (1995). Safety skills in vocational rehabilitation: A qualitative analysis. *Journal of Vocational Rehabilitation, 5*, 25–31.

Martin, J. E., & Marshall, L. H. (1996). *ChoiceMaker self-determination transition assessment.* Longmont, CO: Sopris West.

Martin, J. E., Marshall, L. H., & De Pry, R. L. (2005). Participatory decision-making: Innovative practices that increase student self-determination. In R. W. Flexer, T. J. Simmons, P. Luft, & R. M. Baer (Eds.), *Transition planning for secondary students with disabilities* (2nd ed., pp. 246–275). Columbus, OH: Merrill Prentice Hall.

Martin, J. E., Marshall, L. H., Maxson, L., & Jerman, P. (1997). *Self-directed IEP.* Longmont, CO: Sopris West.

Martin, J. E., Van Dycke, J., Greene, B. A., Gardner, J. E., & Christensen, W. R. (2006). Direct observation of teacher-directed IEP meetings: Establishing the need for student IEP meeting instruction. *Exceptional Children, 72*, 187–200.

Martin, J. E., Van Dycke, J., D'Ottavio, M., & Erickson, A. G. (2007). The student-directed summary of performance: Increasing student and family involvement in the transition planning process. *Career Development for Exceptional Individuals, 30*, 13–26.

Massachusetts Department of Developmental Services. (2013). Blueprint for success: Employee individuals with developmental disabilities in Massachusetts. Retrieved from *www.addp. org/images/Nov2013Conference/blueprint%20for%20success%20full%20version%20final%20 11.6.13.pdf.*

Mastropieri, M. A., & Scruggs, T. E. (1997). Best practices in promoting reading comprehension in students with learning disabilities 1976 to 1996. *Remedial and Special Education, 18*, 198–213.

Mattie, H. D. (2000). The suitability of Holland's self-directed search for non-readers with learning disabilities or mild mental retardation. *Career Development for Exceptional Individuals, 23*, 57–72.

Mazzotti, V. L., Rowe, D. A., Kelley, K. R., Test, D. W., Fowler, C. H., Kohler, P. D., et al. (2009). Linking transition assessment and post-secondary goals: Key elements in the secondary transition planning process. *Teaching Exceptional Children, 42*, 44–51.

McCormick, S., & Cooper, J. O. (1991). Can SQ3R facilitate secondary learning disabled students' literal comprehension of expository test?: Three experiments. *Reading Psychology, 12*, 239–271.

McDonald, L., MacPherson-Court, L., Frank, S., Uditsky, B., & Symons, F. (1997). An inclusive university program for students with moderate to severe developmental disabilities: Student, parent, and faculty perspectives. *Developmental Disabilities Bulletin, 25*, 43–67.

McDonnell, J. (2010). Employment training. In J. McDonnell (Ed.), *Successful transition programs: Pathways for students with intellectual and developmental disabilities* (pp. 241–256). Thousand Oaks, CA: Sage.

McGahee, M., Mason, C., Wallace, T., & Jones, B. (2001). *Student-led IEPs: A guide for student involvement.* Arlington, VA: Council for Exceptional Children.

McGlashing-Johnson, J., Agran, M., Sitlington, P., Cavin, M., & Wehmeyer, M. (2003). Enhancing the job performance of youth with moderate to severe cognitive disabilities using the self-determined model of instruction. *Research and Practice for Persons with Severe Disabilities, 28*(4), 194–204.

McLoughlin, J. A., & Lewis, R. B. (2008). *Assessing students with special needs* (7th ed.). Upper Saddle River, NJ: Pearson.

McPherson, M., Arango, P., Fox, H., Lauver, C., McManus, M., Newacheck, P. W., et al. (1998). A new definition of children with special health care needs. *Pediatrics, 102*, 137–140.

Mechling, L. C. (2006). Comparison of the effects of three approaches on the frequency of stimulus activations, via a single switch, by students who have profound intellectual disabilities. *Journal of Special Education, 40*, 94–102.

Merikangas, K. R., He, J., Burstein, J., Swendsen, J., Avenevoli, S., Case, B., et al. (2011). Service utilization for lifetime mental disorders in U.S. adolescents: Results of the National Comorbidity Survey—Adolescent Supplement (NCS-A). *Journal of the American Academy of Child and Adolescent Psychiatry, 50*(1), 32–45.

Migliore, A., Timmons, A., Butterworth, J., & Lugas, J. (2012). Predictors of employment and postsecondary education of youth with autism. *Rehabilitation Counseling Bulletin, 55*, 176–184.

Mills v. Board of Education of the District of Columbia (1972), 384 F. Supp. 866 (D.D.C. 1972).

Moon, M. S., Luedtke, E. M., & Halloron-Tornquist, E. (2010). *Getting around town: Teaching community mobility skills to students with disabilities.* Arlington, VA: Council for Exceptional Children.

Moore, E. J., & Schelling, A. (2015). Postsecondary inclusion for individuals with an intellectual disability and its effects on employment. *Journal of Intellectual Disabilities, 19*(2), 130–148.

Morgan, R. L., & Alexander, M. (2005). The employer's perception: Employment of individuals with disabilities. *Journal of Vocational Rehabilitation, 23*, 39–49.

Morgan, R. L., Kupferman, S., & Sheen, J. (2012, September). Frequently asked questions about postsecondary education options for young adults with significant disabilities. Available at *http://essentialeducator.org/?p=13696.*

Morgan, R. L., & Salzberg, C. L. (1992). The effects of video-assisted training on employment related social skills of adults with severe mental retardation. *Journal of Applied Behavior Analysis, 25*, 365–383.

Morgan, R. L., & Schultz, J. C. (2012). Towards a multi-modal, ecological approach to increase employment for young adults with autism spectrum disorder. *Journal of Applied Rehabilitation Counseling, 43*, 27–35.

Morgan, R. L., Schultz, J. C., & Woolstenhulme, T. (2011). Transition to adulthood: Bringing special education and vocational rehabilitation together to assist youth with disabilities. *Utah Special Educator, 33*(3), 50–53.

Morningstar, M. E., & Clark, G. M. (2003). The status of personnel preparation for transition education and services: What is the critical content? How can it be offered? *Career Development for Exceptional Individuals, 26*, 227–237.

Mount, B., & Zwernik, K. (1998). *It's never too early, it's never too late: An overview of personal futures planning.* St. Paul, MN: Governor's Planning Council on Developmental Disabilities.

Murphy, S. T., Rogan, P. M., Olney, M., Sures, M., Dague, B., & Kalina, N. (1994). *Developing natural supports in the workplace: A practitioner's guide.* St. Augustine, FL: Training Resources Network.

Nangle, D. W., Erdley, C., Carpenter, E. M., & Newman, J. E. (2002). Social skills training as a treatment for aggressive children and adolescents: A developmental–clinical integration. *Aggression and Violent Behavior, 7*, 169–199.

National Center on Secondary Education and Transition. (2005). *Essential tools: Handbook for implementing a comprehensive work-based learning program according to the Fair Labor Standards Act* (3rd ed.). Minneapolis: University of Minnesota.

National Collaborative on Workforce and Disability for Youth. (n.d.). *Guideposts for success* (2nd ed.). The National Collaborative on Workforce and Disability for Youth. Washington, DC: Author. Retrieved from *www.ncwd-youth.info/guideposts.*

National Collaborative on Workforce and Disability for Youth. (2005). *411 on disability disclosure: A workbook for youth with disabilities.* Washington, DC: Author.

National Collaborative on Workforce and Disability for Youth. (2010). *Making the move to managing your own personal assistance service (PAS): A toolkit for youth with disabilities transitioning to adulthood.* Washington, DC: Author.

National Collaborative on Workforce and Disability for Youth. (2012, September). *Transition's missing link: Health care transition.* Washington, DC: Author.

National Commission on Excellence in Education. (1983). *A nation at risk: The imperative for educational reform.* Washington: U.S. Government Printing Office.

National Council on Disability. (2010). *Workforce infrastructure in support of people with disabilities: Matching human resources to service needs.* Washington, DC: Author.

National Organization on Disability. (2004). *NOD Harris Survey.* Washington, DC: Author.

National Organization to End the Waitlists. (2013). We can, we will, we must end the waitlist—together! Retrieved from *www.noewait.net.*

National Secondary Transition Technical Assistance Center. (2010). *Evidence-based practices and predictors in secondary transition: What we know and what we still need to know.* Charlotte, NC: Author.

National Secondary Transition Technical Assistance Center. (2012). College and career ready standards and secondary transition planning for students with disabilities: 101. Retrieved from *http://nsttac.org/sites/default/files/CCR101.updatedFall2012.pdf.*

National Secondary Transition Technical Assistance Center. (2014). Evidence-based practices. Retrieved from *www.nsttac.org/content/evidence-based-practices.*

Neubert, D. A. (2003). The role of assessment in the transition to adult life process for students with disabilities. *Exceptionality, 11,* 63–75.

Newman, L., Wagner, M., Knokey, A.-M., Marder, C., Nagle, K., Shaver, D., et al. (2011). *The post-high school outcomes of young adults with disabilities up to 8 years after high school: A report from the National Longitudinal Transition Study–2 (NLTS2).* Menlo Park, CA: SRI International.

Nielsen, J. (2013). *Starting early: Perceptions of parents and teachers on 6th to 12th grade transition timeline for students with high-incidence disabilities.* Unpublished master's thesis, Utah State University, Logan, UT.

Niles, S. G., & Harris-Bowlsbey, J. (2005). *Career development interventions in the 21st century* (2nd ed.). Upper Saddle River, NJ: Pearson.

No Child Left Behind (NCLB) Act of 2001, Public Law No. 107-110, § 115, Stat. 1425 (2002).

Nolet, V., & McLaughlin, M. J. (2005). *Accessing the general education curriculum: Including students with disabilities in standards-based reform* (2nd ed.). Thousand Oaks, CA: Corwin Press.

Nollan, K. A., Horn, M., Downs, A. C., Pecora, P. J., & Bressani, R. V. (2002). *Ansell–Casey Life Skills Assessment (ACLSA) and lifeskills guidebook manual.* Seattle, WA: Casey Family Programs.

Noonan, P. M., Gaumer Erickson, A. G., & Morningstar, M. E. (2013). Effects of community transition teams on interagency collaboration for school and adult agency staff. *Career Development and Transition for Exceptional Individuals, 35*(2), 96–104.

Noonan, P. M., McCall, Z. A., Zheng, C., & Gaumer Erickson, A. S. (2012). An analysis of collaboration in a state-level interagency transition team. *Career Development and Transition for Exceptional Individuals, 35,* 143–154.

Noonan, P. M., Morningstar, M. E., & Gaumer Erickson, A. G. (2008). Improving interagency collaboration: Effective strategies used by high-performing local districts and communities. *Career Development for Exceptional Individuals, 31,* 132–143.

O'Brien, J. (2002). Numbers and faces: The ethics of person-centered planning. In S. Holburn & P. M. Vietze (Eds.), *Person-centered planning: Research, practice, and future directions* (pp. 399–414). Baltimore: Brookes.

O'Brien, J., & Lyle, C. (1987). *Framework for accomplishment*. Decatur, GA: Responsive Systems Associates.

Olmstead Commissioner, Georgia Department of Human Resources v. L.C. (1999), 527 U.S. 581.

Osgood, D. W., Foster, E. M., & Courtney, M. E. (2010). Vulnerable populations and the transition to adulthood. *The Future of Children, 20*, 209–229.

Page, T. J., Iwata, B. A., & Neef, N. A. (1976). Teaching pedestrian skills to retarded persons: Generalization from the classroom to the natural environment. *Journal of Applied Behavior Analysis, 9*, 433–444.

Paiewonsky, M., & Roach Ostergard, J. (2010). Local school system perspectives. In M. Grigal & D. Hart, *Think college!: Postsecondary education options for students with intellectual disabilities* (pp. 87–159). Baltimore: Brookes.

Palisano, R. J., Copeland, W. P., & Galuppi, B. E. (2007). Performance of physical activities by adolescents with cerebral palsy. *Physical Therapy, 87*, 77–87.

Parker, D. R., Field, S., & Hoffman, A. (2012). *Self-determination strategies: Case studies of adolescents in transition* (2nd ed.). Austin, TX: PRO-ED.

Parsons, F. (1909). *Choosing a vocation*. Boston: Houghton Mifflin.

Patrick Holschuh, J., & Nist-Olejnik, S. L. (2011). *Effective college learning* (2nd ed.). Boston: Longman.

Pennsylvania Association of Retarded Children v. Commonwealth of Pennsylvania et al. (1972). 343 F. Supp. 279

Pérez Carreón, G., Drake, C., & Calabrese Barton, A. (2005). The importance of presence: Immigrant parents' school engagement experiences. *American Educational Research Journal, 42*, 465–498.

Perske, R. (1972). The dignity of risk. In W. Wolfensberger (Ed.), *Normalization: The principle of normalization in human services* (pp. 194–200). Toronto: National Institute on Mental Retardation.

Peterson, L. Y., Burden, J. P., Sedaghat, J. M., Gothberg, J. E., Kohler, P. D., & Coyle, J. L. (2013). Triangulated IEP transition goals: Developing relevant and genuine annual goals. *Teaching Exceptional Children, 45*, 46–47.

Peterson, L. Y., Sedaghat, J. M., Burden, J. P., Van Dycke, J. L., & Pomeroy, B. (2013, November). *Developing student self-determination across grades 6–12*. Division on Career Development and Transition 17th International Conference, Williamsburg, VA.

Pierangelo, R., & Giuliani, G. A. (2004). *Transition services in special education: A practical approach*. Boston: Pearson.

Polychronis, S., & McDonnell, J. (2010). Developing IEPs/transition plans. In J. McDonnell (Ed.), *Successful transition programs: Pathways for students with intellectual and developmental disabilities* (2nd ed., pp. 81–100). Thousand Oaks, CA: Sage.

Power, P. W. (2013). *A guide to vocational assessment* (5th ed.). Austin, TX: PRO-ED.

Powers, L. E. Turner, A., Westwood, D., Matuszewski, J., & Phillips, A. (2001). TAKE CHARGE for the future: A controlled field-test of a model to promote student involvement in transition planning. *Career Development for Exceptional Individuals, 24*, 89–104.

Prentice, M. (2002). *Serving students with disabilities at the community college* (Report No. EDO-JC-0202). Los Angeles: ERIC Clearinghouse for Community Colleges. (ERIC Document Reproduction Service No. ED467984)

Pyle, N., & Wexler, J. (2012). Preventing students with disabilities from dropping out. *Intervention in School and Clinic, 47*, 283–289.

Quality Indicators for Assistive Technology. (2012). Quality indicators to guide the consideration of assistive technology during the transition process. Retrieved from *http://indicators.knowbility.org/indicators.html*.

Rabren, K., Dunn, C., & Chambers, D. (2002). Predictors of post-high school employment among young adults with disabilities. *Career Development for Exceptional Individuals, 25*, 25–40.

Rehabilitation Act of 1973, 29 U.S.C. § 705 et seq.

Rehabilitation Act of 1973, Public Law 93-112, 87 Stat. 355.

Reid, D. H., & Green, C. (2002). Person-centered planning with people who have severe multiple disabilities. In S. Holburn & P. Vietze (Eds.), *Person-centered planning: Research, practice, and future directions* (pp. 183–202). Baltimore: Brookes.

Richter, S. M., & Mazzotti, V. L. (2011). A comprehensive review of the literature on summary of performance. *Career Development for Exceptional Individuals, 34,* 176–186.

Rizzolo, M. C., Friedman C., Lulinski-Norris, A., & Braddock, D. (2013). Home and community based services (HCBS) waivers: A national study of the states. *Intellectual and Developmental Disabilities, 51,* 1–12.

Robin, A. L., & Foster, S. L. (1989). *Negotiating parent–adolescent conflict: A behavioral–family systems approach.* New York: Guilford Press.

Rueda, R., Monzo, L., Shapiro, J., Gomez, J., & Blacher, J. (2005). Cultural models of transition: Latina mothers of young adults with disabilities. *Exceptional Children, 71,* 401–414.

Ruthowski, S., Datson, M., Van Kuiken, D., & Riehle, E. (2006). Project SEARCH: A demand-side model of high school transition. *Journal of Vocational Rehabilitation, 25,* 85–96.

Salvia, J., Ysseldyke, J. E., & Bolt, S. (2007). *Assessment in special and inclusive education* (10th ed.). Boston: Houghton Mifflin.

Scal, P., & Ireland, M. (2005). Addressing transition to adult health care for adolescents with special health care needs. *Pediatrics, 115,* 1607–1612.

Schalock, R. L., Holl, C., Elliott, B., & Ross, I. (1992). A longitudinal follow-up of graduates from a rural special education program. *Learning Disability Quarterly, 15,* 29–38.

Sharpe, M. N., Johnson, D. R., Izzo, M., & Murray, A. (2005). An analysis of instructional accommodations and assistive technologies used by postsecondary graduates with disabilities. *Journal of Vocational Rehabilitation, 22,* 3–11.

Silverstein, R. (2000). Emerging disability policy framework: A guidepost for analyzing disability policy. *Iowa Law Review, 85,* 1691–1796.

Simon, J. A. (2011). Legal issues in serving students with disabilities in postsecondary education. *New Directions for Student Services, 134,* 95–107.

Sitlington, P. L., & Clark, G. M. (2007). The transition assessment process and IDEIA 2004. *Assessment for Effective Intervention, 32,* 133–142.

Sitlington, P. L., Neubert, D. A., & Leconte, P. J. (1997). Transition assessment: The position of the Division for Career Development and Transition. *Career Development for Exceptional Individuals, 20,* 69–79.

Sparrow, S. S., Cicchetti, D. V., & Balla, D. A. (2005). *Vineland Adaptive Behavior Scales, Second Edition.* Minneapolis, MN: Pearson Assessments.

Spence, S. H. (2003). Social skills training with children and young people: Theory, evidence, and practice. *Child and Adolescent Mental Health, 8,* 84–96.

Stancliffe, R. J., & Lakin, K. C. (2007). Independent living. In S. L. Odom, R. H. Horner, M. E. Snell, & J. B. Blacher (Eds.), *Handbook of developmental disabilities* (pp. 429–448). New York: Guilford Press.

Steere, D. E., Rose, E., & Cavaiuolo, D. (2007). *Growing up: Transition to adult life for students with disabilities.* Boston: Pearson.

Steere, D. E., Wood, R., Pancsofar, E., & Butterworth, J. (1990). Outcomes-based school-to-work transition planning for students with severe disabilities. *Career Development for Exceptional Individuals, 13,* 57–69.

Stewart, D. A., Law, M. C., & Willms, D. G. (2002). A qualitative study of the transition to adulthood for youth with physical disabilities. *Physical and Occupational Therapy in Pediatrics, 21,* 3–21.

Stokes, T. F., & Baer, D. M. (1977). An implicit technology of generalization. *Journal of Applied Behavior Analysis, 10,* 349–367.

Storey, K., & Montgomery, J. (2013). Teaching skills to students. In K. Storey & D. Hunter (Eds.), *The road ahead: Transition to adult life for persons with disabilities* (pp. 85–106). Amsterdam: IOS Press.

Stringham, C. (2013). *Technology and the self-directed IEP: Improving meeting participation for students with severe disabilities.* Unpublished master's thesis, Utah State University, Logan, UT.

Super, D. E. (1957). *The psychology of careers.* New York: Harper & Row.

Super, D. E. (1980). A life-span, life-space approach to career development. *Journal of Vocational Behavior, 16*, 282–298.

Szymanski, E. M., & Hershenson, D. B. (2005). An ecological approach to vocational behavior and career development of people with disabilities. In R. M. Parker, E. M. Szymanski, & J. B. Patterson (Eds.), *Rehabilitation counseling: Basics and beyond* (4th ed., pp. 225–280). Austin, TX: PRO-ED.

Tarleton, B., & Ward, L. (2005). Changes and choices: Finding out what information young people with learning disabilities, their parents and supporters need at transition. *British Journal of Learning Disabilities, 33*, 70–76.

Taylor, J. E., & Averitt Taylor, J. (2013). Person-centered planning: Evidence-based practice, challenges, and potential for the 21st century. *Journal of Social Work in Disability and Rehabilitation, 12*, 213–235.

Technology-Related Assistance for Individuals with Disabilities Act. (1988). (Public Law 100-407), 29 USC 2201.

Test, D. W., Aspel, N. P., & Everson, J. M. (2006). *Transition methods for youth with disabilities*. Upper Saddle River, NJ: Pearson.

Test, D. W., Mason, C., Hughes, C., Konrad, M., Neale, M., & Wood, W. M. (2004). Student involvement in individualized education program meetings. *Exceptional Children, 70*, 391–412.

Test, D. W., Mazzotti, V. L., Mustian, A. L., Fowler, C. H., Kortering, L., & Kohler, P. (2009). Evidence-based secondary transition predictors for improving post-school outcomes for students with disabilities. *Career Development for Exceptional Individuals, 32*, 160–181.

Test, D. W., Richter, S., & Walker, A. R. (2012). Life skills and community-based instruction. In M. L. Wehmeyer & K. W. Webb (Eds.), *Handbook of adolescent transition education for youth with disabilities* (pp. 121–138). New York: Routledge.

Thoma, C., Rogan, R., & Baker, S. R. (2001). Student involvement in transition planning: Unheard voices. *Education and Training in Mental Retardation and Developmental Disabilities, 36*, 16–29.

Thomson, A. M., Perry, J. L., & Miller, T. K. (2007). Conceptualizing and measuring collaboration. *Journal of Public Administration Research and Theory, 19*, 23–56.

Ticket to Work and Work Incentives Improvement Act of 1999, Public Law 106-170.

Townsend, S. (2007). *Transition and your adolescent with learning disabilities: Moving from high school to postsecondary education, training, and employment—parent handbook*. Shawnee Mission, KS: Shawnee Mission School District.

Tullis, C. A., Cannella-Malone, H. I., Basbigill, A. R., Yeager, A., Fleming, C. V., Payne, D., et al. (2011). Review of the choice and preference assessment literature for individuals with severe to profound disabilities. *Education and Training in Autism and Developmental Disabilities, 46*, 576–595.

Turnbull, H. R., Turnbull, A. P., Wehmeyer, M. L., & Park, J. (2003). A quality of life framework for special education outcomes. *Remedial and Special Education, 24*, 67–74.

Uditsky, B., & Hughson, A. (2008). *Inclusive postsecondary education for adults with developmental disorders: A promising path to an inclusive life*. Calgary, Alberta, Canada: Alberta Association for Community Living.

U.S. Census Bureau (2012). Americans with disabilities: 2010. Household economic studies. Current population reports. Retrieved from *www.census.gov/prod/2012pubs/p70-131.pdf*.

U.S. Department of Education Office of Civil Rights (1998). Auxiliary aids and services for postsecondary students with disabilities: Higher education responsibility under Section 504 and Title II of the ADA. Retrieved from *www2.ed.gov/about/offices/list/ocr/docs/auxaids. html*.

U.S. Department of Education Office of Special Education Programs. (2010). *29th annual report to Congress on the implementation of the Individuals with Disabilities Education Act, 2007* (Vol. 1). Washington, DC: Author.

U.S. Department of Education Office of Special Education and Rehabilitative Services. (2002). *A new era: revitalizing special education for children and their families*. Washington, DC: Author.

U.S. Department of Justice. (2012). Letter of finding. Retrieved from *www.ada.gov/olmstead/documents/oregon_findings_letter.pdf*.

U.S. Department of Labor. (n.d.). Field operations handbook. Section 64c04: Unpaid volunteers. Retrieved from *www.dol.gov/whd/FOH/ch64/64c04.htm*.

U.S. Department of Labor. (1991). *What work requires of schools: A SCANS report for America 2000*. Washington, DC: Author.

U.S. Department of Labor. (2002). *O*Net Career Interest Inventory*. St. Paul: JIST Works.

U.S. Equal Opportunity Commission. (2002). EEOC enforcement guidance on reasonable accommodation and undue hardship under the Americans with Disabilities Act. Retrieved from *www.eeoc.gov/policy/docs/accommodation.html*.

U.S. Government Accountability Office. (2003). *College completion: Additional efforts could help with its completion goals* (GAO-03-568). Washington, DC: U.S. Government Printing Office.

U.S. v. Rhode Island and City of Providence 1:13-cv-00442 (D.R.I. 2013).

Vander Stoep, A., Weiss, N. S., Saldanha Kuo, E., Cheney, D., & Cohen, P. (2003). What proportion of failure to complete secondary school in the U.S. population is attributable to adolescent psychiatric disorder? *Journal of Behavioral Health Services and Research, 30,* 119–124.

Vinovskis, M. A. (2009). *From a nation at risk to No Child Left Behind: National education goals and the creation of federal education policy*. New York: Teachers College Press.

Wagner, M., Newman, L., Cameto, R., Javitz, H., & Valdes, K. (2012). A national picture of parent and youth participation in IEP and transition planning. *Journal of Disability Policy Studies, 23,* 140–155.

Wagner, M., Newman, L., Cameto, R., & Levine, P. (2007a). *Changes over time in the early postschool outcomes of youth with disabilities: A report of findings from the National Longitudinal Transition Study (NLTS) and the National Longitudinal Transition Study–2 (NLTS2)*. Menlo Park, CA: SRI International.

Wagner, M., Newman, L., Cameto, R., Levine, P., & Marder, C. (2007b). *Perceptions and expectations of youth with disabilities: A special topic report of findings from the National Longitudinal Transition Study–2 (NLTS2)*. Menlo Park, CA: SRI International.

Walsh, E., Hooven, C., & Kronick, B. (2013). School-wide staff and faculty training in suicide risk awareness: Successes and challenges. *Journal of Child and Adolescent Psychiatric Nursing, 26,* 53–61.

Wandry, D., Wehmeyer, M., & Glor-Scheib, S. (2013). Life-centered education: The teacher's guide. Retrieved from *www.cec.sped.org/Publications/LCE-Transition-Curriculum*.

Webb, K. W., Patterson, K. B., Syverud, S. M., & Seabrooks-Blackmore, J. J. (2008). Evidence based practices that promote transition to postsecondary education: Listening to a decade of expert voices. *Exceptionality, 16,* 192–206.

Wechsler, D. (2003). *Wechsler Intelligence Scale for Children (WISC-IV)*. San Antonio, TX: Psychological Corporation.

Wechsler, D. (2008). *Wechsler Adult Intelligence Scale—Fourth Edition (WAIS-IV)*. San Antonio, TX: Pearson Clinical.

Wehman, P. (1998). Editorial. *Journal of Vocational Rehabilitation, 10,* 1–2.

Wehman, P. (2011). *Essentials of transition planning*. Baltimore: Brookes.

Wehman, P., Schall, C., McDonough, J., Molinelli, A., Riehle, E., Ham, W., et al. (2012). Project SEARCH for youth with autism spectrum disorder: Increasing competitive employment on transition from high school. *Journal of Positive Behavior Interventions, 15,* 144–155.

Wehmeyer, M. L. (2002). The confluence of person-centered planning and self-determination. In S. Holburn & P. Vietze (Eds.), *Person-centered planning: Research, practice, and future directions* (pp. 51–69). Baltimore: Brookes.

Wehmeyer, M. L. (2005). Self-determination and individuals with severe disabilities: Re-examining meanings and misinterpretations. *Research and Practice for Persons with Severe Disabilities, 30,* 113–120.

Wehmeyer, M. L. (2007). *Promoting self-determination in students with developmental disabilities*. New York: Guilford Press.

Wehmeyer, M. L., Agran, M., & Hughes, C. (1998). *Teaching self-determination to students with disabilities: Basic skills for successful transition.* Baltimore: Brookes.

Wehmeyer, M. L., Agran, M., & Hughes, C. (2000). A national survey of teachers' promotion of self-determination and self-directed learning. *Journal of Special Education, 34,* 58–60.

Wehmeyer, M. L., Garner, N., Yeager, D., Lawrence, M., & Davis, A. K. (2006). Infusing self-determination into 18–21 services for students with intellectual or developmental disabilities: A multi-stage, multiple component model. *Education and Training in Development Disabilities, 41,* 3–13.

Wehmeyer, M. L., & Gragoudas, S. (2004). Centers for independent living and transition-age youth: Empowerment and self-determination. *Journal of Vocational Rehabilitation, 20,* 53–58.

Wehmeyer, M. L., & Kelchner, K. (1995). *The Arc's Self-Determination Scale.* Arlington, TX: The Arc National Headquarters.

Wehmeyer, M. [L.] & Lawrence, M. (1995). Whose future is it anyway?: Promoting student involvement in transition planning. *Career Development for Exceptional Individuals, 18,* 69–83.

Wehmeyer, M. L., Lawrence, M., Garner, N., Soukup, J., & Palmer, S., (2004). Whose future is it anyway?: A student-directed transition planning process (2nd ed.). Retrieved from *www. ou.edu/content/dam/Education/documents/wfc-guide-final.pdf.*

Wehmeyer, M. L., & Palmer, S. B. (2003). Adult outcomes for students with cognitive disabilities three years after high school: The impact of self-determination. *Education and Training in Developmental Disabilities, 38,* 131–144.

Wehmeyer, M. L., Palmer, S. B., Agran, M., Mithaug, D., & Martin, J. (2000). Promoting causal agency: The self-determined learning model of instruction. *Exceptional Children, 66,* 439–453.

Weir, C., Fialka, J., Timmons, J., Nord, D., & Gaylord, V. (2011, March). Postsecondary education for students with intellectual disabilities: An overview of current program types. *Impact Newsletter,* pp. 1–2.

Weir, C., Grigal, M., Hart. D., & Boyle, M. (2013). *Profiles and promising practices in higher education for students with intellectual disabilities.* Boston: Institute for Community Inclusion, University of Massachusetts Boston.

Westling, D. L., Fox, L., & Carter, E. W. (2015). *Teaching students with severe disabilities* (5th ed.). Boston: Pearson.

White House, Office of the Press Secretary. (2009). President Obama commemorates anniversary of *Olmstead* and announces new initiative to assist Americans with disabilities [Press release]. Retrieved from *www.whitehouse.gov/the_press_office/President-Obama-Commemorates-Anniversary-of-Olmstead-and-Announces-New-Initiatives-to-Assist-Americans-with-Disabilities.*

Whiston, S., & Keller, B. (2004). The influences of the family of origin on career development: A review and analysis. *The Counseling Psychologist, 32,* 493–568.

White, G. W., Simpson, J. L., Gonda, C., Ravesloot, G., & Coble, Z. (2010). Moving from independence to interdependence: A conceptual model for better understanding community participation of centers for independent living. *Journal of Disability Policy Studies, 20,* 233–240.

Will, M. (1984). *OSERS programming for the transition of youth with disabilities: Bridges to working life.* Washington, DC: U.S. Department of Education.

Will, M. (2010). Foreword. In M. Grigal & D. Hart, *Think college!: Postsecondary education options for secondary students with intellectual disabilities* (pp. xi–xii). Baltimore: Brookes.

Williams, K. T. (2007). *Expressive Vocabulary Test* (2nd ed.). San Antonio, TX: Pearson Clinical.

Williams-Diehm, K., Wehmeyer, M. L., Palmer, S. B., Soukup, J. H., & Garner, N. W. (2008). Self-determination and student involvement in transition planning: A multivariate analysis. *Journal on Developmental Disabilities, 14,* 27–39.

Witt, W., Riley, A. W., & Coiro, M. J. (2003). Childhood functional status, family stressors, and psychosocial adjustment among school-aged children with disabilities in the United States. *Archives of Pediatric Adolescence Medicine, 157,* 687–695.

Wolery, M., Ault, M. J., & Doyle, P. M. (1992). *Teaching students with moderate to severe disabilities: Use of response prompting strategies.* New York: Longman.

Wolery, M., Bailey, D. B., & Sugai, G. M. (1988). *Effective teaching: Principles and procedures of applied behavior analysis with exceptional students*. Boston: Allyn & Bacon.

Wolman, J., Campeau, P., Dubois, P., Mithaug, D., & Stolarski, V. (1994). *AIR Self-Determination Scale and user guide*. Palo Alto, CA: American Institute of Research.

Woodcock, R. W., McGrew, K. S., & Mather, N. (2001). *Woodcock–Johnson Psychoeducational Battery—Revised*. Chicago: Riverside.

Woods, L., Sylvester, L., & Martin, J. E. (2010). Student-directed transition planning: Increasing student knowledge and self-efficacy in the transition planning process. *Career Development for Exceptional Individuals, 33*, 106–114.

Workforce Innovation and Opportunity Act, H.R. 803, 113 Cong. (2014).

World Health Organization. (1997). WHOQOL: Measuring the quality of life. Retrieved from *www.who.int/mental_health/media/68.pdf*.

World Institute on Disability. (n.d.). Individual development account question and answer sheet: A guided for IDA consumers with disabilities. World Institute on Disability. Retrieved from *www.wid.org/publications/individual-development-account-question-and-answer-sheet-a-guide-for-ida-consumers-with-disabilities*.

Young, J., Morgan, R. L., Callow-Heusser, C. A., & Lindstrom, L. (2014, September 18). The effects of parent training on knowledge of transition services for students with disabilities. *Career Development and Transition for Exceptional Individuals*. Published online before print.

Zablocki, M., & Krezmien, M. P. (2012). Drop-out predictors among students with high-incidence disabilities: A National Longitudinal and Transitional study 2 analysis. *Journal of Disability Policy Studies, 24*, 53–64.

Index

Page numbers followed by *f* indicate figure; *t* indicate table